Psychopharmacology

This new, and heavily revised, edition of *Psychopharmacology*, provides a comprehensive scientific study of the effects of drugs on the mind and behavior. With the growing prevalence of psychiatric and behavioral disorders and the rapid advances in the development of new drug therapies, this textbook offers an essential understanding of the necessary details of drug action.

The book presents its coverage in the context of the behavioral disorders they are designed to treat, rather than by traditional drug classifications, to strengthen understanding of the underlying physiology and neurochemistry, as well as the approaches to treatment. Each disorder from the major diagnostic categories is discussed from a historical context along with diagnostic criteria and descriptions of typical cases. In addition, what we presently know about the underlying pathology of each disorder is carefully described. Providing a solid foundation in psychology, neuroanatomy and physiology, the book also offers a critical examination of drug claims, as well as coverage of evidence-based alternatives to traditional drug therapies. Throughout, this text discusses how drug effectiveness is measured in both human and animal studies.

Topics new to this edition include: a stronger emphasis on the environmental impacts on drug effectiveness; more on the mechanisms of adverse reactions to drugs and information on managing drug side effects; the risks and benefits of using "mood stabilizing drugs" to address behavior in youth with ADHD or ASD; and discussion of the research-to-practice gap in pharmacological care for children and adolescents.

Accompanied by a robust selection of support material, this textbook is ideal for undergraduate and pre-professional students on courses in Psychopharmacology, Clinical Psychopharmacology, Drugs and Behavior. It is a valuable contribution to highlight the symbiotic relationship between psychopharmacology and the neural and behavioral sciences.

R. H. Ettinger is Professor of Psychology at Eastern Oregon University. His research focuses on psychopharmacology and includes investigations of the neural mechanisms underlying feeding and addiction. Notably, it has led to the development of an anti-cocaine antibody and an understanding of the role of Pavlovian conditioning in drug tolerance and addiction.

Psychopharmacology

Third Edition

R. H. Ettinger

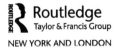

Routledge
Taylor & Francis Group

NEW YORK AND LONDON

Designed cover image: © Getty Images

Third edition published 2023
by Routledge
605 Third Avenue, New York, NY 10158

and by Routledge
4 Park Square, Milton Park, Abingdon, Oxon, OX14 4RN

Routledge is an imprint of the Taylor & Francis Group, an informa business

First edition published by Pearson 2011

Second edition published by Routledge 2017

ISBN: 978-1-032-31289-7 (hbk)
ISBN: 978-1-032-31287-3 (pbk)
ISBN: 978-1-003-30901-7 (ebk)

DOI: 10.4324/9781003309017

Typeset in Bembo MT Pro
by Apex CoVantage, LLC

Access the Support Material: www.routledge.com/9781032312873

Contents

1 Organization and Function of the Nervous System

Our behaviors, including our thoughts, sensations, emotions, memories, and even our states of consciousness, are all a result of complex interactions between neurons distributed throughout our brains. These neurons form elaborate systems that communicate their activity by releasing small amounts of transmitter substances, which act both on receiving neurons as well as on the neuron sending the message. In order for us to understand just how drugs act to treat certain psychological conditions, we must first understand the intricate and sometimes subtle ways in which neurons function to regulate our behaviors. We must also appreciate the complex systems of neurons within the brain that specialize in different functions, including movement, emotions, learning and memory, and our motivational states.

The average human brain weighs approximately 1,400 grams (or roughly three pounds) and contains nearly 200 billion neurons. Each of these neurons may in turn communicate with just a few or as many as tens of thousands of other neurons. How the structure and organization of neurons and their surrounding environment allows for such communication will be the topic of the first part of this chapter. I will then describe the structures and functions of systems within the brain that allow humans and other organisms to function in, and adapt to, their continuously changing environments. This background will be necessary for us to understand how psychological disorders may arise and just how drugs might help to alleviate them.

The Structure and Function of Neurons

As mentioned earlier, the brain contains approximately 200 billion individual nerve cells or neurons. These neurons are the basic units of the brain as well as the rest of the nervous system. Neurons vary in shape, size, and other characteristics according to their location and their specific function.

There are three major classes of neurons: sensory neurons, motor neurons, and **interneurons**. Sensory or afferent neurons carry ascending messages to the **central nervous system** (CNS) from receptors in the skin, ears, nose, eyes, as well as some organs, muscles, and joints. The brain and sometimes the spinal cord interpret these messages and send appropriate responses through descending motor or efferent neurons, which lead to sensory organs, muscles, glands, and other peripheral tissues to control movement and the functioning of glands, sensory organs, and other tissues. Interneurons reside only within the CNS and function to bridge communication between sensory and motor neurons. Without these connecting neurons, sensory messages would never result in the appropriate bodily response. Interneurons also communicate with each other throughout the nervous system. Although neurons vary in size, shape, and function, they share four common structures: the cell body, the dendrites, the axon, and the terminal buttons (see Figure 1.1).

DOI: 10.4324/9781003309017-1

Cell Body or Soma

The cell body or soma is the largest part of the neuron. It contains structures that control the cell's metabolic functions (cell respiration and metabolism). It also contains the nucleus, which contains the cell's genetic information encoded in DNA. The membrane of the cell body can have receptors and receive messages from other neurons, although the cell body is not typically the cell's primary receiving target.

Dendrite

Neurons typically receive messages from other cells at a collection of extensions from the cell body called dendrites, which branch out from the cell body like roots of a tree. (The word *dendrite* comes from the Greek word for tree.) Dendrites may receive information from a few to thousands of surrounding neurons. The more extensive the neuron's network of dendrites, the more connections can be made with other neurons. Interneurons in the brain typically contain far more dendritic branches than neurons in the spinal cord or the peripheral nervous system. Signals received by dendrites are passed on to the membrane of the cell body where excitatory and inhibitory signals are integrated and a *decision* is made whether to transmit the signal along its axon.

Axon

The axon is typically an extended branch of the cell that functions to transmit the electrical signal from the surface of the cell body towards receiving cells. The point on the cell body where both the axon and the electrical signal originate is called the **axon hillock**. The electrical signal is transmitted along the entire length of the axon, which may range from several feet in length in spinal cord and **peripheral nervous system** (PNS) neurons to fractions of millimeters in neurons within the brain. The axon may divide into two or more major branches called collaterals, thereby increasing its capacity to communicate with other neurons. Axons may be myelinated or unmyelinated. Myelin is a type of glial cell that wraps around the axon, providing it with insulation. Most peripheral axons are myelinated, and most (but not all) of

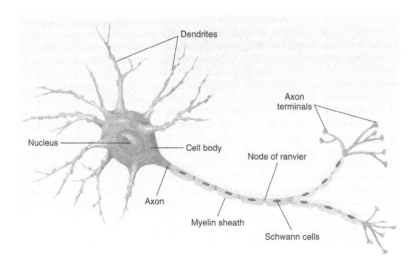

Figure 1.1 Neuron structure.

the axons in the brain are unmyelinated. Myelin serves both to insulate the axon, much like insulation on a wire, and to increase the speed of conduction along the axon. It is myelin that gives brain tissue, which is normally grayish brown, a white color (white vs. gray matter).

Terminal Button

The transmitting end of the axon consists of small bulblike structures known as terminal buttons (see Figure 1.2). The terminal buttons store and release neurotransmitters, which either excite or inhibit adjacent neurons. Terminal buttons are also where neurotransmitter substances are taken back into the cell after their release. The structure that allows for **neurotransmitter reuptake** is a protein called a reuptake transporter. These transporter proteins will be given considerable attention throughout this text, as they are the site where many psychotropic drugs are designed to work.

Once the recycled neurotransmitters, or their precursor chemicals, have been taken back into the terminal button, it is further transported back into synaptic vesicles where it is stored for subsequent release. The amount of neurotransmitter available in synaptic vesicles for release depends on the availability of its metabolic precursors, on the frequency of cell firing, and whether or not it is receiving messages to turn down neurotransmitter synthesis and release by specialized receptors that provide feedback to a neuron abouts its activity.

Neural Transmission

In order for a message to travel from neuron to neuron, it must move from the terminal button at the end of one neuron's axon to the dendrites or cell body of an adjacent neuron. The process by which impulses are transmitted in the CNS is called neural transmission, and it involves both electrical and chemical processes.

Within the PNS, messages are transmitted along the extended axonal fibers of both motor and sensory neurons that are contained within bundles of neural fibers called nerves.

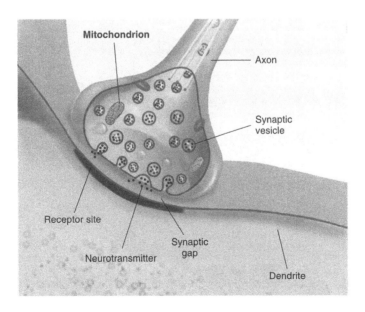

Figure 1.2 Terminal button of axon.

The multitudes of neural circuits or pathways within the CNS are made up of perhaps hundreds of thousands of individual neurons. These fibers extend as continuous structures from sensory receptors or muscles to the CNS. For example, a sensory message from a pain receptor in the skin of your finger is transmitted along a single axonal fiber that extends the length of your arm to a point at which it enters the spinal cord and transfers its message to an interneuron.

Neuron Electrical Activity

All cells, including neurons, are enclosed in a lipid membrane composed of two layers of lipid molecules called a lipid bilayer (see Figure 1.3). This membrane acts as a kind of skin that permits the cell to maintain an internal environment different from the fluid outside of the membrane. The membrane communicates with its external environment through specialized integrated proteins that are distributed throughout the lipid structure. These proteins function to carry glucose to internal cell structures and to carry metabolic waste back out. They also serve to carry chemical ions back and forth across the membrane. These ions carry either a positive or a negative electrical charge and therefore change the membrane's electrical potential. Ions that are particularly important in neural transmission are negatively charged organic ions (An^-), chlorine ions (Cl^-), positively charged sodium ions (Na^+), and potassium ions (K^+). If the cell membrane did not act as a barrier, these ions would be equally distributed both inside and outside of the neuron. However, the negative organic ions do not pass through the cell membrane to the surrounding fluid and the membrane is only semi permeable to other ions. For instance, sodium, potassium, and chlorine ions pass through only when gates are open for them. These gates, called **ion channels**, are actually proteins embedded in the cell's membrane and they become activated by changes in the membrane potential or by the presence of specific chemicals on their surface.

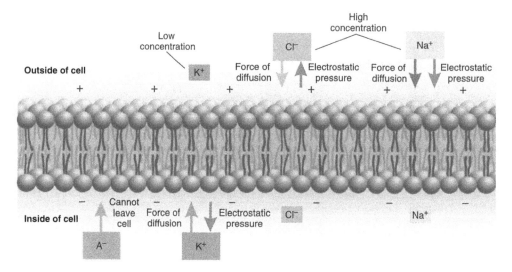

Figure 1.3 Electrostatic and diffusion pressures act on charged ions. At rest the membrane is impermeable to Na^+, so it is not at equilibrium. The concentration of Na^+ is greater on the outside and it is attracted towards the negative inside charge. Although K^+ is relatively free to pass through the membrane, the positive electrical charge outside keeps it from escaping. K^+ ions are at equilibrium, as these forces are balanced at rest.

Resting Potentials

There are essentially two forces acting on these charged ions. The first force is diffusion, which is the pressure on ions to distribute themselves equally in a medium. That is, to move from high to lower concentrations. Perfume diffuses from an open bottle throughout a room. The second force is electrostatic. Ions of similar charge repel each other, as do similarly charged sides of a magnet. This electrostatic force acts to move ions towards the opposite charge and away from a similar charge. When these two forces are at equilibrium the neuron is said to be in its resting state. The distribution of negatively and positively charged ions on either side of the membrane determines the cell's electrical potential during this resting state. This **resting potential** is therefore mostly determined by the concentrations of charged ions in the fluids on both sides of the cell membrane. The ion transport proteins that are embedded in the cell membrane can also contribute to the resting potential to some extent because they also carry an electric charge.

The negative and positive charges are unequal on either side of the membrane when the two forces are in equilibrium, so its interior has a negative electrical potential with respect to its exterior. This phenomenon is due primarily to the negatively charged organic ions on the inside and a high concentration of positively charged sodium ions outside the membrane. Most neurons at rest (that is, when their membrane potential is not changing) have a net negative charge of about -70 millivolts (70/1,000 of a volt) relative to their outside environment. The membrane is said to be in a polarized state when the neuron is at rest (see Figure 1.4).

This differential charge gives the resting neuron a state of potential energy known as the resting potential. In other words, it is in a state of readiness to be activated by an impulse from an adjacent neuron. Maintaining this resting potential allows the neuron to store the energy that it utilizes when it transmits an impulse. The resting potential is maintained because the membrane is relatively impermeable to the positively charged sodium (Na^+) ions concentrated on the outside of the neuron and to the negatively charged organic ions on the inside. A potassium ion can move relatively freely until the two forces operating on it are at equilibrium. That is, the diffusion force trying to expel it from the neuron is counteracted by the higher positive charge outside. Chlorine is also essentially at equilibrium and cannot enter the more negatively charged inside of the cell.

Graded Potentials

The resting potential is disturbed when an impulse is received from another neuron. This disturbance is referred to as a **graded potential**, and its strength varies with the intensity and frequency of stimulation. If we were to measure the charge on the axon during a graded potential, we would observe a change from -70 millivolts to perhaps -60 millivolts, depending on the amount of excitatory stimulation the cell receives (see Figure 1.5). A graded potential by itself is of little consequence. However, when several graded potentials occur simultaneously or in rapid succession, together they may be sufficient enough to depolarize the neuron to a threshold value (the minimum voltage change sufficient to allow Na^+ ions to enter the cell) of about -55 millivolts.

The determination of whether a graded potential is sufficient to bring the axon to its threshold level is made at the axon hillock, a specialized region of the cell body near the base of the axon. The axon hillock integrates all the graded potentials, both excitatory and inhibitory, that reach it. If the sum of these graded potentials reaches a sufficient magnitude or threshold, the voltage gated Na^+ channels open and a sudden depolarization begins. This depolarization is referred to as an action potential.

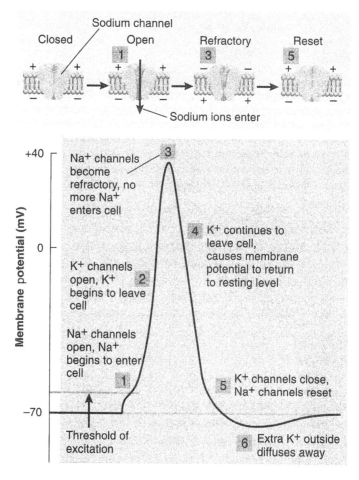

Figure 1.4 The action potential. Once the membrane reaches its threshold voltage of about −55mV, Na$^+$ channels open and begin to depolarize the membrane further. Because K$^+$ is no longer at equilibrium, after Na$^+$ influx, it begins to leave the cell. Na$^+$ channels close and the membrane returns to its resting potential. Na$^+$ −K$^+$ transporters reinstate the resting concentrations of these charged ions.

Action Potentials

An **action potential** is initiated when the axon is depolarized to its threshold level (approximately −55 millivolts). When the membrane reaches this threshold level, a sudden complete depolarization results—that is, the axon goes from about −55 millivolts to approximately +30 millivolts (see Figure 1.4). This rapid depolarization is the result of the membrane changing its permeability to sodium (Na$^+$) ions. When the membrane is no longer impermeable to Na$^+$, it enters the cell, bringing the charge on the inside of the membrane to a positive value (about +30 millivolts). Some potassium ions begin to leave the axon at this time because the electrostatic gradient inside the axon becomes weakened as sodium ions enter. However, the number of potassium ions that leave the inside of the axon is far outweighed by the number of sodium ions that enter.

The change in permeability to Na$^+$ is extremely brief, and the resting potential is quickly restored by the closing of the Na$^+$ gates and the rapid expulsion of K$^+$ from within the axon.

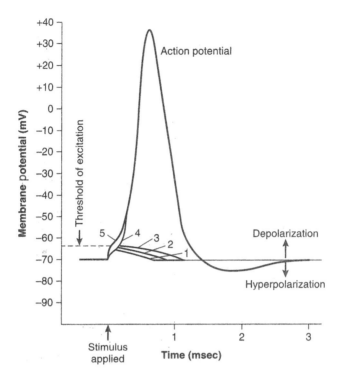

Figure 1.5 Graded potentials (1–2) are not sufficient to open Na$^+$ channels and initiate an action potential. At position 3 the graded potential reaches threshold.

Potassium ions are repelled because of the positive charge now inside the membrane. As potassium ions leave, the charge across the membrane returns to its resting state. In fact, an excess of potassium outflow briefly hyperpolarizes the membrane. This complete process for an action potential takes about 1 millisecond (1/1,000 of a second). Some drugs disrupt this process and prevent the propagation of action potentials by blocking Na$^+$ channels. Local anesthetics, such as lidocaine, block pain messages this way.

Once an action potential occurs at the axon hillock it causes sufficient depolarization further down the axon to reach threshold and initiate another. This process is rapidly repeated as the action potential flows (or propagates) along the entire surface of the axon to the terminal button. Once the action potential reaches the terminal button it initiates processes that lead to the release of neurotransmitter substances, which carry the message to adjacent neurons. I will discuss this process in some detail later on.

Unlike the graded potential, the strength of an action potential does not vary according to the degree of stimulation. Once an action potential is triggered it is transmitted the entire length of the axon with no loss of intensity. Partial action potentials or nerve impulses do not occur; thus, an axon is said to conduct without decrement. Because of this, the action potential is said to follow the all-or-none law: If the sum of the graded potentials reaches a threshold, there will be an action potential; if the threshold is not reached, however, no action potential will occur.

According to the all-or-none law, a neuron fires at only one level of intensity. The fact that, even though a single neuron's impulse level is always the same, two important variables may still change: the number of neurons affected by stimulation and the frequency with which neurons fire. Very weak stimuli may trigger graded potentials in only a few neurons, whereas very strong stimuli may cause thousands of neurons to fire. The frequency in which neurons fire can also vary greatly, from fewer than 100 times per second for weak stimuli to as often as 1,000 times per second for strong stimuli. Thus, the combination of how many neurons fire and how often they fire allows us to distinguish different intensities of stimuli.

The speed with which an impulse propagates along a neuron varies with the properties of the axon, ranging from less than 1 meter per second to as fast as 100 meters per second (roughly 224 miles per hour). At least two important factors affect speed. One is the resistance to current along the axon—there is an inverse relationship between resistance and conduction speed so that speed is reduced as resistance increases. Resistance is most effectively decreased by an increase in axon size, which helps explain why large axons, such as those in PNS neurons, tend to conduct impulses at a faster rate than do small axons.

However, if the nervous system had to depend only on axon size to transmit impulses quickly, there would not be enough room in our bodies for all the large axons we would need. Fortunately, a second property also helps to increase the speed of transmission of nerve impulses. Specialized cells, called glial cells, wrap around some axons, forming an insulating cover called a myelin sheath. (One type of glial cell, the oligodendrocyte, forms the myelin within the CNS. In the PNS the insulating sheaths are built from another type of glial cell known as the Schwann cell.) Between each glial cell the axon membrane is exposed by a small gap called a **node of Ranvier**. It is at these small gaps in the myelin where Na^+ influx occurs. So, an action potential at one **node of Ranvier** can sufficiently depolarize the membrane at the next node further along the neuron (see Figure 1.6).

In these myelinated neurons, action potential does not propagate smoothly down the axon. Instead, they jump from node to node, in a process called *saltatory conduction* (from the Latin *saltare*, meaning to leap). Saltatory conduction is so efficient that a small myelinated axon can conduct a nerve impulse just as quickly as an unmyelinated axon 30 times larger. Because myelin plays such a critical role in the nervous system, it follows that the effects of certain diseases (such as multiple sclerosis [MS]) that involve progressive breakdown in these insulating sheaths can be devastating. In MS, the loss of myelination may short-circuit or delay the

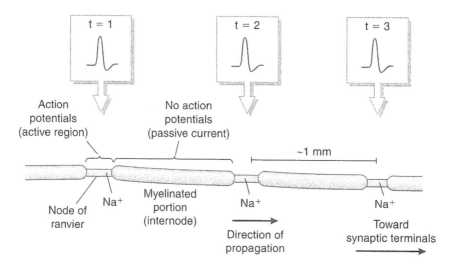

Figure 1.6 Myelinated axon. The passive current beneath the myelin remains above the threshold, so sodium channels at times t = 1–3 open almost simultaneously and depolarize the membrane quickly. A myelinated axon can transmit signals about 200 times faster than an unmyelinated neuron.

transmission of signals from the brain to the muscles of the arms and legs. As a consequence, a person with MS experiences a weakness or loss of control over the limbs. As the disease progresses, more and more neurons become disrupted by demyelination.

Glial cells appear to play numerous other significant roles in the development and function of the nervous system. For instance, astrocytes (named after their star-like structure) form long processes that guide developing neurons to their final destinations. Once these neurons develop and form connections these glial processes disappear. Other astrocytes are involved in the formation of synaptic connections between neurons. They essentially form the "glue" that holds synapses together. These astrocytes do not merely assist in the formation and structure of synapses; they may also be involved in other essential neuronal functions, such as the synthesis of neurotransmitter substances and neurotransmitter removal after it has been released. Astrocytes are also involved in subtitle neuronal communication in what are termed **tripartite synapses** that may function to regulate neuronal activity. They are mentioned here because drugs of the future may actually target glial functioning, and some forms of depression appear to be associated with glial cell loss.

The transmission of an electrical impulse from one neuron to another (or to other types of cells) involves a series of events beginning with the arrival of the action potential at the terminal button. Neurons communicate primarily through the release of neurotransmitters. Far less common is the electrical synapse, in which an electrical potential is conducted from one neuron to the next because of a tight junction between them. These rare electrical synapses will not be discussed here. Because there are several steps in synaptic transmission, and pharmacologists can take advantage of each of them in designing drugs, I will discuss these processes in some detail.

Synaptic Transmission

Neurotransmitter Release

When the axon fires, the action potential travels along the axon to the terminal button. When it arrives at the terminal button, the membrane there changes its permeability to another ion, calcium (Ca^{++}). Calcium then enters the terminal button and allows the synaptic vesicles to migrate to the presynaptic membrane, where they fuse with the membrane and release their contents into the synapse (the fusing of synaptic vesicles to the postsynaptic membrane can be seen in Figure 1.7). The total amount of neurotransmitter released depends on how much Ca^{++} enters the terminal button. More intense stimulation produces a greater frequency of action potentials, which in turn allows more Ca^{++} to enter, thus increasing the amount of neurotransmitter released. The Ca^{++} channel proteins control how much calcium enters the terminal button, but these proteins themselves can be regulated by other proteins that can be activated by both endogenous substances as well as by specific drugs that target them. For example, THC in marijuana attaches to a specific cannabinoid receptor (CB2) that controls Ca^{++} channel protein activity.

Receptors

Once a neurotransmitter is released into the synaptic gap, it diffuses towards the postsynaptic membrane of a receiving cell. The postsynaptic membrane contains sites on specific proteins or chains of amino acids called receptors. These receptors are composed of highly specific molecular structures on the end of an amino acid string exposed in the synaptic gap. The specific molecular configuration of the receptor determines which substances can bind temporarily with it. When a neurotransmitter binds with the receptor complex the postsynaptic

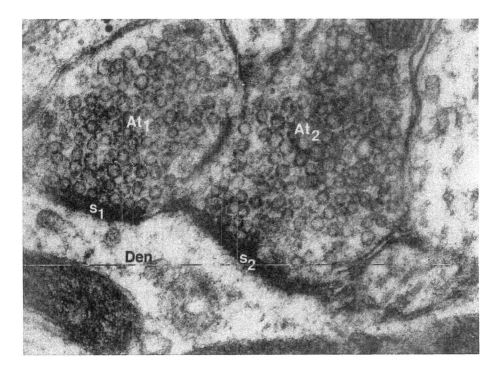

Figure 1.7 Electron micrograph of active synapse. At1 and At2 refer to axon terminals with synaptic vesicles, S1 and S2 are active synapses on a cell dendrite (Den).

membrane's permeability to ions changes briefly, allowing them to flow either in or out depending on the synapse. Drugs may also be designed to bind with receptors, and their effects can either be to mimic the neurotransmitter or they may be to block or prevent the neurotransmitter from binding. These drug effects will be discussed throughout the remaining chapters of this text.

Not only do synapses vary in which ions flow either in or out of the cell, they also vary in how their receptors are configured and how they ultimately control an ion channel. When a receptor directly controls an ion channel, often because it is part of the same protein, it is called an **ionotropic receptor**. When the receptor is not part of the **ion channel**, and other proteins are involved in controlling an ion channel, it is classified as a **metabotropic receptor**.

Ionotropic Receptors

Ionotropic receptors are made up of several proteins called subunits (see Figure 1.8). These subunits span across the cell membrane and form an ion channel for a specific ion such as Cl^-. These subunits also contain binding sites for specific neurotransmitters and for additional substances that can facilitate or inhibit neurotransmitter binding. Upon binding with the neurotransmitter, the receptor protein undergoes a change in configuration, opening the ion channel. The passage of ions either in or out of the cell membrane results in a graded membrane potential. Ionotropic receptors operate quickly to depolarize the postsynaptic membrane. The ion channels controlled by them remain open for only a few milliseconds as the neurotransmitter is quickly released from the binding site and degraded by a breakdown enzyme.

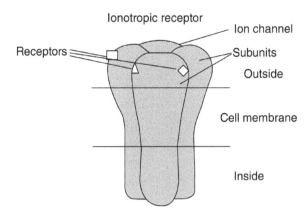

Figure 1.8 Ionotropic receptors contain several membrane-spanning proteins called subunits. Receptors for neurotransmitters and other substances are located on these subunits. The configuration of these subunits form the ion channel. Ionotropic receptors allow the rapid influx of either Na^+ (excitatory), Cl^- (inhibitory), or the outflow of K^+ (also inhibitory).

Metabotropic Receptors

Unlike ionotropic receptors that are relatively simple and quite fast, metabotropic receptors do not directly control ion channels. Rather, when a neurotransmitter is bound to the receptor site a series of events requiring cellular energy is initiated—thus the term metabotropic. Metabotropic receptors are located in close proximity to another membrane protein called a G-protein, short for guanine nucleotide binding protein. When the receptor is activated by a neurotransmitter the G-protein undergoes a change in conformation and a subunit of the protein dissociates or breaks away. The detached subunit of the G-protein is called an ɑ subunit. This dissociated G-protein can affect the cell in one of two specific ways. The first way is similar to an ionotropic receptor. The ɑ subunit attaches to an ion channel and directly opens it. These are called G-protein-gated receptors, and they operate quickly to either depolarize or hyperpolarize the cell membrane, depending on which ions are allowed through the ion channel.

The ɑ subunit may act in a second way by activating an enzyme that facilitates the formation of cyclic AMP (cAMP) from ATP. Cyclic AMP acts as a **second messenger** by activating a third protein called protein kinase. Protein kinase facilitates the **phosphoralation** of a protein that forms an ion channel. Once phosphoralated, this ion channel opens or closes. Metabotropic receptors can both open and close ion channels for all three of the polarizing ions (Cl^-, K^+, and Na^+). Because these receptors require several steps involving enzyme action, the formation of a second messenger, and the activation of an ion channel protein, these receptors are relatively slow when compared to ionotropic receptors. In addition, the ion channels controlled by metabotropic receptors remain in their open or closed state for much longer. In fact, they may remain in their altered state for as long as several minutes. Finally, metabotropic receptors may be located on the neuron releasing the neurotransmitter and thereby control the amount of neurotransmitter released. I have more to say about these receptors later on. Many of the drugs discussed in later chapters alter the functioning of metabolic receptors. Because there are numerous steps and these receptors control the functioning of several cell processes, they provide pharmacologists with more options for altering receptor functioning with drugs (see Figure 1.9).

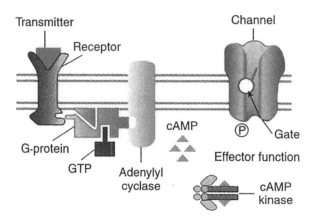

Figure 1.9 When the metabotropic receptor is activated by neurotransmitter, the G-protein undergoes a change in conformation and a subunit of the protein dissociates. The dissociated subunit then activates an enzyme that facilitates the formation of cAMP from ATP. The cAMP acts as a second messenger by activating protein kinase, which phosphoralates the ion channel. These metabotropic receptors can be either excitatory or inhibitory, depending on the ion channel they control.

Neurotransmitter Reuptake

Some neurotransmitters are broken down by enzyme action once they have accomplished their function. The enzymes that function to break down neurotransmitter substances are manufactured and released by the same neuron releasing the neurotransmitter. One such enzyme, acetylcholinesterase, breaks down the neurotransmitter acetylcholine into acetate and choline molecules. These break down products then reenter the terminal buttons to be recycled for further use. In some cases, the neurotransmitter substance is retrieved into the terminal button intact without enzyme degradation. The reuptake process is controlled by specialized membrane proteins called transporters. The density and availability of these transporter proteins determines how quickly neurotransmitter is cleared from the synapse (see Figure 1.10).

These breakdown and reuptake processes, which are essential for normal neuronal functioning, can be influenced by a number of drugs. For example, drugs such as amphetamine and cocaine inhibit the reuptake of several neurotransmitters, resulting in heightened alertness and activity. Other drugs may block the breakdown process resulting in prolonged neurotransmitter action. Some of the antidepressants I discuss later on work in this manner.

Excitatory and Inhibitory Synapses

The postsynaptic membrane of the receiving neuron contains specialized receptor sites that respond to a variety of neurotransmitters. Neurotransmitters act on these receptor sites to produce a change in the permeability of the postsynaptic membrane. Depending on the receptor site and the type of neurotransmitter, this change in permeability can either excite or inhibit action potentials in the receiving neuron.

As stated earlier, neurotransmitters exert their effects by opening ion channels in the postsynaptic membrane, letting either positively or negatively charged ions pass through. If positively charged sodium ions enter, the membrane is excited or depolarized. Neurotransmitters that cause these changes are called excitatory neurotransmitters, and their effects are referred to as **excitatory postsynaptic potentials**, or EPSPs. Conversely, if positively charged potassium

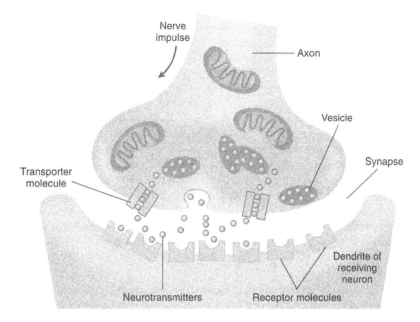

Figure 1.10 Reuptake transporter. Reuptake transporters transport neurotransmitter in the synaptic cleft back into the terminal button. Once in the terminal button, it is transported again into the synaptic vesicles by vesicular transport.

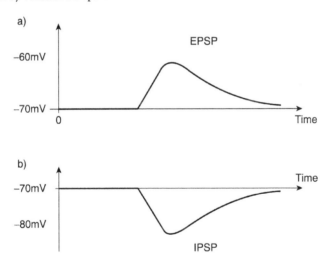

Figure 1.11 Comparison of EPSPs and IPSPs. An EPSP depolarizes the membrane while an IPSP hyperpolarizes it, moving it further from its threshold.

ions pass to the outside of the postsynaptic membrane, or negatively charged chloride ions enter, the membrane inhibited and the graded potential results in making the membrane more negative—a process called hyperpolarization. Neurotransmitters that act in this way are called inhibitory neurotransmitters, and their effects are called **inhibitory postsynaptic potentials**, or IPSPs (see Figure 1.11).

Since hundreds or even thousands of axon terminals may form synapses with any one neuron, EPSPs and IPSPs may be present at the same time. The combination of all these

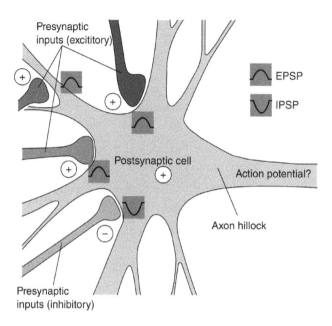

Figure 1.12 Neural integration of excitatory and inhibitory graded potentials. An action potential will only occur whenever the excitatory input exceeds the inhibitory input by the threshold amount.

excitatory and inhibitory signals determines whether the receiving neuron will fire. This is referred to as **neural integration** (see Figure 1.12). For an action potential to occur, EPSPs must not only predominate, they must do so to the extent of reaching the neuron's threshold. To prevent this from happening, there needs to be a sufficient number of IPSPs present to prevent the summation of EPSPs and IPSPs from reaching the threshold of depolarization.

Some neurotransmitters seem to be exclusively excitatory or inhibitory; others seem capable of producing either effect depending on which ion channel it opens in a specific pathway or neural structure. When transmitters have both excitatory and inhibitory capabilities, the postsynaptic receptor protein determines what the effect will be. Thus, these neurotransmitters may have an inhibitory effect at one synapse and an excitatory effect at another.

Neurotransmitters interact with receptors on the postsynaptic cell membrane to change its electrical potential. If the change is sufficient to depolarize the cell membrane, a graded potential is initiated, thus beginning the cycle outlined earlier.

Autoreceptors

As briefly mentioned, some receptors for neurotransmitters are located on the sending cell itself. These receptors are called **autoreceptors**, and they function to regulate the activity of the sending neuron (see Figure 1.13). Autoreceptors can either excite or inhibit the neuron's activity, and thus the amount of neurotransmitter it produces and releases, but it does not do this by controlling ion channels. Instead, autoreceptors regulate internal processes of the cell through the activity of second messenger systems. Most often autoreceptors are proteins of a distinct subset of metabotropic receptors for a specific neurotransmitter. That is, for each known neurotransmitter there are several subtypes of receptor proteins that it binds with. For example, the neurotransmitter serotonin (5-HT) has three main receptor subfamilies: 5-HT1, 5-HT2, and the subfamily for 5-HT 4, 5-HT 6, and 5-HT7. Each of these subfamilies contains additional variants, such as 5-HT1A, 5-HT1B, 5HT2A, etc., building a family of

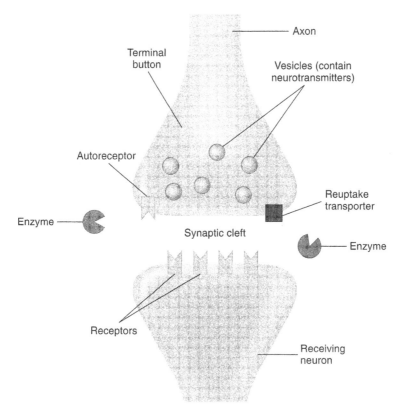

Figure 1.13 Neurotransmitter binds to an autoreceptor, which regulates the amount of neurotransmitter
synthesized and released.

approximately 17 receptor subtypes. These receptor subtypes have unique functions, such as the autoreceptor, and are located on different regions of the cell or even different neural pathways or structures. Interestingly, drugs designed to alter the function of a particular neurotransmitter system may actually only be targeting a specific subtype of receptor. This approach can often result in drugs that alter behavior appropriately without producing undesirable side effects.

Heteroreceptors

These function nearly the same as autoreceptors, with the exception that these receptors receive neurotransmitter released by another neuron. These receptors may either excite or inhibit internal processes that control the synthesis and release of a neurotransmitter. As with autoreceptors, heteroreceptors are metabotropic and it is the activity of a second messenger, not the control of ion channels that determine its effects.

Presynaptic Effects

So far, our discussion has focused on synapses between terminal buttons and receptor sites located on either dendrites or cell bodies of receiving neurons. Synapses between axon terminal buttons and the axons of receiving neurons (axoaxonal synapses) are also common. These synapses differ in one significant way, however. Recall from our discussion of neural transmission that a receiving cell integrates the excitatory and inhibitory influences it is receiving at any given moment. If the neuron is receiving sufficient excitatory input to reach threshold, an action potential will occur. With axoaxonic synapses there is no contribution to neural integration but an effect that contributes to the amount of neurotransmitter released. If the axoaxonal synapse is facilitatory it is called **presynaptic facilitation**, and when it is inhibitory it is called **presynaptic inhibition**. Some analgesics reduce pain by presynaptic inhibition of pain-signaling neurotransmitters. The pain-signaling neuron is still producing action potentials, but the amount of neurotransmitter released is significantly reduced.

Neurotransmitter Substances

Since the discovery of the first neurotransmitter by Otto Loewi in the 1920s, about 50 additional substances have been identified as neurotransmitters. A large number of other neuroactive substances called **neuromodulators** have also been described that modulate the effects of neurotransmitters but do not themselves meet all of the identifying criteria. For a substance to be considered a neurotransmitter it must: (1) be synthesized and stored in the presynaptic neuron, (2) be released into the synapse when the neuron fires, (3) cause a postsynaptic effect after it interacts with a receptor, and (4) there must be some mechanism for degradation or reuptake. Table 1.1 presents a list of several important substances known to be neurotransmitters, as well as the functions they are thought to perform.

Table 1.1 Chemicals known to be major neurotransmitters or neuromodulators.

Neurotransmitter-neuromodulator effects	*Location*	*Functions*
Acetylcholine (ACh) excitatory	Cortex, spinal cord, target organs activated by the parasympathetic nervous system	Excitation in brain. Either excitation or inhibition in target organs of PNS. Involved in learning, movement, and memory.
Norepinephrine (NE) excitatory, inhibitory	Spinal cord, limbic system, cortex, target organs of the sympathetic nervous system	Arousal of reticular system. Involved in eating, emotional behavior, learning, and memory.
Dopamine (DA) inhibitory	Limbic system, basal ganglia, cerebellum	Involved in movement, emotional behavior, attention, learning, memory, and reward.
Serotonin (SE) inhibitory	Brainstem, most of brain	Involved in emotional behavior, arousal, and sleep.
Gama-amino-butyric acid (GABA) inhibitory	Most of brain and spinal cord	Involved in regulating arousal and anxiety. It is the major inhibitory neurotransmitter in the brain.
Endorphins inhibitory	Spinal cord, most of brain	Functions as a natural analgesic for pain reduction. It is also involved in emotional behavior, eating, and learning.
Glutamate excitatory	Brain and spinal cord	Major excitatory neurotransmitter in the brain. Most neurons in the brain receive excitatory input from glutamate.
Glycine inhibitory	Brain and spinal cord	Co-located on glutamate receptors, widespread inhibitory effects throughout the brain.
Substance P excitatory	Spinal cord	Released by pain-transmitting neurons in the dorsal horn of the spinal cord.
Anandamide inhibitory	Brain, spinal cord, and peripheral nervous system	Neuromodulator that acts on heteroreceptors to regulate neurotransmitter release.
Adenosine inhibitory	Brain and peripheral nervous system	Neuromodulator released by neurons and glia. Plays significant roles in sleep and wakefulness, controls vasodilation.

Although the list of substances so far identified as neurotransmitters is quite large, I will discuss a few that are well understood and play important roles in the psychological disorders that will be discussed in later chapters.

Acetylcholine (ACh)

Acetylcholine was the first neurotransmitter discovered. Its discovery by Otto Loewi in 1921 was rather serendipitous and through its many retellings may only slightly resemble the real occasion. However, prior to Loewi's discovery it was unknown whether neuron signaling was electrical or chemical. There was considerable speculation about possible chemical agents that might be neurotransmitters, but no one had yet discovered them. Loewi apparently awoke from a dream about an experiment that would demonstrate chemical signaling. He quickly scribbled it down and went back to sleep. The next morning he found, to his dismay, that he could not read his scribbles, although he could recall that he had dreamt something important. The next night the dream returned, and Loewi rushed to his laboratory to complete it. His experiment involved removing the hearts from two frogs. One heart was dissected with the vagus nerve, which controls heart rate, intact. The other was removed without the vagus nerve. Next, he placed the hearts in separate dishes filled with saline solution and he then stimulated the vagus nerve of his first frog. After demonstrating a reduction in heart rate he removed some of the saline solution and applied it to the heart of his second frog. Heart rate decreased in this frog as well, demonstrating that a chemical released from the vagus nerve controlled heart rate. In 1936, Loewi was the co-recipient of the Nobel Prize in Physiology or Medicine for this work.

In addition to controlling heart rate, acetylcholine plays an important role in motor movement, as it is the neurotransmitter released from motor neurons onto muscle fibers to make them contract. Several toxins, such as botulin, nerve gas, and black widow spider venom, interfere with acetylcholine transmission and produce paralysis in their victims. This form of paralysis is a consequence of sustained muscle contraction, which can also disrupt respiratory muscles and result in suffocation. A common disorder that involves acetylcholine is Alzheimer's disease, which involves a degeneration of acetylcholine neurons in the basal forebrain. Although the causes of Alzheimer's disease are not well understood, and at the present there is no treatment, drugs that increase the availability of acetylcholine are being used to treat the symptoms of this debilitating disease (Tabet, 2006).

There are two subtypes of acetylcholine receptors, named after substances that are known to bind to them. Muscarinic receptors are metabotropic receptors named after an alkaloid found in the mushroom *Amanita muscaria*. These receptors are distributed throughout the brain, but particularly in the cortex, thalamus, hippocampus, mesolimbic system, and the basal ganglia. They play important roles in cognitive and motor functions as well as in opiate reward. Muscarinic receptors in the ventral tegmental area regulate the release of dopamine in the nucleus accumbens. It is this effect that may contribute to opiate addiction.

The other receptor subtype is called nicotinic, named after the alkaloid nicotine found in tobacco plants. Nicotinic receptors are all ionotropic and are found on all muscle cells at neuromuscular junctions. When bound with acetylcholine these receptors control calcium channels, which leads to muscle contraction. On other non-muscular synapses, nicotinic receptors are associated with EPSPs. Often nicotinic receptors are located on axon terminals (axoaxonal synapses), and they contribute to neurotransmitter release by presynaptic facilitation. Nicotinic receptors also contribute to increased dopamine activity in the ventral tegmental area.

Acetylcholine is synthesized in cholinergic neurons from two precursor compounds: choline and acetyl coenzyme A (acetyl-CoA) (see Figure 1.14). Choline is made available from dietary fat, and acetyl-CoA results from glucose metabolism in most cells. Acetylcholine neurons

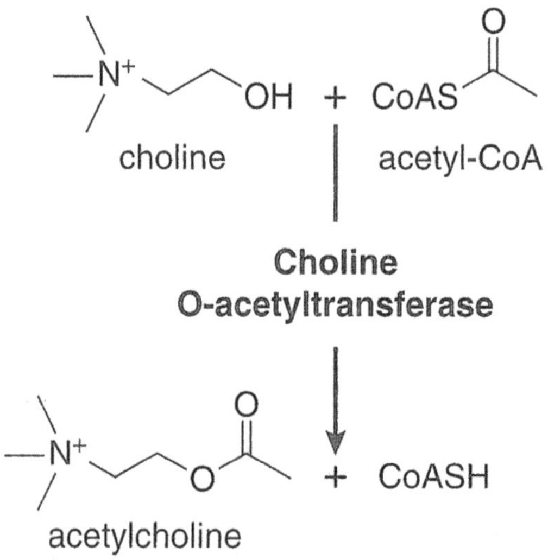

Figure 1.14 Synthesis of ACh from choline and acetyl coenzyme A.

themselves produce choline acetyltransferase (CoASH), the enzyme required to synthesize acetylcholine from these precursors. How much acetylcholine is produced depends both on the availability of its precursors (not typically a problem) and how active these neurons are. Adjusting diet to increase acetylcholine production or ingesting choline has little or no effect.

Acetylcholine Synthesis and Breakdown

Once acetylcholine has been released into the synapse it is quickly broken down by the enzyme acetylcholinesterase (AChE). Acetylcholinesterase not only breaks down acetylcholine that is free in the synapse, it also breaks down acetylcholine that is within the terminal buttons, and not within synaptic vesicles, and the acetylcholine attached to postsynaptic receptors. The breakdown of acetylcholine into choline and acetic acid helps to regulate the amount of acetylcholine available in the neuron as well as to terminate its effects on receiving neurons quickly. Choline is taken back into the neuron by activating the choline transporter protein located on the terminal button. I will have more to say about the synthesis and breakdown of acetylcholine in later chapters when drugs that alter these processes are discussed. The distribution of acetylcholinergic neurons throughout the brain is illustrated in Figure 1.15.

Norepinephrine (NE)

Norepinephrine is distributed throughout the central and peripheral nervous systems. The noradrenergic neurons originate in the pons of the brainstem in a region called the locus coeruleus. They form an excitatory pathway to the cortex known as the **reticular activating system** (RAS). This system is primarily responsible for maintaining cortical arousal. Structures that are innervated along the way include the thalamus, the hypothalamus, and all other limbic structures where it is involved in controlling attention, emotion, and eating. Noradrenergic neurons also play important roles in the PNS-regulating organs, such as the heart. Deficiencies in norepinephrine activity are linked to depression and to attention–deficit disorders (Biederman, 2005).

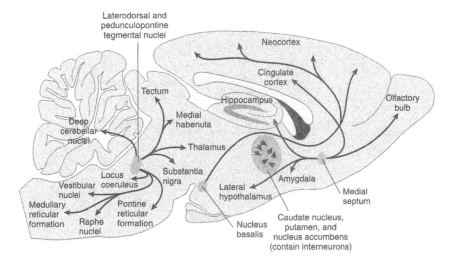

Figure 1.15 Major acetylcholinergic pathways originate in several brainstem regions and the nucleus basalis. They project throughout the brainstem, the limbic system, the basal ganglia, and the cortex.

Norepinephrine binds to several different receptor subtypes that control widely different functions. Norepinephrine α and β subtypes are each separated into two further subtypes: $_1$ and $_2$. All four of these receptor types are found in the brain and in the PNS where they control various organs. The α_2 receptor is also an autoreceptor regulating the synthesis and release of norepinephrine from sending neurons. All noradrenergic receptors are metabotropic and they activate second messenger systems in these neurons. Noradrenergic receptors can produce both excitatory and inhibitory effects depending on the specific receptor. The α_1 and both β_1 and β_2 receptors are excitatory while the α_2 receptors are inhibitory.

Norepinephrine Synthesis and Breakdown

Norepinephrine belongs to a family of neurotransmitters and hormones called catecholamines, a name that describes their primary molecular structure. All catecholamines are synthesized from the same precursor compound, tyrosine, which is made available from dietary proteins. The synthesis of norepinephrine from tyrosine involves several enzymes produced by noradrenergic neurons (see Figure 1.16).

The first phase of the synthesis involves the conversion of tyrosine into DOPA by the enzyme tyrosine hydroxylase. As you might expect by its name, this enzyme facilitates the reaction that adds two hydroxyl groups to tyrosine. The second phase of synthesis from DOPA to dopamine involves the enzyme aromatic amino acid decarboxylase, which cleaves a carbon and several oxygen molecules from DOPA. Finally, dopamine is converted into norepinephrine with the aid of a third enzyme dopamine β-hydroxylase, which adds another hydroxyl group to the molecule. The rate of synthesis depends both on the availability of tyrosine and tyrosine hydroxylase, which is termed a rate-limiting enzyme. When norepinephrine levels are high in the terminal button tyrosine hydroxylase is inhibited, thus decreasing synthesis. When noradrenergic neurons are firing at a high rate, this enzyme is facilitated. As long as there is a sufficient source of tyrosine in one's diet there is no other way to alter norepinephrine levels without drugs. And because the pathways to NE synthesis are complex there are numerous opportunities to alter its synthesis pharmacologically.

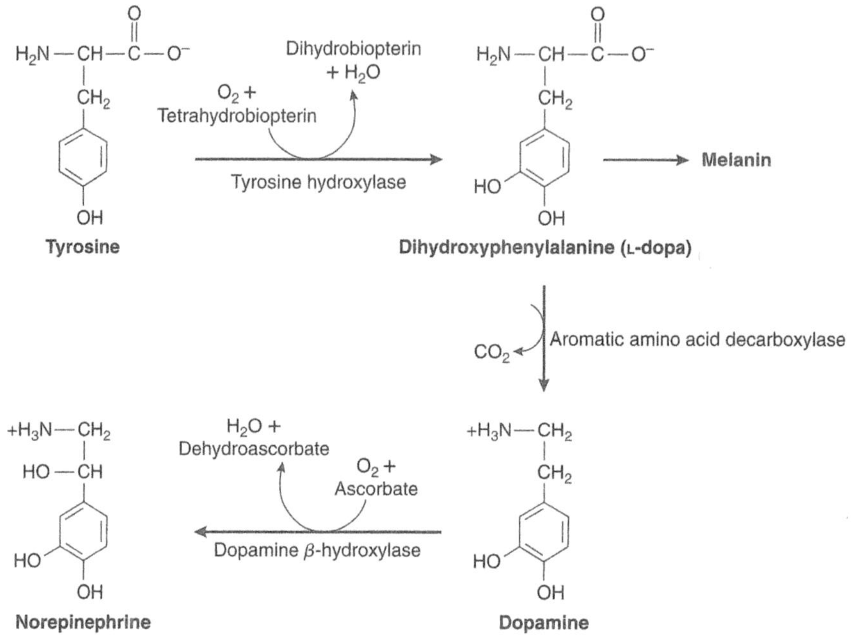

Figure 1.16 Norepinephrine and dopamine are synthesized from dietary tyrosine. Synthesis is terminated at dopamine in dopaminergic neurons.

Norepinephrine is quickly removed from the synapse by two processes: reuptake and break-down by the enzyme monoamine oxydase (MAO). Much of the available norepinephrine in the synapse is transported back into the terminal button intact through the NE transporter protein. The remaining transmitter is broken down by MAO. I will be discussing drugs that block the NE transporter and the activity of MAO later on in our discussions of depression. The major pathways of noradrenergic neurons are illustrated in Figure 1.17.

Dopamine (DA)

Dopamine is located in three distinct pathways that all begin in the brainstem. First, the **nigrostriatal pathway** begins in the brainstem area called the substantia nigra, meaning dark substance, as its color appears somewhat darker than surrounding neural tissues. Axons extending from the cell bodies of dopamine neurons in this region terminate in all regions of the basal ganglia. The primary function of these structures involves voluntary movement, particularly the initiation of movement. Degeneration of dopamine neurons in the nigrostriatal pathway cause Parkinson's disease, which is a severe motor disorder. Parkinson's disease is at the present most effectively treated with a drug (l-DOPA) that readily crosses the blood–brain barrier and is converted into dopamine in the brain (Hurley & Jenner, 2006).

The second major dopamine pathway originates in the ventral tegmental area adjacent to the pons. Axons projecting from the cell bodies of these dopamine neurons form the **meso-limbic system** and project to the nucleus accumbens, the septum, the amygdala, and the hippocampus. Other axons from the ventral tegmental area form the third pathway and project to the frontal cortex. This system is sometimes referred to as the **mesocortical system**, or the reward system (see Figure 1.18). As the name implies, these neurons and their targets have been implicated in reinforcement and they are activated by all addictive drugs. I will have much

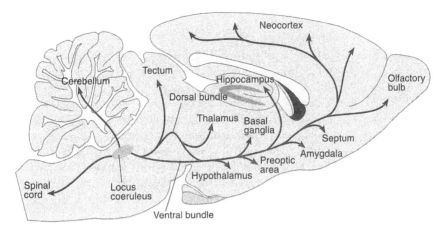

Figure 1.17 Major noradrenergic pathways originate in the locus coeruleus of the brainstem and project throughout the limbic system and cortex.

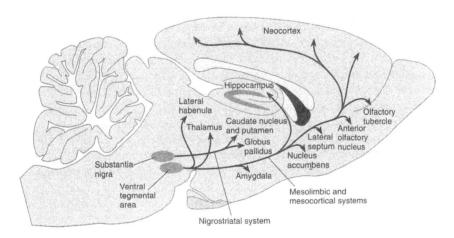

Figure 1.18 Major dopamine pathways originate in the brainstem and midbrain. The mesolimbic system originates in the ventral tegmental area of the midbrain (VTA). The nigrostriatal system originates in the substantia nigra.

more to say about this pathway in discussions of drug abuse. The dopamine pathways are also implicated in the psychotic disorder schizophrenia.

The receptors for dopamine fall into five subfamilies, D_1–D_5. D_1 and D_2 receptors are the most common and they are distributed throughout the basal ganglia, the mesolimbic system, and the cortex. Both of these receptors are metabotropic and regulate the activity of **second messenger systems**, but they have opposite effects. D_1 receptors activate the formation of the second messenger cyclic AMP (cAMP), while D_2 receptors inhibit it. D_2 receptors are primarily inhibitory, resulting in hyperpolarization of the receiving neuron. Because dopamine receptors differ widely in their functions and their distributions they control a large number of important functions. Modern pharmacology attempts to target specific receptor subtypes to produce the desired effects while minimizing unwanted side effects that may also be mediated by dopamine receptors.

Dopamine Synthesis and Breakdown

Dopamine, a catecholamine related to norepinephrine, is also synthesized from dietary tyrosine. The major difference between dopamine and norepinephrine synthesis is that dopamine neurons do not produce the enzyme dopamine β-hydroxylase, which converts dopamine into norepinephrine. Like norepinephrine, the rate-limiting enzyme for dopamine production is tyrosine hydroxylase. Dopamine is quickly removed from the synaptic gap by both reuptake and breakdown. The dopamine transporter protein (DAT), located on the presynaptic membrane, transports dopamine back into the terminal button intact where it can be integrated back into synaptic vesicles and released again. Other dopamine is metabolized by the enzyme MAO. There are two subtypes of monoamine oxidase, MAO-A and MAO-B. Which one plays the major role in breakdown depends on brain location and which neurotransmitter is involved. MAO-A has greater specificity for norepinephrine and serotonin, while both MAO-A and MAO-B metabolize dopamine. Drugs that block the activity of MAO are referred to as monoamine oxidase inhibitors (MAOIs) and they have been widely used to treat depression.

Serotonin (SE)

Serotonin, or 5-hydroxytryptamine (5-HT), belongs to a class of compounds known as monoamines because of their single amine molecular structure. It is distributed throughout the brain and spinal cord and is involved in the control of the sleep/wake cycle, mood, aggressive behavior, and appetite. In fact, since its discovery in the 1970s, it has been implicated in numerous behavioral problems, including sleep disorders, aggression, obesity, anorexia, and depression. A common myth is that simply increasing or decreasing the levels of this neurotransmitter may be the cure to any of these problems. The treatment of behavioral disorders is never this simple.

Serotonin neurons also originate in the brainstem in a region of cell bodies called the raphe nuclei (the term nucleus refers to brain regions that are predominantly cell bodies of a specific neuron type). Two of the regions of greatest interest are the dorsal raphe nucleus and the median raphe nucleus. Axons from these cells travel throughout the cortex and other main brain structures, including the basal ganglia, the thalamus, the hypothalamus, and the mesolimbic system. Receptors for serotonin include both ionotropic and, more predominantly, metabotropic types. As mentioned earlier, they are classified into several subgroups or families, including the 5-HT_1, 5-HT_2, 5-HT_4, etc., through 5-HT_7. These are further divided into 5-HT_{1A} and 5-HT_{1B} for this subgroup. Each of these receptor types seems to have specific functions, and they are distributed in different regions of the brain. I will only discuss a few of these as they have been main targets for pharmacological research. The 5-HT_{1A} subtype function as autoreceptors on serotonin cell bodies regulating the synthesis and release of serotonin, and they are mainly located in the hippocampus and amygdala. 5-HT_{1B} receptors, also autoreceptors, are found predominantly on serotonin axon terminals, and 5-HT_{2A} receptors are located throughout the cortex, the basal ganglia, and the mesolimbic system. The 5-HT_{2A} receptors are metabotropic receptors that activate a second messenger system within the receiving cell.

Serotonin Synthesis and Breakdown

Serotonin is synthesized from tryptophan, an amino acid found in a variety of foods, including dairy products, meats, fish, and poultry. Tryptophan is converted into 5-hydroxytryptophan by the enzyme tryptophan hydroxylase, which is produced by sertotonergic neurons (see Figure 1.19).

This intermediate is converted into 5-HT by amino acid decarboxylase. The amount of serotonin produced is dependent on both the availability of tryptophan and the rate-limiting

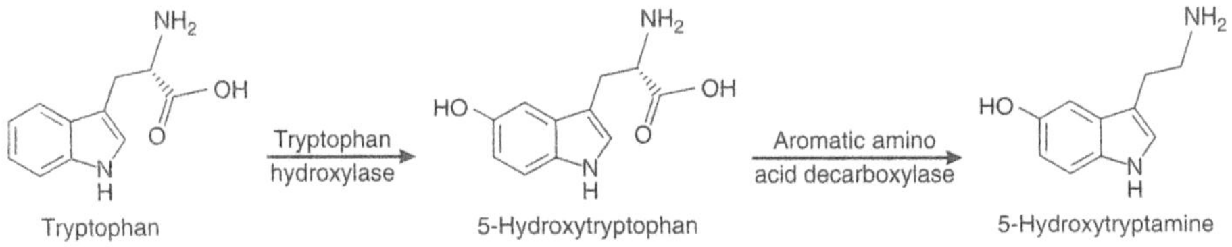

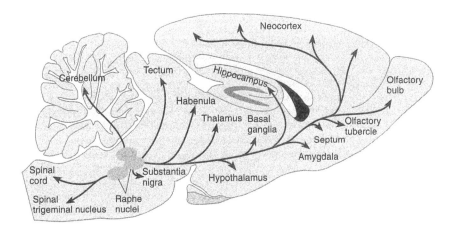

Figure 1.19 Serotonin (5-hydroxytryptamine) is synthesized from dietary tryptophan.

Figure 1.20 Major serotonergic pathways in the brain originate in the raphe nuclei and project throughout the limbic system and cortex.

enzyme tryptophan hydroxylase. However, eating foods rich in tryptophan or taking the supplement may be sufficient to increase serotonin levels only slightly. It is interesting that serotonin levels may actually be increased to a greater extent by eating carbohydrate-rich food. Apparently the amount of tryptophan that can cross from the blood into serotonergic neurons depends on the ratio of carbohydrate to tryptophan-rich protein. This may be why some people are soothed by chocolate!

Serotonin, as with norepinephrine and dopamine, is removed from activity by both reuptake and by enzymatic breakdown. Reuptake is accomplished through the serotonin transporter protein imbedded in the presynaptic membrane. Once inside the terminal button, serotonin can be transported further into the synaptic vesicles for later release. The remaining serotonin is rapidly degraded by monoamine oxidase (MAO), which breaks serotonin into its metabolite 5-hydroxyindolacetic acid. The amount of this metabolite is an index of serotonin activity and it can be easily measured. Both of these processes are targets for drug development and some the most popular antidepressants used today are designed to block the reuptake process. These drugs are called serotonin specific reuptake inhibitors (SSRIs). The major serotonergic pathways are illustrated in Figure 1.20.

Glutamate

Glutamate or glutamic acid is an amino acid derived from glutamine. Not only is it used by cells for protein synthesis and other cellular functions, it is one of the most important excitatory neurotransmitters in the brain. It is known to play an important role in a process called long-term potentiation, which is a change in neuronal functioning that mediates some forms of learning and memory (Robbins & Murphy, 2006). Because of its ubiquitous presence throughout the brain, we should not be surprised to find that its activity will play a role in several of the disorders discussed in later chapters. Unlike the neurotransmitters acetylcholine, norepinephrine, dopamine, and serotonin, glutamate neurons do not originate in the brainstem and form pathways through the limbic and cortical areas of the brain. Rather, glutamate neurons are found in most brain regions with large projections throughout the cerebral cortex, the hippocampus, and the cerebellum.

Glutamate receptors can be either ionotropic or metabotropic. Ionotropic receptors have been classified as either **AMPA** (α-amino 3-hydroxy 5-methyl 4-isoxazole propionic acid), **kainate** (after kainic acid, which binds to it), or **NMDA** (N-methyl D-aspartate). All of these ionotropic receptors control sodium influx, which produces fast depolarization of postsynaptic membranes. In addition to controlling sodium influx, the NMDA receptor also controls calcium (Ca^{2+}) influx, which contributes to both fast depolarization and also initiates a slower and prolonged acting second messenger system. In this sense, the NMDA receptor has both ionotropic and metabotropic properties. Of these three receptor types, it is the NMDA receptor that has received the most attention because of its role in mediating the cellular changes that underlie learning and memory. The NMDA receptor has several unique properties, including functioning as both an ionotropic and a metabotropic receptor. In its resting, polarized state, the glutamate receptor channel is occupied by a magnesium ion (Mg^{2+}) that prevents the influx of Ca^{2+}. In order for the membrane to become permeable to Ca^{2+}, it must be sufficiently depolarized by high-frequency stimulation to eject Mg^{2+}. Finally, this receptor requires the presence of a second neurotransmitter, glycine (an inhibitory neurotransmitter), before the ion channel for Ca^{2+} is opened. In summary, the NMDA receptor controls both Na^+ and Ca^{2+} channels. The Ca^{2+} channel is only opened when both glutamate and glycine are bound to it and the postsynaptic membrane is sufficiently depolarized to eject Mg^{2+}, which is blocking the Ca^{2+} channel. Once Ca^{2+} enters, it initiates a second messenger system, which leads to cellular changes that underlie learning and memory (see Figure 1.21). This cellular change

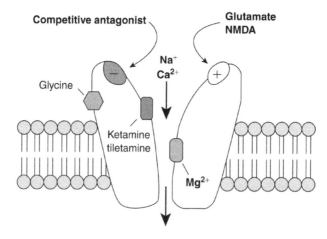

Figure 1.21 Glutamate receptor. Normally the ion channel is blocked by Mg^{2+}. Activation of the receptor displaces Mg2+ and allows either Na^+ or Ca^{2+} to enter. The glutamate receptor requires the presence of glycine (an inhibitory neurotransmitter) before the ion channel for Ca^{2+} is opened.

is called **long-term potentiation**, referring to the fact that the postsynaptic membrane can now more readily depolarize when stimulated. Long-term potentiation is believed to be one of several important kinds of long-term synaptic changes that mediate learning. Drugs that disrupt NMDA receptors can interfere with learning and memory.

There are at least eight metabotropic glutamate receptors that have been identified. These metabotropic receptors mediate second messenger systems that lead to synaptic and cellular changes that contribute to a host of physiological functions, including learning, motor control, and pain.

Glutamate Synthesis and Breakdown

Glutamate is synthesized from glutamine, an abundant nonessential amino acid in all cells that is readily available from proteins in meats, fish, eggs, and dairy products. The synthesis of glutamate from glutamine is facilitated by the enzyme glutaminase. Because all cells can synthesize glutamate, cells that, in addition, store it in synaptic vesicles and release it when the cell is activated are called glutaminergic neurons. Glutamate can also be ingested directly. The food preservative monosodium glutamate (MSG) contains glutamate. Eating foods containing large amounts of glutamate, including the food preservative monosodium glutamate (MSG), may produce symptoms of dizziness and numbness. In large amounts glutamate is known to be neurotoxic and can lead to cell death. Excessive exposure of postsynaptic neurons to glutamate is referred to as **excitotoxicity**, and we will see later that this may contribute to symptoms of schizophrenia.

Glutamate is removed from the synapse by several reuptake mechanisms. All of these are mediated by a glutamate transporter found either on the presynaptic terminal button or on surrounding glial cells. If glutamate is taken up by glial cells it is converted back to glutamine before its transport back to a glutaminergic neuron. Once inside the terminal button, glutamine is converted into glutamate and transported into synaptic vesicles for storage and later release.

Gamma-Amino-Butyric Acid (GABA)

GABA is the major inhibitory neurotransmitter in the brain and spinal cord. Like neural excitation, neural inhibition is critical for the regulation and control of all physiological and behavior functions. Alterations in GABA functioning result from a variety of drugs, including alcohol, and they all have profound effects on behavior and mood. GABAergic neurons are distributed throughout the cortex, the hippocampus, limbic structures, the basal ganglia, and the brainstem and cerebellum. Often GABA neurons are interneurons, but GABAergic neurons may also project along pathways between brain structures. The receptors for GABA can be either ionotropic or metabotropic. The **ionotropic receptor** is classified as GABA$_A$ and the **metabotropic receptor** GABA$_B$. GABA produces neural inhibition by opening Cl$^-$ channels so chlorine can move from the outside of the membrane to the inside. This movement of negatively charged ions to the inside hyperpolarizes the membrane from about -70 mv to an even greater negative charge, making it more difficult for an action potential to occur. The GABA$_A$ receptor is composed of a membrane-spanning protein that contains at least five different binding sites. The primary site is for GABA, but there are additional sites for barbiturates, benzodiazapines, steroids, Picrotoxin, and alcohol. These binding sites are named after compounds or classes of drugs that specifically bind to them. For example, the benzodiazepine drugs all appear to bind specifically to the benzodiazepine site. Each of these other compounds or classes of drugs can cause the Cl$^-$ channel to open on its own and they can facilitate and prolong GABA binding (see Figure 1.22).

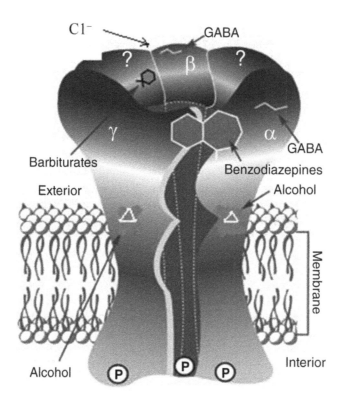

Figure 1.22 GABA$_A$ receptor complex. Contains binding sites for GABA, barbiturate, benzodiazepine, and alcohol.

The GABA$_B$ receptor is a metabotropic receptor that facilitates the opening of K^+ channels, also hyperpolarizing the postsynaptic membrane. The GABA$_B$ receptor is less widely distributed than the GABA$_A$ receptor, and it functions both as a postsynaptic receptor and as an autoreceptor that functions to regulate the synthesis and release of GABA. Most of the GABA drugs discussed in this text primarily affect the GABA$_A$ receptor.

GABA Synthesis and Breakdown

Ironically GABA is synthesized from the excitatory neurotransmitter glutamate discussed earlier by neurons that produce the enzyme glutamic acid decarboxylase. The amount synthesized is regulated by this enzyme, not necessarily the amount of glutamate present within the cell. Drugs that block the synthesis of GABA can produce excessive neural excitation and even seizures.

GABA is removed from the synapse in a manner similar to that of glutamate. That is, GABA is either transported intact back into the terminal button or it is taken up by glial cells and converted first into glutamate, then into glutamine. Glutamine is transported into the terminals of GABA cells for resynthesis and reintegration into synaptic vesicles for storage and release. Excess GABA within the terminal button is degraded by the enzyme GABA aminotransferase, which breaks GABA into its precursor glutamate. Drugs that block the activity of this enzyme may be useful for the treatment of seizures as they can result in increased amounts of GABA available for release. Drugs that increase the activity of GABA are used to treat anxiety, insomnia, and seizures associated with epilepsy and some forms of depression.

Endorphins

Endorphins are a family of peptide neurotransmitters chemically similar to opiates, such as morphine. Their name is derived from endo (for endogenous) and orphin (from morphine). They are widely distributed throughout most of the brain and spinal cord. Extensive research has linked the endorphins to an array of behavioral and physiological processes, including inducing analgesia, a sense of euphoria, counteracting the influence of stress, and modulating food and liquid intake. There are high concentrations of endorphin neurons distributed throughout the cortex, the thalamus, the limbic system, the spinal cord, and in the pituitary gland, which controls the release of the stress hormone corticotrophin releasing factor (CRF). Receptors for the endorphins fall into three subtypes; μ (mu), κ (kappa), and δ (delta). All of the endorphin receptors are inhibitory metabotropic receptors. They control mechanisms within the postsynaptic cell that regulate either K^+ or Ca^{++} influx, or second messenger systems that inhibit cell excitability. I discuss several drugs that bind selectively to these opiate receptors, including the opiate morphine, later on.

Substance P

Substance P belongs to the peptide class of neurotransmitters, hence its name. Its primary function appears to be signaling messages from pain receptors called **nocioceptors** to the dorsal horn of the spinal cord. Substance P activates ascending pain neurons that comprise the spinothalamic pain pathway. Opiates and other drugs can inhibit pain signaling by decreasing the release of Substance P.

The preceding discussion is only a brief review of several of the most important neurotransmitters and neuromodulators that will be further discussed in later chapters. New neurotransmitters and other neuroactive substances are still being discovered and investigated. Such discoveries have been central to the development of psychopharmacology. At present, the number of substances identified and believed to be either neurotransmitters or neuromodulators exceeds 150.

The Organization and Structure of the Nervous System and Brain

Our nervous system is separated into two distinct components: the **central nervous system** (CNS), which consists of the brain and spinal cord, and the **peripheral nervous system** (PNS), which transmits and receives information to and from our muscles, glands, and internal organs and to our skin (see Figure 1.23).

Both of these systems must work in synchrony for normal, adaptive behavior. For instance, information from our stomach (PNS) communicates to the CNS its state of fullness. Although peripheral signals from the stomach are only part of the complex regulation of hunger and eating, they are critical for normal eating behavior. Communication can also originate in the CNS without an eliciting stimulus. A decision to stop reading this text and go outside might originate within the CNS and direct motivational and motor systems to initiate the movement. Drugs used to treat psychological disorders may have both central and peripheral effects. While it is often the CNS effects that are critical for therapy, a drug's peripheral effects (side effects) may be even more salient. Some drugs used to treat schizophrenia, for example, can produce sexual dysfunction, dry mouth, blurred vision, and high heart rate. In the following sections,

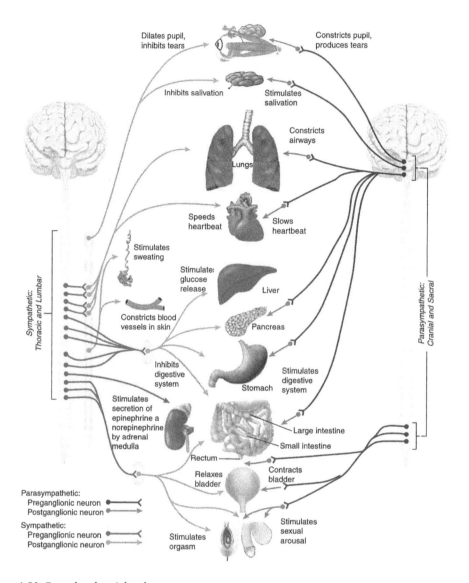

Figure 1.23 Central and peripheral nervous systems.

we will review the major components of the CNS and examine the structure and function of the cells that it is composed of.

Central Nervous System

As stated in the beginning, the average human brain weighs approximately 1,400 grams (or roughly three pounds) and contains nearly 200 billion neurons. The brain is organized into numerous structures that interact to regulate eating and drinking, produce movement, emotion, learning and memory, and allow us to experience the world through our senses. We will examine some of these structures and their functions in this section.

If a person's skull were removed so that you could look at the surface of the brain you would be looking at the surface of the cerebral cortex (see Figure 1.24). In its natural state, the human

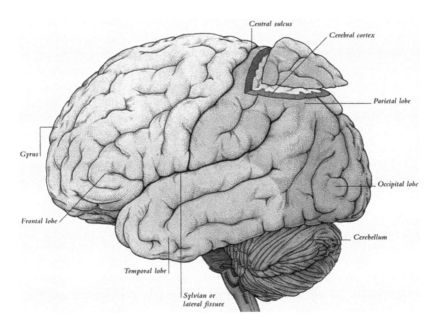

Figure 1.24 Cortex with major fissures and gyri and lobes identified.

cortex looks much like a soft, wrinkled walnut, its outer surface filled with crevices and folds. The left and right sides appear to be separated by a long, deep fissure (called the longitudinal sulcus). The cortex is divided into two sides or cerebral hemispheres that, while not identical, are almost mirror images of each other. Under the cortex are many other structures. Starting from the spinal cord and working roughly upward through the base of the brain, these include the medulla, the pons, the cerebellum, the hypothalamus and other structures of the limbic system, the thalamus, and the structures of the basal ganglia, including the substantia nigra, the caudate nucleus, and the putamen.

Cerebral Cortex

The cerebral cortex consists of the thin outer layer of the brain. Its average thickness is about 3 mm, and its surface area is estimated to be about 2,400 cm². The Latin *cortex* means bark, and the cortex covers the brain in much the same way as bark covers a tree trunk. This portion of the brain is also called the **neocortex**, or new cortex, since it was the last part of the brain to develop during evolution. A deep grove in the cortex is referred to as a fissure or sulcus and a protuberance is called a gyrus. Names for specific regions of the cortex include these terms as identifiers to distinguish and locate them.

The wrinkled and convoluted appearance of the cortex is nature's solution to the problem of cramming the huge neocortical area into a relatively small space within the skull. The size of the skull is essentially fixed because increases in skull size would require commensurate increases in the size of female pelvic structures to allow for full-term childbirth. As this example illustrates, evolutionary changes to one structure often require changes to others.

The cortex is divided into four lobes named after the bones of the skull that cover them. The frontal lobes include everything in front of (rostral to) the central sulcus, the temporal lobes on either hemisphere are located below the lateral fissure, the parietal lobes are behind (caudal to) the central sulcus, and the occipital lobes are at the caudal tip of each hemisphere.

These lobes are further separated into functional areas. Three of these areas receive and process sensory information: the primary auditory cortex, the primary visual cortex, and the primary somatosensory cortex. Adjacent to each of these sensory areas is an association cortex where sensory processing, perception, and memories occur. In addition to sensory processing, the cortex includes large areas for motor control and movement. The primary motor cortex is located within the frontal lobes in the gyrus immediately rostral to the central sulcus. Areas for processing emotion are located in both of the prefrontal regions of the frontal lobes and in the cingulate cortex, which lies deep within the longitudinal sulcus that separates the two hemispheres. In addition to processing emotion, the prefrontal areas are involved, along with the sensory association cortices, in the processing of short-term memories (see Figure 1.24).

We will be discussing many of these cortical areas in later chapters, as they are implicated in several psychological disorders and are sites of action for a number of psychotropic drugs.

Spinal Cord

Because the brain occupies the commanding position in the CNS, the spinal cord is often overlooked in discussions of the biological bases of behavior. However, the spinal cord fills the very important function of conveying messages to and from the brain. In addition, the spinal cord controls reflexes, which are simple circuits of sensory and motor neurons that initiate responses to specific stimuli.

All complex behaviors require integration and coordination at the level of the brain. However, certain basic reflexive behaviors (such as a leg jerk in response to a tap on the kneecap or the quick withdrawal of a hand from a hot stove) do not require brain processing. Different parts of the spinal cord control different reflexes: Hand withdrawal is controlled by the upper spinal cord, whereas the knee jerk response is controlled by an area in the lower cord. The brain is not directly involved in controlling these simple reflexive responses, but it is clearly aware of what action has transpired. The top of the spinal cord and the brainstem are illustrated in Figure 1.25.

Before beginning our discussion of the CNS and its various structures and systems, we need to review the terms that describe how the brain is dissected and the locations of structures relative to these dissections. Anatomists typically describe the brain from one of several transections through it. Sections along the axis from front to back are referred to as sagittal sections. The most common of these sections is a mid-sagittal section through the midline of the brain. Another way of observing structures within the brain that do not fall along the midline is to take a series of sections horizontally through the brain. These horizontal sections reveal the relative positions of structures that do not lie along the mid-sagittal plane. Finally, sections may be taken vertically through the brain. These views of the internal structures of the brain are referred to as coronal sections (see Figure 1.26).

These anatomical terms will be used throughout this chapter to describe various structures and systems of the brain.

Medulla

The medulla is the lowest part of the brain, located just above (superior to) the spinal cord. This structure is in a well-protected location, deep and low within the brain. It contains centers that control many vital life-support functions, such as breathing, heart rate, and blood pressure. The medulla also plays an important role in consciousness and in regulating other reflexive functions, such as sneezing, coughing, and vomiting. The medulla forms the base of the RAS, which is discussed later (see Figure 1.25). Opiates, and alcohol at high doses, can disrupt the medulla's response to CO_2, leading to respiratory depression and death.

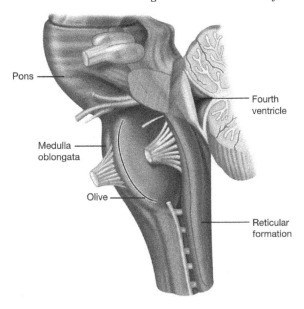

Figure 1.25 Brainstem section showing the pons and the medulla. The reticular formation is a complex array of neurons that ascend through the midline of the brainstem and project to the thalamus. These neurons are essential for vital functions such as respiration, heart rate, blood pressure, as well as cortical arousal.

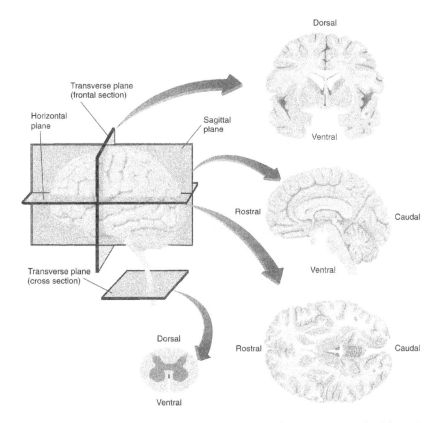

Figure 1.26 Sections of the human brain from different anatomical perspectives. Each of these views reveals the relative positions of various structures within the brain.

Pons

The pons is a large bulge in the lower brain core, dorsal to the medulla. The pons plays an important role in fine-tuning motor messages as they travel from the motor area of the cerebral cortex down to the cerebellum. Species-typical behaviors (such as fear and feeding behaviors) and facial expressions are mediated by the pons, which appears to program the patterns of muscle movement required for them.

The pons also plays a role in processing some sensory information, particularly visual information. In addition, the pons contains specialized nuclei that help control respiration and mediate pain and analgesia.

Cerebellum

The cerebellum is a distinctive structure about the size of a fist, tucked beneath the posterior part of the cerebral hemispheres. It consists of two wrinkled hemispheres covered by an outer cortex. The cerebellum's primary function is to coordinate and regulate motor movements that are broadly controlled by higher brain centers, including the cortex and structures of the basal ganglia, to be discussed later. The cerebellum fine-tunes and smooths out movements, particularly those required for rapid changes in direction. For example, when you reach out to catch a moving ball, your cerebellum is involved in the timing of your movements. This kind of timed movement clearly involves learning. Experiments with animals have shown that the activity of specific cells in the cerebellum change during the course of learning, and that blocking projections from cells within the cerebellum disrupts learned responses (Wikgren et al., 2006).

Damage to the cerebellum results in awkward, jerky, uncoordinated movements and may even affect speech. Professional boxers are especially susceptible to slight damage to the cerebellum, which results in a condition called punch-drunk syndrome. Motor impairment following alcohol intoxication may also be related to alcohol's effects on cells in the cerebellum.

Reticular Formation

The reticular formation consists of a set of neural structures that extend from the medulla up to the thalamus. Research has demonstrated that the reticular formation plays a critical role in consciousness and in controlling arousal and alertness. For this reason, it has become common to refer to this collection of structures as the **reticular activating system**, or RAS (see Figure 1.25). Attention-deficit/hyperactivity disorder (ADHD) may result from insufficient, rather than excessive, arousal produced by the reticular system, explaining why treatment with psychostimulants is often successful. I will discuss this in more detail in our chapter on attention disorders.

Some of the neural circuits that carry sensory messages from the lower regions of the brain to the higher brain areas have ancillary or detouring fibers that connect with the reticular system. Impulses from these fibers prompt the reticular formation to send signals upward, making us more responsive and alert to our environment. Experiments have shown that mild electrical stimulation of certain areas within this network causes sleeping animals to awaken slowly, whereas stronger stimulation causes animals to awaken rapidly, with greater alertness.

The reticular formation also seems to be linked to sleep cycles. When we fall asleep, our reticular systems cease to send alerting messages to our brains. While sleeping, we may screen out our extraneous stimuli, with the possible exception of critical messages, such as the sounds of a squeaking floor or a baby's cry. Although the role of the reticular formation in sleep is still not fully understood, we do know that reticular neurons inhibit sleep-active neurons during wakefulness (Osaka & Matsumura, 1994) and that serious damage to this structure may cause a person to be extremely lethargic or to enter into a prolonged coma. Recent evidence also suggests that patients in a severe coma may be aroused by electrical stimulation of the reticular system (Cooper et al., 1999).

Limbic System

The **limbic system** is the portion of the brain most closely associated with emotional expression and motivation; it also plays a significant role in learning and memory. The limbic system is a collection of structures located around the central core of the brain, along the innermost edge of the cerebral hemispheres. The key structures of the limbic system include the amygdala, the hippocampus, the nucleus accumbens, parts of the hypothalamus, and the bundles of axons that connect these structures. The limbic system also includes the cingulate gyrus, which is located above the corpus callosum within the fissure that separates the two cerebral hemispheres. Damage to, or stimulation of, sites within this system may profoundly affect emotional expression, either by causing excessive reactions to situations or by greatly reducing emotional responses. Limbic structures are also implicated in major depression, and drugs we discuss later on will act on some of these structures. Structures of the limbic system are illustrated in Figure 1.27.

Amygdala

The amygdala, a small structure located in the inferior temporal lobe, plays an important role in the expression of anger, rage, aggression, and fear-motivated behavior. Electrical stimulation or surgical damage to areas within the amygdala may cause an animal to go into a blind rage, whereas in other parts of the amygdala the same procedures may produce extreme passivity. The amygdala also plays a significant role in social cognition and in decision-making. Amygdala damage in humans results in the inability of memories to trigger emotional states. These emotional states are essential to normal social functioning and decision-making. For example, when you make a decision to invest a large sum of money, an emotional state induced by the

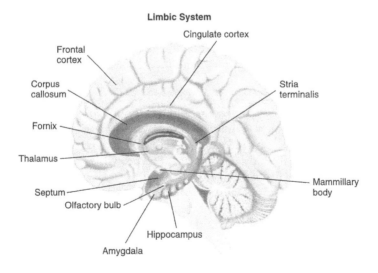

Figure 1.27 Limbic structures revealed from a sagittal section of the brain.

thought of either making more or losing it all guides your decision to invest or not. People with amygdala damage lose these functions, making normal decisions difficult (Adolphs et al., 1995; Bechara & Damasio, 2002; Bechara et al., 2003).

Nucleus Accumbens

The nucleus accumbens, located near the amygdala, is part of a group of structures that form the pathway for dopamine neurons originating in the upper pons and terminating in the frontal cortex. This pathway, referred to as the **mesolimbic-cortical system**, begins in the ventral tegmental area of the pons and passes through the nucleus accumbens, where it is routed to the frontal cortex. The nucleus accumbens is associated with the reinforcing properties of a category of highly valued stimuli, including food, sex, and addictive drugs. The dopamine-containing neurons of the mesolimbic system have an excitatory effect on the frontal cortex.

Hippocampus

The hippocampus is also located in the inferior temporal lobe. This structure plays a significant role in the formation of new memories. Individuals who experience damage to this structure have difficulty storing new information in memory. Recent evidence suggests that the hippocampus may also undergo significant alterations as a result of stress and its size may be smaller in patients who have experienced prolonged periods of stress, have post-traumatic stress disorder, or who may have schizophrenia. The stress hormone cortisol, a glucocorticoid, can cause neuronal atrophy in the hippocampus, as well as inhibit the growth of new neurons in adults. Both of these consequences result in a decline in memory.

Hypothalamus

The hypothalamus is a grape-sized structure that lies inferior to the thalamus and above the optic chiasm. Although it is relatively small, it is essential for many physiological functions and for the motivation of behavior. The hypothalamus integrates information from a number of neurotransmitters and hormones that indicate changes in body states. The maintenance of a relatively constant internal environment, including fluid and nutrient levels, requires the integration of information about the status of these systems as well as the initiation of motivational systems to ensure they remain relatively stable. For example, neurons in the lateral hypothalamus secrete the peptide neurotransmitter **orexin** in response to signals indicating depletion in energy stores. Orexin, in turn, stimulates appetite and a reduction in metabolic rate to conserve remaining energy.

Shivering when we are cold and perspiring when we are hot are both homeostatic processes that act to restore normal body temperature and are controlled by neurons in the anterior hypothalamus. The hypothalamus is also critical to sexual motivation, and it contains distinct nuclei for males and females. The medial preoptic nucleus of the hypothalamus contains a greater number of cells in males than in females. The growth of these neurons depends on androgens during development, and they are responsible for normal male sexual behaviors. In females it is the ventromedial hypothalamus that controls sexual motivation, and this region contains large numbers of estrogen receptors (see Figure 1.28).

The hypothalamus is also the center of the neuroendocrine system, which controls the activity of the pituitary gland and various other hormone-secreting endocrine glands. The hypothalamus contains specialized secretory cells that produce and release hormones that stimulate the **pituitary gland**. The pituitary gland produces and secretes a variety of essential hormones, including male and female sex hormones, growth hormone, adrenocorticotropic

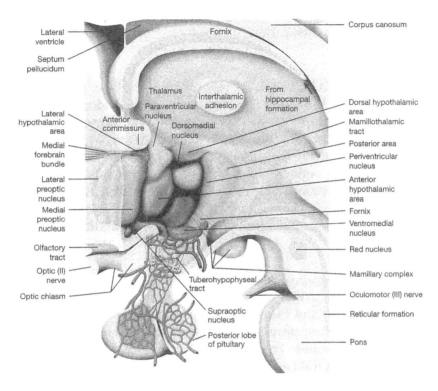

Figure 1.28 Hypothalamus and thalamus revealed from an animated sagittal section.

hormone, antidiuretic hormone, and oxytocin. Figure 1.28 illustrates the hypothalamus and many of its nuclei.

Thalamus

The thalamus is located above the hypothalamus in the center of the cerebral hemispheres. It is composed of two oval-shaped lobes that lie side by side, one in each hemisphere. Sensory input to the cortex is routed through specific regions within the thalamus with the sole exception of the sense of smell. These distinct regions are specialized for certain kinds of sensory information. Auditory messages from the inner ear travel to the medial geniculate nucleus of the thalamus before being routed to the primary auditory cortex, and visual messages transmitted from your eyes pass through the lateral geniculate nucleus in route to the primary visual cortex. In addition to this function, the thalamus also appears to work in conjunction with the reticular formation to help regulate sleep cycles and to control the excitability of all regions of the cortex. I will have more to say about the thalamus and its control over the excitability of the cortex in the chapter on attention disorders.

Basal Ganglia

The basal ganglia consist of several subcortical brain structures, including the caudate nucleus, the putamen, and the substantia nigra (see Figure 1.29). These structures receive messages from the cortex and the thalamus. The primary function of the basal ganglia is in the control and initiation of motor movement. One of the most common disorders of the basal ganglia is

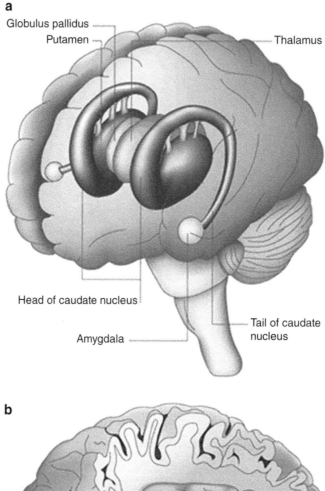

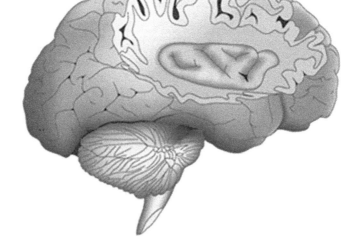

Figure 1.29 The structures of the basal ganglia include the caudate nucleus, the putamen, and the globus pallidus.

Parkinson's disease, which results from the progressive destruction of the dopamine-containing neurons of the substantia nigra. This destruction leads to decreased activity of other structures within the basal ganglia, including the caudate nucleus and putamen. This disease occurs most often in the elderly; however, it may occur in individuals in their late forties or fifties,

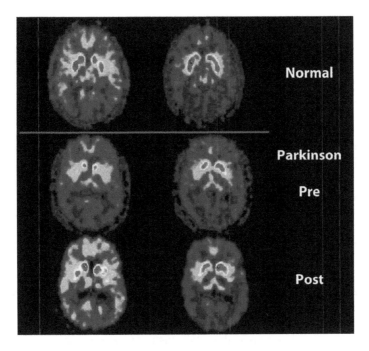

Figure 1.30 PET scans revealing the activity of neurons within the caudate nucleus in normal subjects, as well a patient with Parkinson's disease before (pre) and after (post) L-DOPA treatment. Red and yellow colors indicate more neural activity than green and blue colored areas.

like Michael J. Fox. Parkinson's disease is characterized by difficulty in initiating movement, rigidity, and tremors often in the hands. Parkinson's disease is commonly treated with drugs that increase dopamine neural transmission such as L-DOPA, but embryonic and stem cell transplants into the substantia nigra are perhaps the most promising treatments for the future (Brederlau et al., 2006).

A related movement disorder, **tardive dyskinesia**, may result from long-term use of anti-psychotic medication. These drugs block a subset of dopamine receptors referred to as D_2 receptors. As a result, these dopamine receptors may become sensitized, causing the excessive movement associated with this disease. In a sense, Parkinson's and tardive dyskinesia are opposite diseases—Parkinson's occurring when dopamine pathways begin to degenerate in the basal ganglia, and tardive dyskinesia when dopamine receptors in the same region become too sensitive (see Figure 1.30). I will have more to say about tardive dyskinesia in the chapter on antipsychotic medication.

Glossary

Action potential complete depolarization of the neuronal membrane from −70 mV to approximately +40 mV.

Autoreceptors receptors located on the terminal button or cell body that receive neurotransmitter released from its terminal button. Autoreceptors control neurotransmitter synthesis and release.

Central nervous system (CNS) consists of the entire brain and the spinal cord.

Excitatory postsynaptic potentials graded membrane potentials that depolarize the neuron, bringing it closer to its firing threshold.

Excitotoxicity a consequence of a high rate of presynaptic activity on a neuron resulting in excessive Ca^{++} influx and eventual cell death.

Graded potential small changes in a membrane's resting potential. Graded potentials may be excitatory and depolarize the membrane from -70 mV to -60 mV, or they may be inhibitory and hyperpolarize the membrane to -75 or -80 mV. See also **Excitatory** and **Inhibitory postsynaptic potentials**.

Heteroreceptors receptors located on the terminal button or cell body that receive neurotransmitter released from another neuron. Heteroreceptors control neurotransmitter synthesis and release.

Inhibitory postsynaptic potentials graded membrane potentials that hyperpolarize the neuron, making it less likely to fire.

Interneurons reside only within the central nervous system and function to bridge communication between sensory and motor neurons.

Ion channel a protein embedded in the cell membrane that controls the movement of charged ions across the cell's membrane.

Ionotropic receptor a receptor that directly controls an ion channel on the cell membrane.

Neocortex Latin for new cortex, since it was the last part of the brain to develop during evolution. It consists of the outer layers of the cerebral cortex.

Neural integration the process of summation of all excitatory and inhibitory potentials on the cell of receiving neurons.

Neuromodulator a substance produced and released by neurons or glia that alters cell functioning. Neuromodulators may alter the effects of neurotransmitters at synapses and, unlike neurotransmitters, they may act at greater distances from the releasing cell.

Neurotransmitter reuptake the process of removing neurotransmitter substance from the synaptic gap back into the terminal button by a transporter protein.

Nigrostriatal pathway dopamine neurons originating in the substantia nigra of the brainstem and project to the striatum or basal ganglia.

Node of Ranvier a small gap in the myelin that surrounds the axon of a neuron. The membrane of the axon is exposed to the extracellular environment at these gaps.

Orexin a peptide neurotransmitter produced by cells within the lateral hypothalamus. Orexin is a powerful appetite stimulant and plays a significant role in sleep–wake cycles.

Peripheral nervous system (PNS) transmits and receives information to and from our muscles, glands, and internal organs and to our skin.

Phosphoralation the adding of a phosphate molecule to the ion channel protein. Phosphoralation results in a change in the protein configuration, allowing for charged ions to pass through it.

Pituitary gland attached to the base of the hypothalamus by the pituitary stalk, the pituitary gland is responsible for the production and secretion of a variety of essential hormones.

Resting potential the state of a neuron when the ionic electrostatic and diffusion forces are at equilibrium. The resting potential may vary between -60 and -70 mV depending on the neuron and its location.

Reticular activating system noradrenergic and cholinergic neurons originating in the brainstem and projecting via the thalamus to the cortex.

Second messenger a substance within the cell that becomes activated during cell signaling. Second messengers initiate biochemical processes that result in opening or closing ion channels, the activation of cell enzymes or hormones, and the expression of genes.

Tardive dyskinesia a severe motor disorder characterized by facial tics, lip smacking, tongue extensions, and rapid eye blinking. Can be caused by long-term use of antipsychotic medication.

2 Psychopharmacology
Pharmacokinetics and Pharmacodynamics

Have you ever wondered whether getting that morning coffee might work just a little bit better if you could hook yourself up to an IV? While being tied to a drip bag with a long thin tube might get caffeine into your blood stream much more quickly, missing out on the sensory aspects of this morning ritual would make your experience much less pleasant. As we will see in this chapter the action of a drug can, and often does, depend not only on its pharmacological properties, but on how rapidly it enters the brain, the context in which it is administered, and our expectations of its effects. We begin by examining how routes of administration and drug dose affect how much and for how long drugs are available at target sites. We will also explore how repeated exposure to a drug alters its effectiveness. These are all topics of **pharmacokinetics**, the science of how drugs are absorbed, distributed to body tissues, and eliminated from the body after metabolism.

Drug Names

Before we discuss pharmacokinetics, however, a brief discussion of the drug naming convention is in order. Students are often appropriately confused over drug names, as most drugs have several. For example, drugs can be named after their chemical structure, which may be useful to a chemist, but these names are far too awkward to use in any other context. The **chemical name** for the popular antidepressant Prozac is N-methyl-3-phenyl-3-[4-(trifluoromethyl)phenoxy]-propan-1-amine. A drug's chemical name reveals its chemical composition and molecular structure. Pharmaceutical companies may also patent **brand names** or trade names for their product. These brand names reveal little if anything about the drug's makeup or structure. Most of us are familiar with drug brand names because these are the names that are used in advertising the drug. When drugs are marketed in different countries they may have several brand names. The name Prozac is a brand or trade name. Pharmaceutical companies typically receive exclusive rights to manufacture and distribute brand name drugs that they have developed. Once this exclusivity has expired (typically after five to seven years) a drug can be manufactured and distributed by other drug manufacturers as a **generic drug**. The generic drug name can be used by any number of companies who market and distribute the same generic drug. The generic name for Prozac is fluoxetine. Generic drugs must contain the same active ingredients as the original brand name drug and they must be pharmacologically equivalent. Because several manufacturers may compete to produce and market generic drugs, their cost is often considerably less than their equivalent brand name drug. Table 2.1 presents several common drugs and their respective brand and generic names.

DOI: 10.4324/9781003309017-2

Table 2.1 Examples of several common drug names.

Chemical name	Brand (trade) name	Generic name
N-methyl-3-phenyl-3-[4-(trifluoromethyl) phenoxy]-propan-1-amine	Prozac	fluoxetine
methyl alpha-phenyl-2-piperidineacetate	Ritalin	methylphenidate
N,N,*6-trimethyl-2-(4-methylphenyl)-imidazo(1,2-a) pyridine-3-acetamide*	Ambien	zolpidem
7-chloro-1-methyl-5-phenyl-1,3-dihydro-2*H*-1, 4-benzodiazepin-2-one	Valium	diazepam
4, 5-epoxy-14-hydroxy-3- methoxy-17- methylmorphinan-6-one	Percocet, Percodan	oxycodone

Note: The drug brand name is always capitalized while the generic name is not.

Pharmacokinetics: Drug Absorption, Metabolism, and Tolerance

Drug absorption refers to the mechanisms by which drugs get into the blood stream and are distributed throughout the body. Because our focus in this text is on psychopharmacology, we are particularly interested in how drugs get into the brain. How quickly and how much of a drug reaches the brain depends on several factors, including how it is administered and how readily molecules of the drug pass from the blood stream into neural tissues. We first examine routes of administration, and then we will look at factors that influence a drug's passage from the blood into the brain.

Oral Administration (PO)

Perhaps the most common route of drug administration is the ingestion of a pill or tablet, but it would also include the oral ingestion of liquids. If taken orally a drug must be both soluble in gastric fluids and not destroyed or broken down by them so it can cross from the lining of the stomach and upper intestine into the blood stream. In order to pass through the tissues lining the gastric tract a drug must also be fat soluble to some extent. The greater its solubility in fat the more rapidly it can permeate the mucosal lining into the blood. Fat solubility will also be a factor in determining how rapidly a drug can pass from the blood stream into neural tissues in the brain. The reason fat solubility is important is that the tissues lining the stomach, the upper intestine, blood vessels, and neurons are composed primarily of fats or lipids. Fat-soluble compounds literally dissolve in these tissues and pass through by diffusion. Oral ingestion of drugs is often the most preferred method of administration, but absorption may take between half an hour and three hours depending on a drug's fat solubility and where it is absorbed. For instance, some drugs are designed to quickly dissolve in the mouth and are absorbed through the mucosal lining in the mouth and throat. Other drugs are more slowly absorbed in the lining of the upper intestine. Most of us are familiar with how long it takes an oral analgesic to relieve the pain associated with an extracted tooth. When a drug may not be stable in stomach acids and enzymes, or when it needs to reach the brain more quickly, other methods may be preferred.

Inhalation

A number of both illicit and legal drugs are typically administered by inhalation, including nicotine and marijuana. This method is preferred for drugs of abuse because they are absorbed quickly through the lungs into the blood stream. The lungs have a very large surface area and blood volume, so absorption will take a mere few seconds. Drugs used to administer anesthesia (e.g., halothane) are often administered by inhalation. The level of anesthesia is then carefully monitored and regulated throughout its duration. For drugs used to treat psychological disorders inhalation is not preferred, because therapeutic doses of these drugs require a stable blood level, unlike the rapid spike in levels preferred by drug users. Most of us are familiar with a variety of bronchial and nasal inhalers used to treat asthma and congestion. Other drugs, such as methamphetamine, cocaine, and heroin, vaporize upon heating and these vapors are inhaled. This is often preferable to oral or nasal administration because this method produces an intense state of euphoria, and it is often less risky than intravenous administration when needle sharing may spread diseases such as AIDS.

Intravenous (IV)

An intravenous injection is a rapid and precise way to administer a drug. Drug absorption is rapid because it is delivered directly into venous blood where it is rapidly distributed throughout the circulatory system. Passage of the drug through membranes of the gastric system or the lungs is bypassed completely. Intravenous administration is more precise because the entire amount of the drug administered gets into the blood stream. Following oral administration, unpredictable amounts of the drug get trapped temporarily in fat tissue, making the amount reaching the blood difficult to determine. Because drugs administered intravenously have such rapid onset, they are also much more dangerous. Overdose by intravenous administration can easily cause death by respiratory or heart failure and severe allergic reactions. The intravenous use of recreational drugs is of particular concern because they are often administered in less than aseptic conditions, increasing the risk of infections and diseases spread by shared needles. Additionally, drugs mixed and prepared outside of specialized laboratories often contain contaminants. The soluble contaminants may be toxic, and those that are insoluble actually may lodge in the lungs and blood vessels, causing damage to these and other organs.

Intramuscular (IM)

Drugs can also be delivered into skeletal muscle where they are absorbed more slowly. Absorption typically occurs within one hour, depending on the injection site and the amount of blood flow to the muscle tissue. Often drugs administered intramuscularly are mixed in an oil base to further slow their absorption. Several hormones are commonly administered intramuscularly, including Depo Provera (medroxyprogesterone) as a female contraceptive and testosterone for hormone replacement in men.

Transdermal

Nicotine patches, motion sickness patches, testosterone replacement gel, and some forms of female contraceptives are examples of transdermal drug administration. Because the skin is relatively impermeable to water-soluble substances, these drugs need to be fat soluble in order to pass through the skin. Absorption is quite slow and can be sustained over several days or weeks.

Subcutaneous (SC)

Subcutaneous administration may consist of either a subdermal injection or the implantation of a drug in pellet form. Several hormones are available in pellet form, including the newly approved female contraceptive Implanon. This delivers contraceptive hormones for up to three years per implant.

Intraperitoneal (IP)

The delivery of a drug directly into the abdominal cavity beneath the peritoneum is a common route of administration in small laboratory animals. This method of drug administration is not used for humans because of the risks of contaminating the abdominal cavity and possible damage to internal organs. Drugs are administered to small animals with this procedure when rapid absorption is required. You might wonder why researchers don't prefer intravenous injections in these cases since more accurate dosing can be achieved this way. However, as you might imagine, delivering drugs intravenously in small laboratory rats and mice can be quite difficult. The time course of plasma concentrations of cocaine following different routes of administration are presented in Figure 2.1. Table 2.2 describes advantages and disadvantages of each administration method.

Cell Membrane Permeability

Once a drug is administered it must pass through several membranes before it actually reaches the brain. The first membranes drugs encounter are the cell membranes that make up the linings of the gastric system, skin cells, muscle and fat cells, or the mucosal lining of the lungs. All of these tissues are composed of a phospholipid bilayer made up of complex lipid (fat) molecules arranged in two rows. These phospholipid molecules are composed of a head region that is negatively charged and an uncharged tail region that is split into two segments. These molecules are arranged such that their heads form both the inner and outer surfaces of the membrane and their tails remain in-between these charged segments. The negatively charged heads of these molecules are hydrophilic (attracted to water) and are exposed to both the intra and extra cellular fluids. The uncharged tails are hydrophobic (repel water) and therefore prevent fluid and water-soluble substances from easily passing through the membrane. Embedded in this arrangement of phospholipid molecules are protein molecules that serve a variety of transport functions. In order for substances to pass through the cell membrane they must either be carried through by one of the specialized transporter molecules or be fat soluble and

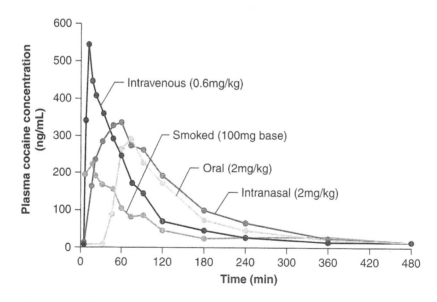

Figure 2.1 Comparison of absorption times for different administration routes.

Source: Adapted from Carlson (2010).

Table 2.2 Routes of drug administration.

Route of administration	Main advantages	Main disadvantages
Oral (PO)	Patient administration, relatively safe	Delayed and variable absorption
Inhalation	Rapid availability, patient administration, reliable absorption, accurate blood levels	Irritation of nasal passages or the throat and lungs, possibility of overdose
Intravenous (IV)	Rapid availability, reliable absorption, accurate blood levels	Patient administration difficult, possibility of contamination and infection from needles, possibility of overdose
Intramuscular (IM)	Prolonged and reliable absorption, easy to administer	Patient administration difficult, possibility of contamination and infection from needles
Transdermal	Prolonged and reliable absorption, easy to self-administer	Local irritation, variable absorption, more difficult to regulate blood levels
Subcutaneous (SC)	Prolonged and reliable absorption, easy to administer	Patient administration difficult, possibility of contamination and infection from needles
Intraperitoneal (IP)	This method is primarily used to administer drugs to smaller laboratory animals when intravenous administration is not feasible	Possibility of damage to internal organs, local irritation at injection site, delayed absorption compared to intravenous injection

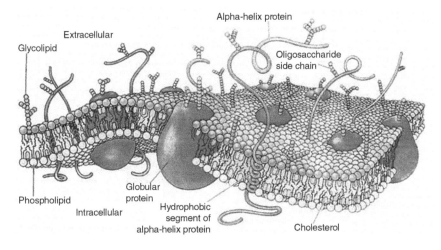

Figure 2.2 Cell membrane. The arrangement of phospholipid molecules into a bilayer with negatively charged hydrophobic heads. This arrangement keeps fluids from passing through the cell membrane. Molecules may pass through the cell membrane if they are carried through by proteins embedded in the cell membrane or if they are fat soluble and enter by diffusion.

essentially dissolve in the membrane and pass through by diffusion. Figure 2.2 shows how the plasma membrane is constructed and how it incorporates various proteins within it.

Substances must also pass through small blood vessels called capillaries to enter and leave the blood stream. Capillary membranes are constructed of a tightly packed single layer of cells that have small gaps between them. Substances that fit through these gaps can enter and leave the blood stream by diffusion. That is, diffusion pressure forces a substance through the membrane down its concentration gradient until the concentration is essentially equal on both sides of the capillary wall. Most drugs easily pass through capillary membranes this way and become distributed throughout the body's tissues. The greater the blood flow to tissue, the greater the concentration of the drug. Because the brain has relatively high blood flow, we would expect higher concentrations of the drug there. However, an additional membrane must be crossed before drugs can enter the brain.

Blood–Brain Barrier

The capillaries that circulate blood throughout most of the brain are constructed differently from capillaries in other tissues. Because the brain requires a very stable and protected environment to function effectively, substances cannot easily pass between small gaps in the capillary membrane. These capillaries are constructed of cells with tight junctions, allowing only very small molecules to pass. Additionally, the capillary walls are surrounded by a type of glial cell called an astrocyte. These astrocytic feet provide an additional barrier by tightly adhering to the capillary endothelial membrane. This impermeable construction is referred to as the **blood–brain barrier (or BBB)** (see Figure 2.3). Some essential substances, such as glucose and some amino acids, are carried through by specialized transporters in the capillary membrane. Fat-soluble substances, including all psychoactive drugs, can dissolve in the membrane and pass through by diffusion. The blood–brain barrier provides an effective means to protect the brain from perturbations in the chemical environment of the blood stream. Additionally, the blood–brain barrier protects the brain from potentially toxic substances, including most viruses and bacteria.

There are a few areas of the brain where the blood–brain barrier is relatively weak, allowing some substances to be detected by specialized neurons in those areas. For example, neurons in the area postrema of the medulla detect some toxic substances and trigger vomiting to rid the body of potentially toxic substances still in the stomach. Other areas, including the subfornical organ located on the underside of the fornix and between the lateral ventricles, has a weak blood–brain barrier and detects the presence of hormones involved in the regulation of fluid balance. The blood–brain barrier poses a significant obstacle to drug development. In order for drugs to reach their target receptors in the brain they must pass through the blood–brain barrier.

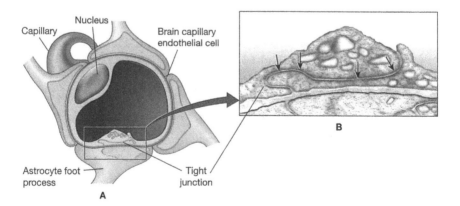

Figure 2.3 Blood–brain barrier. Tight junctions between astrocytic (glial cell) end feet and capillary endothelial cells (A). Electron micrograph showing tight junctions between capillary endothelial cells and astrocytic feet (B).

Source: Adapted from Goldstein and Betz (1986).

Placental Barrier

Pregnant females have an additional barrier that separates the blood system of the mother from that of the fetus. This barrier, however, must allow essential substances, including nutrients and oxygen in the mother's blood, to enter into the fetal blood supply. In addition, it must allow metabolic waste produced by the fetus to be eliminated through the mother's circulatory system. The placenta is an ineffective barrier to drugs ingested by the mother and the fetus can have drug levels that are equally high. This is why it is critical to avoid potentially harmful drugs, such as alcohol, during pregnancy. Fetuses exposed to addictive drugs such as heroin, methamphetamine, and cocaine show symptoms of withdrawal during maternal abstinence. It is important to keep in mind, however, that most drugs used to treat psychological disorders are not necessarily harmful to a developing fetus.

Drug Metabolism

Once a drug has entered the blood stream and begins to circulate throughout the body, much of it is becoming attached to inactive proteins or dissolved in fat tissue and some of it begins to undergo metabolism and excretion. The drug bound to inactive sites is referred to as **depot binding**. As the blood concentration of the drug begins to drop, some of the drug bound to depot sites reenters the bloodstream (down its concentration gradient), thereby prolonging its activity. The drug remaining in circulation begins to be excreted. The concentration of a drug in the blood and surrounding tissues begins to reach an equilibrium after administration depending on how fat soluble the drug is. When the concentrations in the blood and tissues are essentially the same, this is referred to as **tissue equilibrium**. Drugs that are more fat soluble reach tissue equilibrium more quickly than less fat-soluble drugs. As concentrations of the drug in the blood begin to decrease because of metabolism or elimination, the drug in surrounding tissues begins to move back into blood—down its concentration gradient. Thus, drug concentrations begin to drop.

There are several ways in which drugs and their metabolites leave the body: through exhalation (breathalyzer tests for alcohol rely on this), perspiration through the skin, and excretion through the kidneys. Only small amounts of volatile drugs like alcohol are actually exhaled, but significant amounts are excreted through perspiration and the kidneys after metabolism. If fat-soluble drugs did not undergo metabolism they would continue to be reabsorbed and released by tissues. Metabolism of foreign material by the liver is an essential mechanism to rid our body of potentially toxic substances, and sometimes these substances damage it. For this reason, liver function is routinely monitored in individuals taking certain drugs because the drug or its metabolite may be toxic. And, as you may know, the liver is often severely damaged in alcoholics.

The most important enzymes involved in the metabolism of drugs are primarily produced by cells in the liver. These enzymes are called **cytochrome P450**, or CYP450. There are at least 50 of these enzymes in the liver and other body tissues, including the kidneys, intestines, and lungs. Different members of this CYP450 family of enzymes are involved in the metabolism of different drugs. For example, CYP450 2E1 is important for the conversion of alcohol into acetaldehyde and then to acetic acid.

Drug metabolism by enzymes in the liver typically results in inactive water-soluble metabolites that are filtered out by the kidneys. In some cases, however, the metabolite of a drug may also be as active as, or even more active than, the parent drug. These active metabolites reenter the blood system and are absorbed again. Drugs that have active metabolites have significantly longer durations of action than drugs that do not. The active metabolite is eventually metabolized into inactive water-soluble compounds and filtered out of the blood by the kidneys.

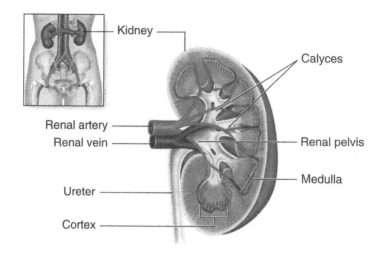

Figure 2.4 Each kidney filters about 1 liter of blood each minute. Drug metabolites are excreted through the kidneys.

The kidneys are located in the back of the abdomen below the ribs. They function to filter and excrete byproducts of metabolism and regulate body fluids. Once a drug is metabolized by liver enzymes, its water-soluble metabolites are captured in the kidneys and excreted in urine. Drug testing for illicit drugs (actually their metabolites) is often conducted on urine samples. Approximately 1 liter of blood plasma is filtered by the kidneys each minute and over 99.5 percent of this fluid is returned into circulation. The remaining fluid is excreted as urine. The structure of the kidney is revealed in Figure 2.4.

Drug Half-Life

As the body continues to metabolize and excrete a drug that is in circulation, its concentrations in the blood and other tissues begin to decline. The time course of this decline can be accurately measured by assays of blood taken at specific intervals after drug administration. One useful measure of the time course of drug elimination is called elimination **half-life**. A drug's half-life is the amount of time it takes for a drug's initial tissue equilibrium level to be decreased by metabolism and elimination by 50 percent (half of its peak level). In Figure 2.5, the drug reaches a peak blood plasma level of approximately 20 mg/l and is quickly redistributed to tissues over the first hour. After one hour, plasma and tissue concentrations fall as the drug is eliminated through metabolism and excretion. From hour two to hour five the plasma concentrations fall by one-half (from 8 mg/l to 4 mg/l) indicating a drug half-life of three hours. This three-hour half-life remains constant for this specific drug. Therefore, in the next three hours the plasma level will be decreased by another 50 percent, or down to 2 mg/l, and to 1 mg/l after 11 hours or three half-lives. Different drugs have different half-lives ranging from hours to days. For example, cocaine has a half-life of about one hour. The popular antidepressant Prozac has a half-life of about 48 hours, but it has an active metabolite that has a half-life of almost six days. Because of its relatively long half-life, missing a daily dose may not be problematic.

The concept of elimination half-life is important for several reasons. First, knowing a drug's half-life will allow us to predict its duration of action. Also, knowledge of a drug's half-life

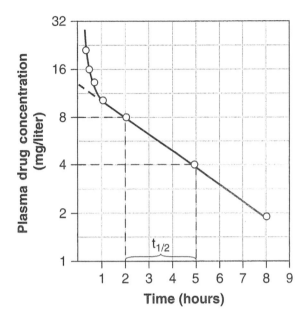

Figure 2.5 Drug half-life. Plasma concentrations of a drug following an intravenous injection. Concentrations were measured every 15 minutes following administration for the first hour, then at hour one, hour five, and hour eight. During the first hour plasma concentrations fell rapidly as the drug was redistributed to tissues. After one hour the plasma concentration was essentially equal to tissue concentrations and levels fell in a linear manner. In this example the half-life ($t_{1/2}$) is three hours.

allows for adjusting dose intervals to achieve a steady blood level of the drug. Drugs used to treat most conditions, including psychological disorders and pain, are most effective when blood levels fall within a narrow range. When blood levels fall below this range the drug response is too low to be effective. When its level is above this level it may be toxic or lethal. If drugs are administered at appropriate intervals, according to their relative half-lives, blood and tissue concentrations remain relatively stable. More frequent dosing with smaller drug doses typically results in more stable steady-state concentrations. Many of us are familiar with the typical four-hour dosing intervals for Vicodin and OxyContin that cycles us through drug stupor and pain! A more effective, but less convenient, dosing schedule might be half the four-hour dose every two hours, as Figure 2.6 reveals.

The relationship between a drug dose and its physiological effects is called a **dose response curve**. As shown in Figure 2.6, there is little physiological response until the dose is increased. Then, as the dose continues to increase there is a sharp rise in its effectiveness until a point at which no further increase in effectiveness is produced. When examining the effectiveness of oxycodone on pain, for instance, we see that below doses of 0.01 ug/ml of blood there is little relief from pain. Above 0.01 to about 0.10 ug/ml there is a sharp rise in analgesia. Above doses of 0.10 ug/ml the analgesic response is essentially flat. Most drugs produce several physiological effects, and this is certainly true for the opiates like oxycodone. In addition to analgesia we can observe its effects on respiration. At low therapeutic doses there is little **respiratory depression** (decrease in respiratory rate). At doses approaching 3 ug/ml, respiratory depression begins to become a concern. And, at blood levels over 4 ug/ml, the drug may be lethal, producing complete respiratory depression (see Figure 2.7). This discussion reveals that drugs may have several dose response curves, one for each physiological response. Furthermore, these dose

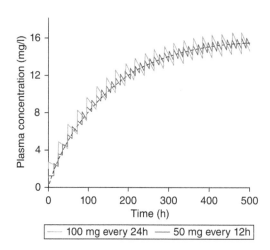

Figure 2.6 Plasma levels of opiate following two different dosing schedules. Relatively stable levels are reached after several days of administration.

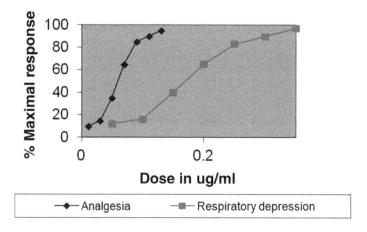

Figure 2.7 Dose response curves for oxycodone. The dose response curve for analgesia rises rapidly from about 0.01 through 0.05 ug/ml. After about 0.10 ug/ml there is little increase in analgesia. The dose response curve for respiratory depression, however, rises gradually from about 0.05 ug/ml through doses of 0.25 ug/ml. At doses exceeding 0.30 ug/ml, respiratory depression is almost certain.

response curves may not overlap. Next, we examine how repeated exposure to a drug can actually shift a dose response curve.

Tolerance

As implied earlier, dose response curves are not static. After repeated administration the effectiveness of a dose of the analgesic oxycodone, for example, diminishes considerably. The decrease in effectiveness of a dose of a drug (a shift to the right in the dose response curve as illustrated in Figure 2.8) following repeated administration is called **tolerance**. Tolerance occurs to all drugs taken over a period of time, but it occurs most rapidly to drugs in the

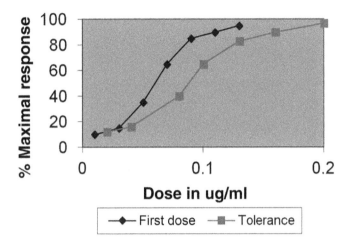

Figure 2.8 Dose response curves for oxycodone. Tolerance to the analgesic effects of oxycodone is expressed as a shift in the dose response curve for analgesia to the right.

opiate family (oxycodone and morphine are opiates). In fact, when an individual experiences tolerance to oxycodone that person will also be tolerant to other opiates, including morphine. This phenomenon is called **cross-tolerance**.

There are a variety of mechanisms that contribute to drug tolerance, and it appears that some mechanisms contribute to tolerance to a greater extent than others for different classes of drugs. For this reason, tolerance may develop at quite different rates to different drugs. In some cases tolerance can develop over the course of a week, and in other cases it may take many months or even years. Furthermore, some changes in drug responsiveness that contribute to tolerance are easily reversed when the drug is discontinued, while other mechanisms may persist long after. We know the most about tolerance to drugs in the opiate and stimulant families, since these families of drugs have been studied most extensively.

Metabolic Tolerance

As I discussed previously, psychoactive drugs must undergo metabolism by enzymes in the liver before they can be excreted. The enzymes responsible for the metabolic enzymes that break drugs into water-soluble compounds actually increase in availability after repeated exposure to a drug. This results in more rapid metabolism as more enzymes are available for degradation. For example, alcohol is metabolized by the liver enzyme alcohol dehydrogenase, which catalyzes the oxidation of alcohol into acetylaldehyde. Acetylaldehyde is further converted into acetic acid by acetyldehyde dehydrogenase. The amounts of these liver enzymes increase with exposure to alcohol, contributing to alcohol tolerance.

Cellular Tolerance

In addition to enzymatic degradation, there appear to be cellular adaptations to some drugs that diminish their effects on target cells. One cellular adaptation that follows drug-induced increases in neurotransmitter availability is **downregulation**. When synaptic activity increases significantly the number of postsynaptic receptors may actually be reduced, making the postsynaptic cell less responsive to chemical transmission (see Figure 2.9). Another mechanism of

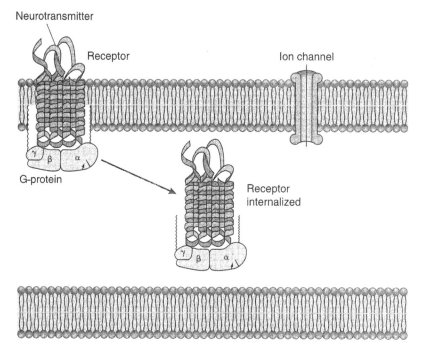

Figure 2.9 Downregulation of receptors. Metabotropic receptors may become internalized during the development of tolerance. The expression or the internalization of receptors may occur rapidly and underlie the dynamics of associative tolerance.

downregulation is an increase in the sensitivity of autoreceptors on the transmitting neuron. Autoreceptors essentially function to slow down the activity of the firing cell, resulting in less neurotransmitter being synthesized and released. Both mechanisms of downregulation contribute to drug tolerance.

Associative Tolerance

Given what we have learned about tolerance so far, it might be quite surprising to observe that an organism could display tolerance to a drug in one context, but not in another. After all, if tolerance results from downregulation and more efficient enzymatic degradation, why would the context where a drug was administered make any difference in how we respond to it? In an experiment conducted by Siegel (1975), rats were administered progressively increasing doses of morphine over a period of several weeks. At the end of this period, all of the animals had developed tolerance and were receiving a dose of morphine that would be lethal to most untreated animals. On the final day of morphine administration, half of the animals received their injections in a novel context, while the remaining half received their injections in the familiar drug environment. Most of the animals that received the drug in the novel context demonstrated signs of overdose, while none of them receiving their drug in the familiar context did. This experiment, and many that have followed, reveals that contextual cues associated with drug onset become conditioned stimuli that can elicit tolerance. When animals received their drug injection in a novel context, tolerance was not expressed. In this case the conditioning is a form of Pavlovian conditioning where contextual cues (conditioned stimuli) associated with drug onset (unconditioned stimulus) come to elicit conditioned tolerance (a conditioned response). The conditioned response in this example is called a compensatory response to the effects of the drug. Compensatory conditioned responses function to maintain relatively stable internal conditions. Tolerance compensates for the large perturbation caused by opiate administration. It is important to point out that this phenomenon is not habituation, which could be defined as a decrease in the effectiveness of a stimulus (in this case a drug) to elicit a response. Since habituation is not an associative form of conditioning it would not be context specific.

In the author's laboratory we have further demonstrated that these contextual cues can undergo extinction of tolerance when animals are exposed to the drug context without drug injections. After extinction, tolerance to morphine is not expressed. Extinction can be reversed, however, when a single morphine dose is administered in the original drug context. This reinstatement of tolerance can even occur months after extinction, suggesting that conditioned tolerance to drugs may never be completely reversed. The neural mechanisms underlying associative tolerance are still unknown but rapid internalization of receptors and **downregulation** are likely to mediate it (results from these experiments are presented in Figures 2.10 and 2.11).

Reinstatement of conditioned tolerance, and other drug responses, may contribute to the high recidivism rates for recovering drug addicts. After treatment, re-exposure to the context where drugs were previously used often elicits drug behaviors, including drug craving and seeking. Drug and alcohol addicts (including smokers) are all too familiar with how powerful contextual and internal cues can be to inducing cravings. A major component of addiction treatment is to get addicts to recognize these triggers in themselves, and in their environment, and learn to control their exposure to them. The mechanisms leading to associative tolerance

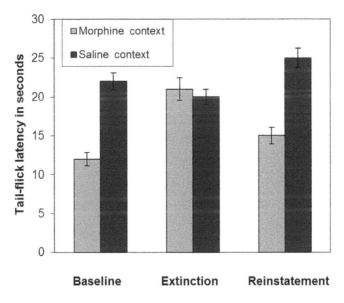

Baseline   Extinction   Reinstatement

Figure 2.10 Conditioned tolerance, extinction, and reinstatement. Animals administered morphine in a distinctive context show tolerance (a decrease in tail-flick latency) in that context but not in a context where saline was administered (longer tail-flick latencies). After several trials where they were exposed to the distinctive morphine context without drug administration, tolerance was extinguished (longer latencies). Tolerance can be reinstated following a single exposure to the morphine context with a morphine injection.

Source: Author's laboratory.

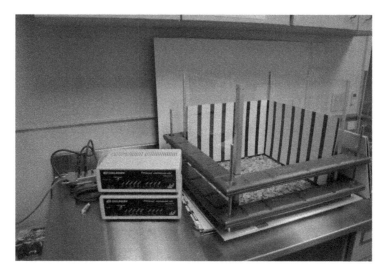

Figure 2.11 The distinctive context for morphine administration.
(Photo from author's laboratory.)

and reinstatement are long lasting and perhaps permanent. Addicts are never completely free from reinstatement if drug use occurs in a specific context or during specific internal states.

Behavioral Tolerance

The associative tolerance described previously involves conditioned associations between a context where drugs are administered and drug onset. This form of conditioning is referred to as Pavlovian conditioning, and it appears to contribute to a rapid decrease in receptor availability. Operant conditioning can also contribute to drug tolerance. For example, if animals are given intoxicating doses of alcohol before learning a complex motor task, they tend to perform that task better when under the influence of alcohol than when in a sober state. Alcohol in this example becomes a discriminative stimulus that occasions a set of behavioral adaptations to motor behavior (Wenger et al., 1981). Behavioral adaptations such as these are referred to as behavioral tolerance or **state-dependent learning**.

Drug Toxicity and Overdose

As we can see in the previous dose response curves, psychoactive drugs often have several distinct effects, and not all of them are desirable. Additionally, some drug effects are caused by the pharmacological actions of the drug and others are not. For example, morphine is well known for its analgesic properties, but it also produces hypothermia, constipation, and, at high doses, respiratory depression. All of these side effects are attributable to its pharmacological actions. It is also possible to have non-pharmacological reactions to drugs, such as an allergic reaction. Although quite rare with morphine, allergic reactions can occur with any drug, and they can be lethal. Other non-pharmacological reactions could include damage to the liver or kidneys where drugs are concentrated, as they are responsible for drug metabolism and excretion. Certain drugs may also be harmful to a developing fetus and cause developmental abnormalities or damage to developing organs. All of these drug reactions are examples of drug toxicity, which is a measure of the potentially harmful effects of a drug. Some toxic reactions may be minimized by carefully adjusting drug dosages, but others, such as allergic reactions, can occur with any dose.

At high doses all drugs can produce toxic reactions and even death. When a drug's toxic reactions are attributable to an excessive dose it is called an *overdose* reaction. Overdose reactions can be lethal, and they are most likely attributable to respiratory, kidney, or liver failure. In experimental animals, where drug toxicity is investigated, the dose that is lethal (LD) to 50 percent of the animals receiving it is called the LD_{50} dose. When the dose is lethal to all of the experimental animals it is the LD_{100} dose. A drug's safety is determined by comparing the drug's therapeutically effective dose (ED) with its lethal dose. The area between these two dose response curves is called the **therapeutic index**. Typically, the wider the range or therapeutic index between a drug's effective and lethal doses, the safer it is.

As cellular and conditioned tolerance to a drug develop, synaptic changes, including down-regulation of receptors, occur and the dose response curve shifts to the right. These changes may not occur at the same rate at all sites of drug action. As a result, tolerance to some drug effects may occur at different rates from others. If tolerance to the therapeutic effect occurs at a faster rate than to a drug's adverse or toxic effects the therapeutic index narrows. For example, tolerance appears to occur more quickly to an opiate's analgesic effects (its ED) than to effects on respiratory centers (its LD). This contributes to the high risk of overdose observed in experienced, tolerant drug users. In Figure 2.12, the effective and lethal dose response curves are shown for the analgesic oxycodone. As tolerance to the analgesic effects begins to develop, the dose response curves for effective and lethal doses merge, considerably increasing the risk of overdose.

Placebo Effects

Not all drug effects are caused by pharmacological properties or even drug interactions with receptors. In fact, recent research on the effectiveness of antidepressant medication has confirmed that about half of the improvement in depression symptoms can be attributed to the **placebo effect**. Just what is the placebo effect, and how can it contribute significantly to the treatment of depression and chronic pain? A placebo is a pharmacologically inert substance administered under the guise of medication. In well-designed clinical studies neither the patients nor the physician know which patient group receives the placebo or the actual medication. This

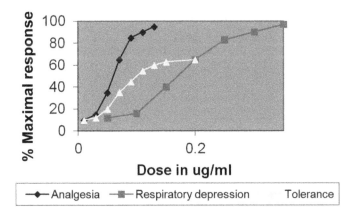

Figure 2.12 Dose response curves for oxycodone. As tolerance develops to oxycodone's analgesic effects the effective dose response curve moves to the right, narrowing the therapeutic index.

double-blind approach is intended to rule out patient compliance as well as physician biases that may flaw the results. As shown in Figure 2.13, the proportion of patients who respond to treatment for depression has increased steadily over the past 20 years. While it would be tempting to say that this increase reflects improvements in antidepressant drugs over these years, how would this account for the same increase in the effectiveness of placebo treatment, which contributes to the same rate of improvement? The figure also reveals that in the year 2000 about 55 percent of the patients treated with medication responded positively, while about 30 percent of the patients receiving placebos improved. In other words, the placebo effect appears to account for more than 50 percent of the improvement in depression symptoms.

Similar results on the effectiveness of placebos are regularly observed in comparisons of placebos with analgesics for postoperative and chronic pain. Also, a number of these studies have further revealed that the placebo effect for analgesia is mediated by the endogenous opiate system (e.g., Zubieta et al., 2005). In fact, the drug naloxone, which blocks opiate activity, also blocks the placebo effect, suggesting that ingesting a placebo can activate the endogenous opiate system and alleviate pain by the very same mechanisms used by opiate analgesics (Levine et al., 1978). Because the neural mechanisms for pain and analgesia are well understood, this has been an ideal model to investigate the neural mechanisms of placebo effects.

Progress has also been made in revealing the mechanisms mediating the antidepressant action of placebos. While investigators have observed neural changes in the cortex of placebo-treated patients, which are similar to the effects observed after antidepressant therapy, the neuro-chemical mechanisms for the placebo effect in the treatment of depression are still unknown

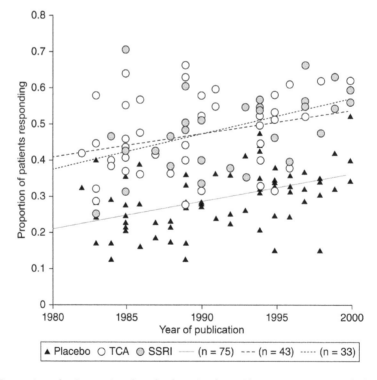

Figure 2.13 Proportion of patients assigned to placebo, tricyclic antidepressants (TCAs), and selective serotonin reuptake inhibitors (SSRIs) who showed a 50 percent or greater improvement on the Hamilton Rating Scale for depression scored by year of publication.

Source: Walsh et al. (2002).

(Benedetti et al., 2005). With this in mind, the placebo effect accounts for a significant amount of the treatment effect observed following drug therapy and must be taken into account in studies of drug effectiveness. Simply comparing the efficacy of drug treatment to non-treated control subjects might lead to flawed conclusions about the value of drug treatment.

In this section, we have examined how the effects of a drug depend on how it is administered, how rapidly and completely it is absorbed, and how repeated exposure and drug administration context can alter drug effectiveness by contributing to the development of tolerance. Additionally, we have examined how to evaluate the safety and effectiveness of a drug by comparing dose response curves for its therapeutic and toxic effects. We have also seen that the placebo effect can contribute significantly to a drug's effects and how well-designed studies can isolate this contribution. We next look at how drugs interact with receptors to produce their effects.

Pharmacodynamics: Mechanisms of Drug Action

Once a drug has passed from the blood supply into the brain it can begin to exert its effects on neuronal functioning. A basic principle of **pharmacodynamics** is that drug effects are mediated by their influence on target cells. While many of these effects are caused by the interaction between a drug and specific receptors, other effects may be mediated by a drug's effects on neurotransmitter synthesis, storage, release, reuptake, or on its metabolism. Ultimately all psychoactive drugs alter neural function by either facilitating or inhibiting neurotransmission. When a drug acts to facilitate neurotransmission it is called an **agonist** and when it acts to inhibit or decrease neurotransmission it is referred to as an **antagonist**. A variety of these mechanisms of action are described in Figure 2.14.

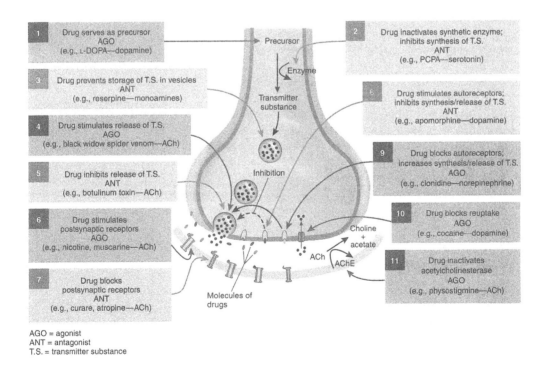

AGO = agonist
ANT = antagonist
T.S. = transmitter substance

Figure 2.14 Mechanisms of drug action.

Source: Adapted from Carlson (2010).

Drug Agonists

Because there is a long chain of events leading to the synthesis, storage, release, and breakdown of neurotransmitter substances, there are numerous opportunities to alter these processes with drugs. Some of these drug effects are transient, lasting only as long as the drug is present. Other effects are longer term, affecting receptor expression and protein synthesis. We will examine some of the most common ways drugs act to facilitate neural communication. Drugs that directly bind to and activate receptor sites are called direct agonists. Drugs that facilitate neurotransmission by increasing neurotransmitter availability or release are called indirect agonists.

Neurotransmitter Synthesis and Availability

Some drugs function as agonists by either increasing the synthesis of a neurotransmitter or by increasing the amount released into the synapse. As you recall, neurotransmitters are synthesized from precursor compounds in the neurons that release them. Increasing the availability of precursor compounds, and/or the rate limiting enzymes necessary for their production, can increase neurotransmitter availability. For example, the dopamine agonist L-DOPA (3, 4-dihydroxy-L-phenylanine), which is commonly used to treat Parkinson's disease, is the metabolic precursor to dopamine. L-DOPA readily crosses the blood–brain barrier, unlike dopamine, and is quickly converted into dopamine by the enzyme aromatic amino acid decarboxylase. Because this enzyme is also found in peripheral tissues, some of the L-DOPA gets converted into dopamine before it reaches dopaminergic neurons. To prevent this from occurring, peripheral inhibitors of aromatic amino acid decarboxylase, such as Carbidopa, are co-administered with L-DOPA.

Neurotransmitter Release

Neurotransmitter is typically released from synaptic vesicles directly into the synaptic gap only after they have fused with the presynaptic membrane. However, some drugs may actually enhance the amount of neurotransmitter released by causing it to be released into the presynaptic terminal, where it is then transported into the synaptic gap. Amphetamine and methamphetamine are examples of dopamine agonists that increase dopamine activity by causing dopamine to leak from the synaptic vesicles into the terminal button. Additionally, these drugs cause the dopamine transporter to operate in reverse and carry this intracellular dopamine outside of the cell where it can activate dopamine receptors.

Although not a drug, the venom from black widow spiders, as well as some poisonous snakes, acts as an acetylcholine agonist by increasing the amount of ACh released into the synapse. This results in over activity of acetylcholine neurons at neuromuscular synapses causing muscular contraction. In humans, black widow spider venom is rarely lethal, but the venom from snakes, which is delivered in much larger quantities, can be.

Neurotransmitter Breakdown and Reuptake

The breakdown and reuptake processes that terminate the activity of neurotransmitter released into the synapse are essential for normal neuronal activity. These processes, however, may also be altered by drug action, resulting in prolonged neurotransmitter activity. The catecholamine neurotransmitters dopamine and norepinephrine, as well as the monoamine serotonin, are degraded by the synaptic enzyme monoamine oxidase (MAO). Drugs that block the activity of this enzyme, called MAO inhibitors (MAOIs), enhance neural activity, preventing the metabolic breakdown of these neurotransmitters. Because all three of these neurotransmitters are degraded by MAO, MAO inhibitors are not selective in agonizing any one of them specifically. MAO inhibitors such as phenelzine (Nardil) are used as antidepressants and will be discussed later on.

Blocking the **reuptake** of intact neurotransmitters is an effective way to enhance neurotransmission either selectively or in combination with other neurotransmitters. Blocking reuptake prolongs the action of neurotransmitters on their receptors. This has the immediate effect of increasing neurotransmission and a delayed effect of prompting downregulation of the receptors. The popular antidepressant fluoxetine (Prozac) acts as a **selective serotonin reuptake inhibitor** (SSRI) by blocking the serotonin transporter. Several new generation antidepressants act to inhibit the reuptake of both serotonin and norepinephrine. These drugs may be as effective as the SSRIs without some of the adverse side effects.

Neurotransmitter Receptor Activation

Some drugs, because of their chemical structure, actually bind selectively with specific receptors and agonize neurotransmission directly (direct agonist). In these cases the drug is said to have a high binding affinity for the receptor. Occasionally, a drug has such high affinity it competes effectively with the natural ligand or neurotransmitter for these receptors. Because there are no reuptake transporters for drugs, and they are not degraded by synaptic enzymes quickly, these drugs may have prolonged effects. The hallucinogenic drug lysergic acid diethylamide (LSD) is an example of such a drug. LSD has a high affinity for most serotonin receptors, but its hallucinogenic effects are believed to be mediated by the 5-HT_2 subtype. Other hallucinogenic drugs have similar agonistic actions on serotonin receptors. Table 2.3 presents several common drugs and their mechanisms of action.

Drug Antagonists

If a heroin overdose victim suffering from respiratory and cardiac failure is fortunate enough to make it to an emergency room, they will likely receive an intravenous injection of naloxone (Narcan). Within a minute, respiration and heart function will return to normal and the patient will again be responsive to pain and to his surroundings. Without the injection of this powerful opiate antagonist this patient may not survive. Drug antagonists function to inhibit or block neurotransmission. In this example, naloxone competes for the same opiate receptors as heroin, but even more effectively. The difference is that naloxone does not activate the

Table 2.3 Common drugs that act as agonists and antagonists.

Drug	Mechanism of action
Cocaine	Dopamine agonist
L-DOPA	Dopamine agonist
Amphetamine	Dopamine/norepinephrine agonist
Prozac	Serotonin agonist
Valium	GABA agonist
Alcohol	GABA agonist
Thorazine	Dopamine antagonist
Atropine	Acetylcholine antagonist
Marijuana	Cannabinoid agonist
LSD	Serotonin agonist
Narcan	Opiate antagonist

receptor; it merely blocks it so that neither heroin nor the endogenous ligand (an endorphin) can exert their effects. Within a few hours, naloxone is metabolized and excreted and opiate receptors may return to normal. Not all antagonists work this directly on receptors. As we saw with drug agonists, there are many steps in the neurotransmission process, and drugs can antagonize them all.

Neurotransmitter Synthesis and Availability

The synthesis of catecholamine neurotransmitters is dependent upon the availability of both dietary tyrosine and the enzyme tyrosine hydroxylase, which converts it into DOPA. The drug α-methyl-para-tyrosine (AMPT) acts as an indirect antagonist by blocking the ability of tyrosine hydroxylase to catalyze this conversion, thus depleting both dopamine and norepinephrine. In animal studies, this depletion causes behavioral depression and movement disorders. In humans, AMPT has been used to treat dyskinesia, a movement disorder, and has been shown to induce relapse of major depression and seasonal affective disorder—a type of depression associated with low levels of ambient light.

Neurotransmitter availability can also be disrupted by drugs. For example, the antihypertensive drug reserpine binds to the vesicular transporter protein preventing newly synthesized or recycled catecholamines and serotonin from being transported into synaptic vesicles. As you may recall from earlier on, neurotransmitter remaining in the terminal button is quickly degraded by MAO. Reserpine nonselectively antagonizes dopamine, norepinephrine and serotonin by depletion, producing behavioral depression and sedation. Because of these central effects, reserpine is only rarely used to treat hypertension today. Reserpine is used in animal studies that are investigating the roles of catecholamine and serotonin depletion in depression.

Neurotransmitter Release

The release of catecholamine neurotransmitters is regulated by presynaptic autoreceptors. The receptor subtypes of these autoreceptors are the α_2 receptor for norepinephrine and the D_2 receptor for dopamine. Drugs that stimulate these receptors actually reduce the amount of neurotransmitter released. Because very few drugs have affinities for specific subtypes of receptors, the effects of drugs can be contradictory. That is, a drug such as apomorphine (derived from morphine) stimulates dopamine receptors, but because it agonizes D_2 receptors it actually decreases dopamine release from neurons containing them. So, apomorphine, although a dopamine agonist, has antagonistic effects on some dopamine neurons.

Botulism toxin (Botox) is another example of a substance that inhibits the release of neurotransmitter. In this case it antagonizes acetylcholine by preventing synaptic vesicles from fusing with the presynaptic membrane. The effect of poisoning is muscle weakness, and in severe cases botulism toxin can cause asphyxiation and death. In extremely small doses botulism toxin is used as a cosmetic to eliminate facial wrinkles. It does this by paralyzing small groups of muscle cells that, in their contracted state, cause wrinkles.

Neurotransmitter Receptor Activation

In the early 1950s, well before the catecholamine neurotransmitters were identified, the drug chlorpromazine (Thorazine) was introduced as the first drug to treat schizophrenia, which is perhaps the most debilitating of all the psychological disorders. While chlorpromazine was rapidly becoming the treatment of choice for severe psychosis, its mechanism of action remained a mystery for nearly a decade. We now know that chlorpromazine acts as a direct antagonist on dopamine receptors. This discovery has led to modern theories describing the molecular basis of schizophrenia as well as to many new drugs for its treatment. By blocking dopamine receptors, chlorpromazine disrupts dopamine neurotransmission in the basal ganglia, the mesolimbic system, and in the cortex.

Drugs that directly antagonize receptors vary in their affinity for specific receptor subtypes. Newer drugs being developed for schizophrenia treatment are focused on minimizing the severe motor side effects associated with older medications by targeting specific dopamine receptors. We will examine this in more detail in the chapter on antipsychotic medication.

In this section we have reviewed examples of how drugs can act to both facilitate and disrupt neurotransmission. Because there are many steps in the neurotransmission process there are many ways to alter neural activity with drugs. Using drugs to alter neurotransmission has led to a greater understanding of just how different neurotransmitter systems contribute to both normal and disordered behavior. It has also led to far more effective treatment for behavior disorders, while at the same time minimizing troubling side effects.

As we will see in the following chapters, modern drug development is going beyond altering drug-receptor interactions and examining ways to alter the expression of genes within specific populations of neurons. These manipulations can affect receptor expression as well and other properties of cell functioning that may contribute to the treatment of psychological disorders.

Glossary

Agonist a substance that facilitates or increases neural transmission.

Antagonist a substance that inhibits or decreases neural transmission.

Associative tolerance a decrease in responsiveness to drugs that is controlled by cues associated with drug use and onset. Conditioned tolerance is a consequence of Pavlovian conditioning.

Behavioral tolerance learned behavioral adaptations that occur in a drug state and contribute to enhanced motor performance. Also referred to as state dependent learning.

Blood–brain barrier (or BBB) a relatively impermeable membrane forming and surrounding capillaries in the brain that prevents most substances from leaving the circulatory system and entering the brain.

Brand name a drug's brand or trade name is a name given by its manufacturer and is used in advertising the drug. A drug brand name is protected by a patent.

Cellular tolerance cellular adaptations to some drugs that diminish their effects on target cells.

Chemical name a drug's chemical name reveals its chemical composition and molecular structure.

Cross-tolerance tolerance to a drug in the same class as the drug administered repeatedly. Tolerance may be observed to codeine after it has already developed to morphine.

Depot binding drug binding to inactive sites.

Dose response curve the relationship between a drug dose and its physiological effects. Often this relationship is sigmoidal.

Double-blind in a double-blind experiment neither the patients nor the physician knows which patient group receives the placebo or the actual medication. This experimental design can eliminate both subject and researcher biases, which may affect the outcome of drug trials.

Downregulation a decrease in neurotransmitter synthesis or release caused by drug action on target receptors. Downregulation may also involve decreases in receptor availability.

Generic drug generic drugs must contain the same active ingredients as the original brand name drug, and they must be pharmacologically equivalent. Because several manufacturers may compete to produce and market generic drugs, their cost is often considerably less than their equivalent brand-named drug.

Half-life the amount of time it takes for a drug's blood level to be decreased by metabolism and elimination by 50 percent (half of its peak blood level).

Metabolic tolerance metabolic enzymes that break drugs into water-soluble compounds actually increase in availability after repeated exposure to a drug. This results in more rapid metabolism as more enzymes are available for degradation.

P450 a class of liver enzymes responsible for the metabolism of many psychoactive drugs.

Pharmacodynamics the science of the mechanisms of drug action or how drugs affect target cells and induce pharmacological effects.

Pharmacokinetics the science of how drugs are absorbed, distributed to body tissues, and eliminated from the body after metabolism.

Placebo a pharmacologically inert substance administered under the guise of medication.

Respiratory depression a decrease in respiratory depth and frequency caused by inhibition of respiratory centers in the brainstem. Often the cause of death from drug or alcohol overdose.

Reuptake a process where neurotransmitter substances are removed from the synaptic gap and returned to the terminal button of the transmitting neuron. Reuptake decreases the availability of the neurotransmitter at receptor sites.

Selective serotonin reuptake inhibitor a class of antidepressant drugs that selectively inhibit serotonin reuptake, leaving serotonin available at receptor sites.

Therapeutic index the range between a drug's therapeutically effective dose and its lethal or toxic dose. The therapeutic index can decrease as tolerance develops.

Tissue equilibrium when the concentrations of a drug in the blood and surrounding tissues are essentially the same.

Tolerance a decrease in the effectiveness of a drug after repeated administration. This is observed as a shift to the right in the dose response curve.

3 Mood Disorders

Major Depression and Bipolar Disorders

Jamie is a 28-year-old woman who was recently divorced after a six-year marriage. She remembers feeling depressed during most of her high school years, especially during her senior year when she sought help following a suicide attempt. Jamie had an unremarkable childhood; her parents both worked but she was rarely alone during her pre–high school years. She has two younger brothers; both appear without symptoms of depression, and she has always had several close friends. After graduating from college with a degree in interior design, Jamie held several jobs and is now employed with an architectural firm. She enjoys her job but feels it is getting more stressful and contributing to her overwhelming fatigue.

After Jamie's suicide attempt, she was prescribed medication, which she took regularly for about a year. The medication appeared to work somewhat, but she still felt depressed and the drug made her drowsy and interfered with her concentration at work. Since her diagnosis Jamie has gained over 50 lbs and she no longer swims or runs, activities she enjoyed throughout college. She now reports that she doesn't look forward to evenings with friends, travel, or even visiting her parents or brothers, all things she did when she was married. She spends her hours after work watching television and talking with girlfriends on the phone. She gets little pleasure from reading and finds she is often distracted by extreme loneliness and sadness. Although Jamie has had no other suicide attempts, she has contemplated it frequently since her divorce as the only solution to her pain. During these periods she finds herself soothed by chocolate, which she blames for her weight problem.

Jamie's case is not untypical. She has done well in her job, has a number of close friends, and is relatively healthy. In fact, most of her coworkers and friends would not consider her to be depressed. She is seeking help again now because she wants more from her life. She is tired of being alone and would like to begin dating and hopefully find another romantic partner. She doesn't like being with herself and feels no one else would like to be with her either. She also hopes that treatment will help her lose weight, since attempts at dieting have failed.

Depression is the most common of the psychological disorders affecting the lives of nearly everyone. It affects us because we are either among the many who live with depression or because it affects family members or close friends. Nearly one out of every ten adults each year is diagnosed with depression, and many more may go undiagnosed. The lifetime prevalence (at least one occurrence during one's lifetime) is as high as 17 percent, affecting about 24 percent of all women and 12 percent of all men, or about 21 million Americans. Depression can occur at any age, but it first appears most frequently in late adolescence and early adulthood. It contributes significantly to suicide risk, which is the third leading cause of death in adolescents and young adults. Depression is considered to be the leading cause of disability in the United States for ages 15–44 (NIMH, 2021a). Depression is also a major contributor to substance use disorders (for instance, alcohol, methamphetamine, cocaine, and opiate abuse) and to eating disorders, including obesity and bulimia. Because depression adversely affects the lives of so many, it is no surprise to learn that the economic impact of depression on the productivity of our workforce and on our healthcare systems is estimated to exceed $40 billion

DOI: 10.4324/9781003309017-3

annually. On the other hand, the sales of prescription drugs to treat depression are escalating and now exceed $20 billion each year.

This chapter discusses several severe mood disorders emphasizing **major depressive disorder** and **bipolar disorder (BPD)**. We will examine their diagnostic criteria, their pathology, and the pharmacological approaches to their treatment. Other depressive disorders, including persistent depressive disorder (dysthymia), are not discussed here because their pathology and treatment do not differ significantly from that of major depressive disorder.

Major Depressive Disorder

Defining and Diagnosing Depression

The point at which someone who is experiencing symptoms of depression becomes diagnosed with major depressive disorder is never clear and will vary depending on who is making the clinical judgment. This is because the symptoms of depression are subjective and assessing them through patient interviews can be challenging. The diagnostic criteria for depression, and for all other psychiatric disorders, are presented in the *Diagnostic and Statistical Manual of Mental Disorders* (DSM). Published by the American Psychiatric Association, this is widely accepted as the standard guide for defining and diagnosing all recognized behavioral and psychological disorders. Presently the DSM is in its fifth text revision (DSM-5TR).

The diagnostic criteria for major depressive disorder (unipolar depression) require that an individual experience at least five of the following symptoms on most days during the two-week period leading to the diagnosis:

1. *A depressed mood for most of the day.* This may be characterized by a persistent sadness or irritability, a tendency to cry easily, and a feeling of hopelessness and discouragement. Some patients describe their mood as "gray," meaning it lacks any change in emotion.
2. *A diminished interest and pleasure in most activities.* This includes recreational activities that were previously enjoyed (e.g., golf, tennis, or skiing), as well as social activities with friends and family. Depression may also contribute to a diminished interest in sexual activity.
3. *A significant change in appetite and weight.* Although appetite and weight often increase during depressive episodes, some may experience a diminished appetite and unwanted weight loss. In some cases, carbohydrate cravings may occur, and this could be associated with serotonin depletion. As we saw in Chapter 1, carbohydrate diets can contribute to increases in serotonin synthesis and availability.
4. *Either insomnia or hypersomnia.* A disruption in normal sleeping patterns is common in all types of depression, as well as in non-depressed individuals. Because sleeping difficulties can be caused by many things, including diet, alcohol consumption, medication, a lack of physical activity, and stress, their prevalence in depression is not surprising. Chronic sleep problems, whether insomnia or hypersomnia, can exacerbate other symptoms of depression, making them even more debilitating.
5. *Motor agitation or retardation that is observable by others.* Often patients don't recognize these changes in their behavior. Increased agitation or lethargy may be more noticeable for others. Pacing, frequent urges to get up and move about, or the inability to complete tasks are examples of behavioral agitation. The inability to initiate activities, excessive sleep, or sitting for hours at a time are examples of behavioral retardation.
6. *Fatigue or diminished energy.* Very common in depression, these symptoms are often described as a lack of motivation or excessive tiredness and are clearly related to other

symptoms listed here. Some patients experience such extreme fatigue they may spend much of their day inactive or in bed.

7. *A diminished ability to think or to concentrate.* Concentration may be frequently disrupted by thoughts of guilt or remorse, or the urge to move. Depression makes most activities and work difficult, contributing to a loss of productivity and the enjoyment most of us get from work and our leisure activities.

8. *Feelings of helplessness, worthlessness, or guilt.* Depressed individuals often describe their lives as worthless and without significant meaning. In addition, they feel that their efforts rarely result in gratification. Efforts to do well in school or work begin to diminish, leading to even less gratification and less future effort.

9. *Recurrent thoughts of suicide or an attempted suicide.* Almost everyone has thought of suicide at some point in their life, but depression is often associated with persistent suicide thoughts and plans. Suicide attempts are a clear sign of depression and must always be taken seriously. Over 30,000 people commit suicide each year, making it the third leading cause of death among our youth.

We all experience these symptoms from time to time throughout our lives. They can be associated with the loss of a significant other, the breakup of a relationship, or with the unexpected termination of employment. Depression associated with significant changes in one's life does not typically escalate into a major depressive disorder, even though it can be disruptive and make normal daily activities difficult. This **reactive depression** is relatively transient, often disappearing on its own within a few weeks or months without treatment. Moreover, reactive depression tends to be intermixed with periods of normal mood. Major depressive disorder is much more persistent and debilitating, and although it can go into a remission, during a depressive episode there is little or no relief from its symptoms.

Major depressive disorder is often accompanied by anxiety. The anxiety may be related to an unrealistic fear of public or open places as in **agoraphobia**, for example, or it may be generalized in that there are no particular contexts or occasions that bring it about. Generalized anxiety can be acute and is often associated with greatly elevated sympathetic activity. In these instances, it is difficult to know whether the feelings of anxiety follow the elevated sympathetic response or contribute to it. We mention anxiety here because when depression occurs with significant anxiety it may be treated differently than when depression is the only or primary feature of the disorder. Anxiety disorders and their treatment will be discussed in a later chapter.

Pathology of Major Depressive Disorder: Monoamine Hypothesis

Most of the evidence available today suggests that abnormalities in the serotonergic and/or noradrenergic systems, including the brain structures that they innervate, underlie severe depression. In the 1960s, researchers began to speculate that these neurotransmitter systems were involved in depression, since drugs that were effective in its treatment altered neurotransmitter availability and breakdown. Likewise, drugs that depleted neurotransmitter availability could cause depression-like symptoms. These observations led to the prominent **monoamine hypothesis** of depression. According to this hypothesis, deficiencies in the monoamine (single amine group in their molecular structure, see Figure 3.1) neurotransmitters dopamine, norepinephrine, and/or serotonin would be sufficient to cause depression.

Some of the earliest evidence for the amine hypothesis came from observations of patients being treated for high blood pressure with the drug Reserpine. Reserpine not only reduces blood pressure, it also blocks the vesicular transport of monoamine neurotransmitters into synaptic vesicles. Left in the terminal button, these monoamines get degraded by MAO, resulting

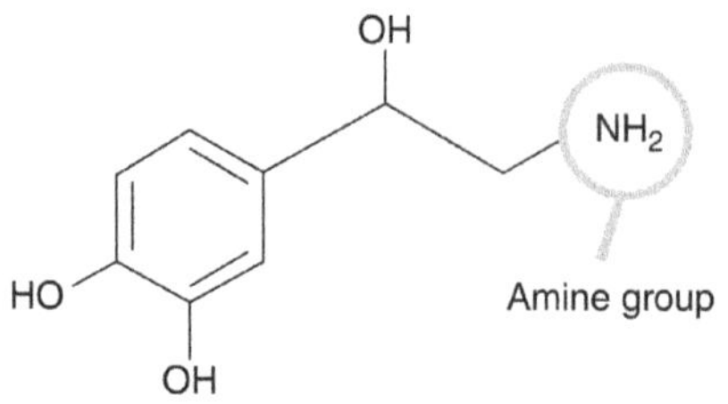

Figure 3.1 Molecular structure of norepinephrine with a single amine group circled.

in a depletion of available neurotransmitters. One serious side effect observed in patients being treated with Reserpine is depression. This drug-induced depression disappears quickly once Reserpine treatment is discontinued. Although Reserpine is not used as an antihypertensive today, it is still used in animal studies to examine the effects of amine depletion on behavior.

The consideration of the monoamine neurotransmitters as factors in depression was also reasonable given their distributions throughout the limbic system and frontal cortex—areas known for their roles in behavioral arousal, emotion, and motivation. Because Reserpine nonspecifically depletes monoamine neurotransmitters, the earliest versions of the monoamine hypothesis could not distinguish which of the monoamine neurotransmitters were involved in behavioral depression, nor could they suggest how these deficiencies caused it.

Since its inception, the monoamine depletion hypothesis has generated considerable support, and it is presently the most widely accepted account of the pathology of depression. And although this hypothesis has undergone revision, there is still no consensus about its details. Depression may actually result from several different alterations in the structure and function of monoamine neurotransmitter systems and in their target neuronal structures. It is becoming increasingly clear, however, that depression is a neurological disease that may be reversible or partially reversible by pharmacotherapy in many patients.

Revised Monoamine Hypothesis of Depression

One observation that has plagued the monoamine hypothesis since its beginning has been that even though antidepressant treatment produces rapid changes in neurotransmitter availability, the symptoms of depression do not disappear as quickly. The **lag time** between drug-induced changes in neurotransmitter availability and any corresponding changes in symptoms may be two weeks or longer. If depression were merely the result of monoamine depletion, we would expect more rapid improvement. What kinds of neuronal changes might take longer to be expressed?

The most recent revisions to the monoamine hypothesis propose that depression may be a consequence of neural degeneration in the hippocampus and in the frontal cortex, caused by monoamine neurons in these areas failing to produce sufficient amounts of tropic or growth factors. One protein that has received considerable attention is **brain-derived neurotropic factor** (BDNF) which is a nerve growth factor essential for normal cell survival, receptor growth, and for the growth of new neurons. Brain-derived neurotropic factor acts within the cell nucleus to maintain normal cell functioning and to facilitate synaptic growth by signaling the expression of new receptor sites. The synthesis of brain-derived neurotropic factor is dependent on a series of cellular events beginning with the influx of Ca^{++} upon activation of monoamine metabotropic receptors. Ca^{++} in turn activates second messengers that regulate the **transcription** of BDNF from the cell's DNA (see Figure 3.2). The second messenger

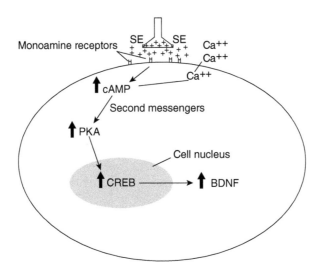

Figure 3.2 The neurotropic factor BDNF regulates receptor growth and expression. Activation of monoamine
metabotropic receptors allows for the influx of Ca^{++}, which activates second messenger systems and
an increase in CREB and BDNF synthesis. BDNF is essential for the expression of new receptors,
cell maintenance, and cell survival.

mediating BDNF transcription appears to be a protein called **CREB**, which stands for cyclic
adenosine monophosphate, or **c**AMP **r**esponse **e**lement **b**inding protein (Tao et al., 1998). In
summary, **downregulation** of monoamine neurons may lead to further downregulation of
an essential growth factor in neurons in the hippocampus and the frontal cortex. This downregulation disrupts neuronal signaling and plasticity and may lead to cellular degeneration.

Downregulation of monoamine activity also occurs as a result of neuronal inhibition by
autoreceptors. As you recall from Chapter 1, autoreceptors both on the soma and on terminal buttons regulate neuron excitability and the amount of neurotransmitter synthesized and
released from the terminal button. Patients with major depression may have increased numbers
of these autoreceptors, which may contribute to decreases in both serotonin and norepinephrine release. Chronic treatment with antidepressants downregulates these autoreceptors,
resulting in increased postsynaptic activity and increased BDNF levels (Lee et al., 2010; Levin
et al., 2007).

How do depressed patients get downregulated BDNF transcription and the cascade of
neuronal consequences resulting from it? There are several possibilities, including genetic
predispositions to autoreceptor expression and to downregulated BDNF transcription or to the
CREB activity that regulates it. Evidence to support this comes primarily from animals that
have been genetically altered to not express the BDNF gene (knockout mice). These animals
demonstrate depression-like behavior and a resistance to antidepressant treatment. Both of
these effects are consistent with the idea that BDNF downregulation contributes to depression
and that antidepressant treatment can reverse it (Castren & Monteggia, 2021; Monteggia et al.,
2007; Yang et al., 2020).

Additionally, environmental stress has been shown to contribute to BDNF downregulation. Animals exposed to stressors, including maternal separation or forced swimming, show
decreased CREB and BDNF activity, suggesting that chronic stress may contribute to behavioral
depression by altering BDNF transcription from DNA (Nair et al., 2007). The stress hormone
contributing to BDNF downregulation and to cell damage appears to be the glucocorticoid,

cortisol (Haynes et al., 2004; Schule et al., 2006; Villanueva, 2013). It appears that stress in humans also leads to cell death in several brain regions, including the hippocampus and the frontal lobes. Chronic stress leads to decreased norepinephrine and serotonin activity and ultimately downregulated BDNF synthesis, as depicted in Figure 3.3. Treatment with antidepressants can reverse both BDNF activity and increase cell growth and survival in these brain regions (Hosang et al., 2014; Lee & Kim, 2010; Licinio & Wong, 2002; Yang et al., 2020).

Further evidence for decreased or downregulated synthesis of BDNF in depression comes from both animal and human studies. For example, as shown in Figure 3.4, patients with

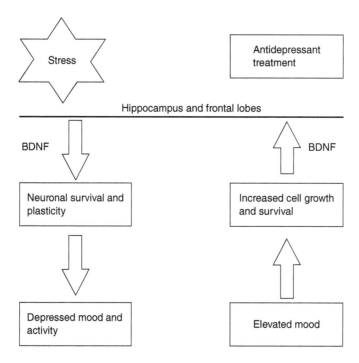

Figure 3.3 BDNF levels. Chronic stress leads to downregulation of BDNF synthesis, resulting in cell degeneration and death in several brain regions. Treatment with antidepressants can reverse this.

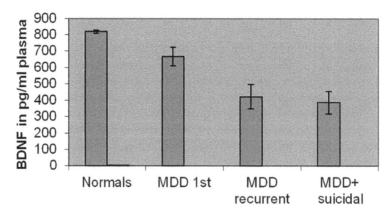

Figure 3.4 BDNF levels in depression (mean pg/mL +/− SE). Blood plasma levels of BDNF decrease as the severity of depression increases.

Source: Lee et al. (2006).

depression have low levels of BDNF in their blood when compared to non-depressed subjects, and those patients with recurring depression have even lower levels (Lee et al., 2006; Park et al., 2014; Post, 2007; Yoshida et al., 2007). Antidepressant therapy acts to both downregulate presynaptic autoreceptors and to stimulate the formation of BDNF, reinstating normal cell functioning and growth. The lag time between the initiation of antidepressant treatment, and the neuronal adaptations resulting from it, correspond well with improvements in mood.

Animal studies continue to play an important role in pharmacology research and drug development. Experimental methods and the measurement of behaviors indicative of depression have also become more standardized. For example, chronic mild stress, forced swimming, and the removal of the olfactory bulbs have all been effectively used to induce behavioral symptoms of depression. These symptoms include decreases in forced swim time, decreases in sexual behavior, depressed appetite, and impairments in learning and memory (see Figure 3.5). In addition to inducing behavioral depression, these manipulations have been shown to suppress the synthesis of BDNF in several brain regions. Chronic, but not acute, treatment with antidepressant drugs appears to reverse both the downregulation of BDNF synthesis and the symptoms of depression in these experimental animals (Grønli et al., 2006; Khundakar & Zetterstom, 2006; Rogóz et al., 2005).

It appears that all antidepressants have the ability to downregulate autoreceptor expression and to activate the second messenger systems that lead to BDNF synthesis. These neuronal adaptations may be the critical mechanisms of antidepressant action (Blom et al., 2002; Casarotto et al., 2021; Lee & Kim, 2010; Nibuya et al., 1996; Thome et al., 2000; Thomas et al., 2003; Tiraboschi et al., 2004; Yang et al., 2020). Antidepressant treatment may act to upregulate BDNF transcription and synthesis by activating CREB directly or by increasing Ca^{++} influx, which then activates CREB. Increases in BDNF activity promote the growth and expression of postsynaptic serotonin receptors, thereby enhancing serotonergic neurotransmission (Altar, 1999; Koponen et al., 2005).

Pharmacological Treatment of Major Depressive Disorder

In the following sections, we begin to review the history and the evolution of drug development and the pharmacological treatment of depression. The first drugs used to treat depression were introduced in the late 1950s, well before their mechanisms of action were understood. As the monoamine neurotransmitters and their pathways were being described in the 1960s, drugs

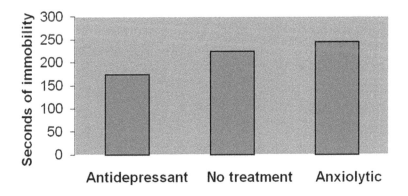

Figure 3.5 Immobility time during forced swim challenge. Antidepressants significantly decrease immobility in a forced swim challenge with laboratory rats.

Source: Data from Porsolt et al. (1977).

were becoming used as research tools to investigate the functions of neurotransmitter systems as well as for therapy for a variety of behavioral disorders. This interrelationship between drug development and neuroscience research continues to the present.

Tricyclic Antidepressants

The tricyclic category of antidepressant drugs all share a common three-ring molecular structure from which they derive their name and classification (see Figure 3.6). Discovered in the late 1950s, these drugs were first used unsuccessfully to treat schizophrenia. Their ability to treat major depression was discovered quite by accident in hospitalized patients. The tricyclic antidepressants include about eight compounds, each marketed under different brand names. Imipramine, the first **tricyclic antidepressant** produced, is currently marketed under several brand names, including Imipramin, Deprinol, and Tofranil. Other tricyclics, their common brand names, and their pharmacokinetics are included in Table 3.1. These drugs differ only slightly in their molecular structure, and their mechanisms of antidepressant action are all essentially the same. They differ only in their relative specificities for different monoamine neurotransmitters and in their side effects on acetylcholine and histamine receptors.

Mechanisms of Tricyclic Antidepressant Action

All tricyclic antidepressants bind effectively to the reuptake transporter proteins for both norepinephrine and serotonin. By competitively binding to transporter proteins, they interfere with the normal reuptake of these neurotransmitters, thereby increasing the duration they

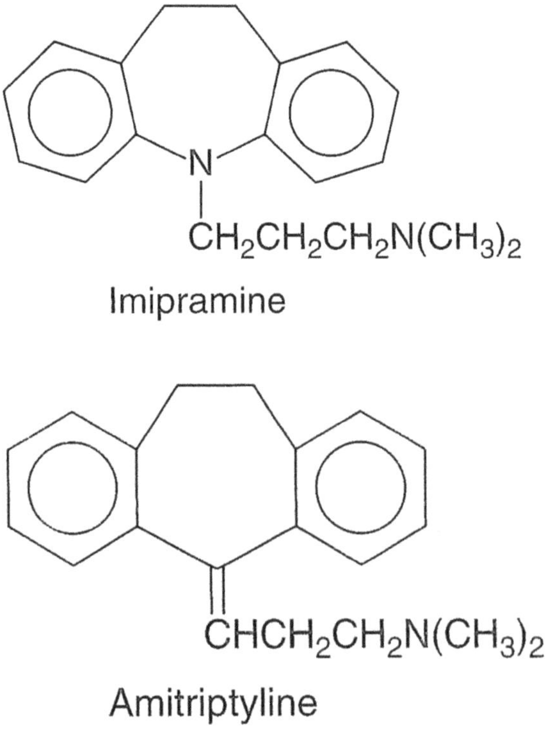

Imipramine

$CH_2CH_2CH_2N(CH_3)_2$

Amitriptyline

$CHCH_2CH_2N(CH_3)_2$

Figure 3.6 Tricyclic antidepressant chemical structure.

remain in the synaptic gap. The longer neurotransmitters remain in the synapse, the longer they may exert their effects on pre- and postsynaptic receptors. Because blocking reuptake of neurotransmitters is an immediate effect of antidepressant treatment, and their effects on symptoms of depression, if they occur at all, are often delayed by several weeks, it is believed that their antidepressant effects result from synaptic adaptations and neuronal growth, following the downregulation of presynaptic autoreceptors and the **upregulation** of BNDF synthesis (see Figure 3.7).

Side Effects of Tricyclic Antidepressants

While the antidepressant action of the tricyclic antidepressants appears to be their effects on reuptake mechanisms, they also block both histamine and acetylcholine receptors to some extent. Histamine blockade (an antihistamine effect) produces drowsiness and fatigue in most patients. This antihistamine effect can be minimized to some degree by taking it at night rather than early in the day. If insomnia and agitation are part of the complex of symptoms this may actually be an attractive side effect. In addition, tricyclic antidepressants block acetylcholine receptors and may cause dry mouth, dizziness, hypotension, constipation, blurred vision, and difficulties with concentration and memory formation. While all of these cholinergic effects are unwanted, they are experienced to varying extents by patients. Some patients may find that their effectiveness and their relatively low cost outweigh their annoying side effects, while others may find them intolerable. Several common tricyclic antidepressants and their respective half-lives are shown in Table 3.1.

Overdosing with tricyclic antidepressants can, and does, occur and may lead to seizures, cardiac arrhythmias, severe hypotension, and even death. Unintentional overdose would be

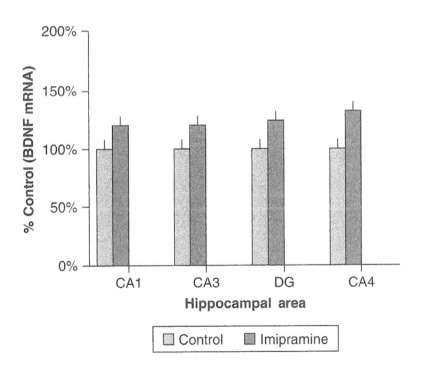

Figure 3.7 Imipramine significantly increased BDNF synthesis in all hippocampal areas examined.
Source: Data from Russo-Neustadt et al. (1999).

Table 3.1 Tricyclic antidepressants.

Drug name	Common trade names	Half-life hours
Amiltriptyline	Elavil	10–28
Desipramine	Norpramin	24
Doxepin	Sinequan	8–24
Imipramine	Tofranil, Imipramin	10–20
Nortriptyline	Pamelor	36
Protriptyline	Triptil, Vivactil	74
Trimipramine	Surmontil	7–23

quite rare, however, since there is a relatively wide therapeutic index (AD_{50} to LD_{50}) for these drugs. The toxic effects of the tricyclic drugs are typically seen at doses exceeding ten times their normal dose (i.e., 1,000 mg or more).

Monoamine Oxidase Inhibitors (MAOIs)

Monoamine oxidase inhibitors (MAOIs) were also developed in the late 1950s and were found by coincidence to function as antidepressants. Iproniazid, the first MAOI, was actually developed to treat tuberculosis. Unexpectedly, Iproniazid was observed to have mood-elevating and **psychostimulant** effects and was soon after recruited to treat major depression. Because of often severe and even life-threatening side effects, and newer alternatives for pharmaco-therapy, these drugs have only limited usefulness today.

Mechanisms of MAOI Antidepressant Action

Monoamine oxidase is produced by all monoamine neurons and functions to **deaminate** (remove the amine group) these neurotransmitters within the terminal button. The amount of monoamine available for storage and release is therefore regulated by MAO. Monoamine oxidase inhibitors (MAOIs) prevent this oxidative reaction, resulting in increased availability of these neurotransmitters for storage and release. There are two subtypes of monoamine oxidase that preferentially deaminate different monoamines: Monoamine oxidase-$_A$ (MAO_A) deaminates norepinephrine, dopamine, and serotonin, while MAO-$_B$ deaminates dopamine and phenylanine but has less specificity for norepinephrine and serotonin. The early MAOIs inhibited both MAO-$_A$ and MAO-$_B$ equally, but newer MAOIs have been developed to be more specific in attempts to reduce their side effects. Monoamine oxidase inhibitors are typically irreversible, meaning that once they have deactivated MAO the enzyme remains unavailable in the terminal button until it has been replaced. The resynthesis of MAO may take as long as several weeks. Reversible MAOIs have been developed, but they are not com-mercially available in the United States. Presumably the MAO inhibiting effect could be more carefully regulated by dose with reversible MAOIs (see Table 3.2).

As with the tricyclic antidepressants, the lag time from initial treatment to the observation of therapeutic effects, if observed, is typically about two weeks, which corresponds to the time for synaptic adaptations resulting from downregulated autoreceptor expression and to upregulated BDNF synthesis.

Side Effects of MAOI Antidepressants

The MAOIs all have significant and sometimes serious side effects, including sedation and fatigue, dizziness, movement disorders such as tremors, blurred vision, decreased libido, dry

Table 3.2 Monoamine oxidase inhibitors (MAOIs).

Drug name	Common trade names	Selectivity
Isocarbazid	Marplan	MAO-$_A$, MAO-$_B$
Phenelzine	Nardil	MAO-$_A$, MAO-$_B$
Selegiline	Eldapril	MAO-$_B$
Tranycypromine	Parnate	MAO-$_A$, MAO-$_B$

Note: Because these MAOIs are irreversible, elimination half-life does not affect their clinical effectiveness.

mouth, and weight gain. A more serious side effect may occur if MAOIs are taken with foods containing tyramine (derived from the amino acid tyrosine), an amine formed as a byproduct of fermentation. Foods such as cheese, yogurt, aged meats, certain breads, wine, and even some fruits contain tyramine, which is normally deaminated in the liver by MAO. However, MAOIs deactivate even liver MAO, resulting in excess levels of tyramine, which may increase norepinephrine storage and release. Excessive norepinephrine activity can cause severe headaches, sweating, nausea, and a hypertensive crisis that can cause a stroke.

A newer selective MAOI called selegiline was approved in an oral formulation by the FDA in 2003 for treating Parkinson's disease, and again in 2006 as a skin patch for treating major depression. Selegiline acts primarily on MAO-$_B$, so it increases dopamine storage and release without interacting with tyramine-containing foods as significantly as do nonselective MAOIs. At higher doses, selegiline also inhibits MAO-$_A$, producing its antidepressant effect. The other side effects associated with nonselective MAOIs, including dry mouth, decreased libido, weight gain, and fatigue, do not appear to be as bothersome with selegiline.

Selective Serotonin Reuptake Inhibitors (SSRIs)

By the late 1970s, researchers were beginning to distinguish between the behavior-stimulating and mood-elevating effects of antidepressants, which acted on both the noradrenergic and serotonergic systems. It was believed that the behavior-stimulating effects were mediated by blocking norepinephrine reuptake while the mood-enhancing effect was mediated by serotonin. In attempts to target these systems individually, research focused on developing drugs to specifically enhance serotonin (or 5-HT) neurotransmission, while at the same time minimizing effects on histamine and acetylcholine receptors, which mediated most of the troublesome side effects. In 1988, after over ten years of pharmacology research, fluoxetine (Prozac) was approved for the treatment of major depression. Since the development of Prozac a number of similar compounds have been developed and approved for the treatment of depression as well as other psychological disorders (see Table 3.3). These drugs are known as **second-generation** antidepressants. These drugs differ considerably from the **first-generation** MAOIs and tricyclics in their mechanisms of antidepressant action, as well as their effects on histamine and acetylcholine receptors. Additionally, second-generation antidepressants were developed specifically for treating depression, unlike the MAOIs and tricyclics, which were developed to treat other diseases and only later identified for their antidepressant effects. With the development of these second-generation compounds came the first significant advance in the 30-year history of treating depression with drugs.

Mechanisms of SSRI Antidepressant Action

As their name implies, SSRIs were developed to specifically inhibit the reuptake of serotonin by competitively binding with the serotonin transporter protein. This competitive binding effectively blocks the reuptake of a significant amount of extracellular serotonin, leaving it available to engage pre- and postsynaptic receptor sites for longer durations. The SSRIs do not specifically target subtypes of serotonin receptors, so they effectively increase serotonin activity at 5-HT$_1$, 5-HT$_2$, and 5-HT$_3$ receptor types. Recall from Chapter 1 that the 5-HT$_1$ receptor types function both as metabotropic postsynaptic receptors and as inhibitory autoreceptors. It is believed that the antidepressant effects of SSRIs are primarily mediated by the 5-HT$_{1A}$ receptor types, while some of their adverse side effects may be mediated by 5-HT$_2$ receptors. Specifically, the 5-HT$_{1A}$ autoreceptor is believed to be overexpressed in major depression, resulting in excessive inhibition of serotonergic neurons in the raphi nucleus, amygdala, and hippocampus. Chronic treatment with SSRIs leads to downregulation of these inhibitory autoreceptors and a corresponding increase in serotonergic activity (Figure 3.8). Selectively blocking the effects of SSRIs on 5-HT$_2$ receptors may enhance the effectiveness of SSRI treatment and decrease some unwanted side effects (Levin et al., 2007; Marek et al., 2005; Parsey et al., 2006).

In summary, SSRIs increase serotonergic activity by blocking the reuptake transporter, leaving serotonin in the synapse for longer durations. Increases in serotonin activity result in neuronal adaptations and downregulation of 5-HT$_{1A}$ autoreceptors (see Figure 3.8). The 5-HT$_2$ type receptors may mediate many of the troubling side effects associated with SSRI use. Research employing selective 5-HT$_2$ antagonists in combination with SSRIs further confirms the role of 5-HT$_1$ receptors in major depression and provides promise for an even

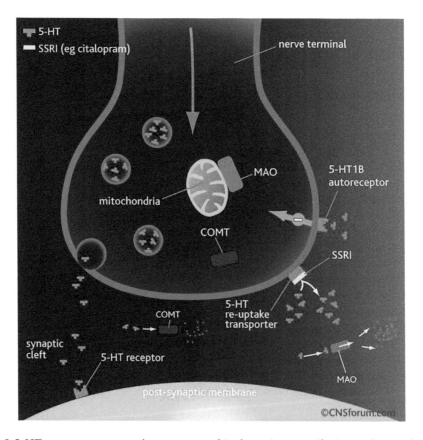

Figure 3.8 5-HT$_{1A}$ autoreceptors may be overexpressed in depression, contributing to decreased serotonin activity. SSRIs downregulate inhibitory 5-HT$_{1A}$ autoreceptors in several regions of the brain, including the hippocampus, raphe nucleus, and the amygdala.

Table 3.3 Serotonin specific reuptake inhibitors (SSRIs).

Drug name	Brand name	Half-life hours
Citalopram	Celexa	23–45
Escitalopram	Lexapro	27–32
Fluoxetine	Prozac	24–48[*]
Fluvoxamine	Luvox	9–28
Paroxetine	Paxil	24
Sertraline	Zoloft	22–36

[*] Active metabolite

more effective therapy with reduced side effects. Drugs with this property will be described in the next section. Several of the most common SSRIs are listed in Table 3.3.

Side Effects of SSRI Antidepressants

All antidepressants thus far have had significant side effects, and the SSRIs are not going to be an exception. As mentioned, most of the side effects—including sexual dysfunction in males, decreased libido, gastrointestinal problems, decreased appetite, insomnia, and agitation—are primarily mediated by the 5-HT_2 receptor types. Additionally, a life-threatening condition referred to as **serotonin syndrome**, which is a toxic reaction caused by excessive serotonin activity, may occur. Symptoms of **serotonin syndrome** include disorientation, confusion, visual disturbances, severe agitation, mania, hypertension, hyperthermia, cold sweats, and diarrhea. In severe cases, serotonin syndrome can lead to a coma and perhaps death. This syndrome is most probable when SSRIs are taken with other medication that can increase serotonin activity, including all non-SSRI antidepressants and St. John's Wort, an herbal remedy for depression (Izzo, 2004). However, serotonin syndrome can also occur as an overdose to any SSRI taken alone.

In recent years, there has been considerable attention surrounding cases of suicide in children and adolescents taking SSRIs. In fact, in early 2004 the Food and Drug Administration (FDA) issued a warning that antidepressant drugs significantly increased the risk of **suicide ideation** and **suicidality** in children and adolescents. In 2007, this warning was revised to include warnings about increased risks of suicide ideation and attempts in young adults aged 18–24. Additional language was added stating that scientific data did not show this increased risk in adults older than age 24, and that adults aged 65 and older taking antidepressants actually have a decreased risk of suicidality. The contribution of SSRIs to suicidality is quite small (e.g., Tiihonen et al., 2006) and not all studies have found it (e.g., Nilsson et al., 2004). In a recent analysis of all research published between 1988 and 2021, investigators found small and inconsistent differences in suicidality between adolescents with major depression taking antidepressants and those taking placebos. Antidepressants were found to be more effective than placebos in treating symptoms of depression in adolescents, however (Bridge et al., 2007; Kuan et al., 2022).

Since the regulatory warning regarding SSRI and suicide risk was issued, SSRI prescription rates for adolescents have dropped significantly. During this same time, as shown in Figure 3.9, researchers report a concerning increase in suicides by this age group. In the United States, suicide rates among youth have increased dramatically since 2005, corresponding with the decrease in prescription rates (Dudley et al., 2010; Gibbons et al., 2007).

Clearly the debate about whether antidepressants can increase suicide ideation and attempts will continue with mixed results well into the future. Suicidality is a common symptom of

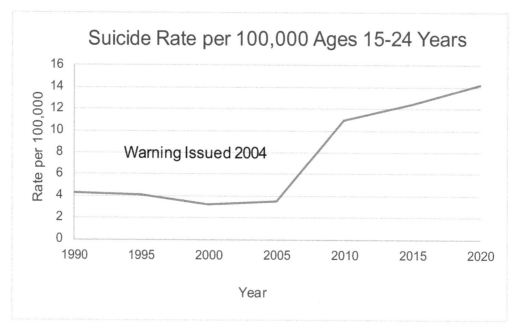

Figure 3.9 Suicide rate among youth in the United States (15–24 years of age).
Source: CDC (2022).

major depression in all age groups and must always be considered sincerely in any treatment program.

Serotonin-Norepinephrine Reuptake Inhibitors (SNRIs)

The most recent additions to the antidepressant arsenal come from attempts to minimize drug side effects, shorten the lag time in therapeutic effectiveness, and increase the range of symptoms treated. Depression often includes both depressed mood and depressed behavior. For instance, overwhelming fatigue, excessive sleepiness, and prolonged sleep duration can be quite common in depressed patients. Increasing noradrenergic activity promotes arousal by enhancing the activity of the reticular activating system. While drugs that target norepinephrine more specifically, such as amphetamine, are not effective in treating depression, the SNRIs, which block the reuptake of both serotonin and norepinephrine, are. Additionally, because the antagonism of acetylcholine and histamine receptors, and increasing the activity of 5-HT_{2-3} receptors, mediate most of the troublesome side effects of antidepressants, new dual-action drugs are being designed to evade these receptor effects.

Mechanisms of SNRI Antidepressant Action

The SNRIs all differ considerably in their effects on serotonin and norepinephrine neurons and several also increase dopamine activity to some extent (see Table 3.4). Duloxetine (Cymbalta) was approved in 2004 for treating depression and **neuropathic pain**. Its mechanisms of action include blockade of the serotonin and norepinephrine reuptake transporters as well as the reuptake transporter for dopamine. Dopamine activity in the frontal cortex may also be increased indirectly by increasing noradrenergic activity to those neurons.

Table 3.4 Serotonin (SE)-norepinephrine (NE) reuptake inhibitors (SNRIs).

Drug name	Brand name	Receptor effects	Half-life hours
Duloxetine	Cymbalta	NE, 5-HT, and DA reuptake blockade	12
Mirtazepine	Remeron	Blocks α-2 NE and 5-HT$_1$ autoreceptors, and 5-HT$_{2-3}$ antagonism	20–40
Nefazodone	Serzone[+]	NE and 5-HT reuptake blockade, and 5-HT$_{2-3}$ antagonism	12★
Venlafaxine	Effexor	NE and SE reuptake blockade, DA reuptake blockade is weak	3–7★

[+] No longer available in the US or Canada
★ Active metabolite
★ Active metabolite

Because duloxetine does not antagonize 5-HT$_2$ and 5-HT$_3$ receptors, as do the other SNRIs, sexual dysfunction in men and decreased libido in both sexes may still occur. In addition, duloxetine can cause nausea, intestinal upset, hypertension, and sedation.

Mirtazepine

Mirtazepine (Remeron) is a unique antidepressant that increases noradrenergic and serotonergic activity by blocking both noradrenergic α-2 and 5-HT$_{1A}$ autoreceptors that normally decrease neurotransmitter synthesis and release. Mirtazepine also antagonizes 5-HT$_{2-3}$ postsynaptic receptors, thereby decreasing some of the most troublesome sexual side effects associated with SSRIs.

Nefazodone

Nefazodone (Serzone) not only blocks the reuptake transporters for both serotonin and norepinephrine but also acts as a 5-HT$_{2-3}$ antagonist. By blocking 5-HT$_{2-3}$ receptors, the side effects associated with SSRI treatment are minimized. In particular, the adverse effects on sexual functioning and libido are reduced with Nefazodone when compared to SSRI antidepressants (Clayton & Montejo, 2006). Because of a risk of liver toxicity, however, Nefazodone was withdrawn in Canada in late 2003, and it was subsequently discontinued in the United States in 2004. Nefazadone is still available under other brand names in some countries.

With the major difference between the SSRIs and the SNRIs being their effects on norepinephrine reuptake, these drugs appear to contribute to the same neuronal adaptations as other antidepressants. And although their side effects may not be as bothersome, they are no more effective than any of the other antidepressants that we have already mentioned. Ultimately, all antidepressants contribute to upregulation of BDNF synthesis and the neuronal growth and adaptation that it promotes. Several additional dual-action antidepressants are listed in Table 3.4.

Atypical Antidepressants

Not all antidepressants alter the availability or the activity of serotonin and norepinephrine as the antidepressants thus far discussed do. Because their mechanisms of action don't follow this traditional approach, these drugs are often referred to as **atypical** antidepressants. Originally, the SNRIs were classified as atypical because of their effects on both norepinephrine and serotonin, but now they are classified by their dual mechanisms of action. There are a few

Table 3.5 Atypical antidepressants.

Drug name	Brand name	Receptor effects	Half-life hours
Amoxapine	Asendin	Blocks norepinephrine reuptake	8★
Bupropion	Wellbutrin Zyban	Blocks dopamine reuptake, partially blocks norepinephrine reuptake, blocks nACh receptors	10–14★
Maprotiline	Ludiomil	Blocks norepinephrine reuptake (NRI)	51
Reboxetine	Norebox, Edronax	Blocks norepinephrine reuptake (NRI)	13
Trazodone	Desyrel	Blocks 5-HT reuptake, blocks 5-HT$_{2A}$ receptors	3–9

★ Active metabolite
★ Active metabolite

atypical antidepressants that are available today. Only two of these, Bupropion and Trazodone, will be discussed in any detail. Others are listed in Table 3.5.

Bupropion (Wellbutrin)

Bupropion has been approved for the treatment of depression (as Wellbutrin) and to diminish cravings associated with smoking cessation (as Zyban). Bupropion is as effective as other antidepressants, but its mechanism of action is quite different. Bupropion acts primarily as a selective dopamine reuptake inhibitor by blocking the dopamine transporter protein. It acts to a lesser extent to inhibit the reuptake of norepinephrine (Stahl et al., 2004). Bupropion also acts as an antagonist on acetylcholine nicotinic receptors. Because Bupropion does not act on serotonergic receptors, it has few of the side effects associated with SSRIs and SNRIs. In fact, Bupropion may act to enhance sexual functioning and libido and may be used with SSRIs to augment their effectiveness and to diminish their side effects (Clayton et al., 2004, 2014). Interestingly, although Bupropion does have stimulant properties, it does not possess the reinforcing properties or the abuse potential associated with other dopamine–norepinephrine agonists, such as amphetamine and cocaine. Perhaps this is due to its relatively slow absorption rate and to its lower occupancy of transporter sites compared to these abused drugs.

Notable side effects caused by Bupropion include restlessness, agitation, motor tics or tremors, decreased appetite and weight loss, abdominal discomfort, and rare seizures. Because of these effects Bupropion is not used with patients exhibiting anxiety, panic disorder, or manic episodes.

Trazodone (Desyrel)

Trazodone was approved by the FDA in 2010 for the treatment of depression. Its mechanisms of action are complex and include both serotonin agonism (via blockade of the serotonin transporter) and antagonism (blockade of 5-HT$_{2A}$ receptors). It belongs to a class of drugs referred to as serotonin antagonist and reuptake inhibitors (SARIs). Trazodone acts as a serotonin receptor antagonist much like other SSRIs. That is, it blocks serotonin reuptake transporters. But, unlike SSRIs, Trazodone also blocks 5-HT$_{2A}$ and 5-HT$_{2C}$ receptors, which are believed to mediate many of the side effects associated with SSRIs (Stahl, 2009). Typical SSRIs and SNRIs agonize other 5-HT receptors causing anxiety, insomnia, overeating, and sexual dysfunction in many patients (Figure 3.6). While the 5-HT$_{2A}$ receptors may desensitize after prolonged use of SSRIs in some patients, these side effects remain problematic for most. Trazodone minimizes these side effects by antagonizing 5-HT$_{2A}$ and 5-HT$_{2C}$ receptors.

Table 3.6 Functions of several serotonin receptors.

$5HT_{1A}$	$5HT_{2A}$	$5HT_{2C}$
Antidepressant Anxiolytic Pro-cognitive Hormone regulation	Sleep Sexual function Anxiety Regulation of dopamine release	Sleep Sexual function Anxiety Appetite, obesity Regulation of dopamine and norepinephrine release
None	Regulation of glutamate release	Regulation of glutamate release
Inhibition of cortical pyramidal neurons	Excitation of cortical pyramidal neurons	None

(From Stahl, 2009).

How Effective Are Antidepressants?

There is little doubt that treating major depression with medication is effective, and literally tens of thousands of scientific articles support their use. However, it is also well known that not all patients respond to medication. Most available research suggests that as many as 40 percent of patients with major depression will not respond to initial antidepressant therapy, and for others the effectiveness of medication can diminish over time. This rate of non-responding is certainly high, but it can be misleading since many patients who, after initial therapy, were labeled as non-responders do in fact respond to a different antidepressant (Rosack, 2002; Ruelaz, 2006).

Another complication in interpreting the effectiveness of antidepressants is the observation that many placebo-treated patients improve throughout their initial treatment period. Well-designed studies on the effectiveness of medication must include placebo controls to rule out effects not attributable to the drugs being investigated. According to Kirsch and Sapirstein (1998), placebos accounted for about 75 percent of antidepressant effectiveness in the 19 clinical trials they investigated. They concluded that the remaining 25 percent might be attributable to **active placebo** effects as opposed to antidepressant effects. Active placebo effects include perceptible side effects of a drug that do not contribute to its clinical effectiveness. For example, sedation, dry mouth, and dizziness may lead patients to believe their medication is working because these side effects are common with antidepressants. Consequently, they might report fewer, less severe symptoms than patients taking inert placebos, which do not cause these effects.

Clearly not all researchers are as critical of antidepressant effectiveness. More recent research comparing the effectiveness of antidepressants vs. placebos in over 7,000 patients found that antidepressants provided a more sustained treatment effect for major depression than did placebos, which tend to lose their effectiveness quickly (Papakostas et al., 2006). In summary, methodological issues continue to plague research on the efficacy of antidepressants, but the vast majority of research confirms their effectiveness when compared for sustained, not merely short-term, outcomes. Clearly the debate on whether antidepressants are significantly more effective than placebos will continue into the future. Urgently needed are better objective methods to measure treatment outcomes and more standardized double-blind research methodologies incorporating active placebos. At present, outcomes are measured in human studies using a number of subjective depression rating scales, which can reveal inconsistent outcomes.

Ketamine and Psilocybin for Treatment-Resistant Depression

As previously stated, as many as 40 percent of depressed patients do not respond to traditional monoamine therapy or the antidepressant effects of these drugs tend to wane over time.

Research with this population of patients suggests that alternative treatment with either ketamine or the psychedelic psilocybin may be more beneficial and longer acting.

Ketamine (Sprayato and Ketanest)

Ketamine is not a new drug. In fact, it has been used for decades for anaesthesia and to calm severely agitated patients in the emergency room. In 2019 the FDA approved a ketamine nasal spray called esketamine named after the S-ketamine isomer. Its brand or trade names include Spravato and Ketanest. S-ketamine is a potent glutamate NMDA agonist and its antidepressant activity appears to be a consequence of rapid increases in glutamate activity which, in turn, increase monoamine release and BDNF synthesis in the medial prefrontal cortex and the hippocampus (Devama & Duman, 2019). As you recall from our earlier discussion, both of these regions reveal decreased BDNF activity and its corresponding neural degeneration in major depression (Lin et al., 2021; Yang et al., 2020).

Although ketamine's FDA approval is quite recent, numerous studies have confirmed its rapid and sustained antidepressant effects. A recent review of over 2,000 treatment-resistant patients from 79 studies revealed substantial and lasting antidepressant effects of ketamine (Alnefeesi et al., 2022). As you recall, monoamine therapies typically reveal antidepressant effects after a lag time of about three weeks of treatment. Ketamine is known to produce antidepressant effects within 24 hours even after a single oral dose. Repeated administration appears to produce long-lasting effects (Kryst et al., 2020). At the time of this writing, it was too early to comment about ketamine's long-term effectiveness and tolerability. Over the next several years researchers will have the opportunity to conduct longer-term studies that will address these concerns.

Psilocybin

The psychedelic psilocybin will be discussed in much more detail in Chapter 9, but evidence for its antidepressant effects will be briefly addressed here. Psilocybin occurs in a family of naturally occurring mushrooms. It is an alkaloid with strong agonistic effects on serotonin receptors, particularly the 5-HT_{2A} receptor. Psilocybin also has indirect and weaker agonist effects on dopamine and glutamine neurons (Ling et al., 2022). The pharmacodynamics of psilocybin's antidepressant effects are still unknown. However, in a number of clinical trials with depressed patients, psilocybin was shown to have significant antidepressant and anxiolytic effects after two doses. These effects were sustained for up to six months without significant adverse effects (Goldberg et al., 2020; Griffiths et al., 2016; Li et al., 2022). Psilocybin has also been shown to be effective in treating treatment-resistant depression (Carhart-Harris et al., 2018). While psilocybin remains to be a restricted substance (Schedule 1), it has been approved for use in clinically supervised settings in the state of Oregon.

St. John's Wort

Are there effective herbal treatments for major depressive disorder? Perhaps the most extensively studied and the most widely used herbal product for the treatment of depression is St. John's Wort, which is the common name for the flowering plant *Hypericum perforatum*. Extracts from the yellow *Hypericum* flower have been used for centuries to treat a variety of conditions, including psychological disorders, pain, and even malaria. More recently the *Hypericum* extract has become available over the counter in tablet form.

St. John's Wort is widely proclaimed to be an effective antidepressant, and a number of studies seem to support its use for the treatment of mild to moderately severe depression. It must be pointed out, however, that research comparing the effectiveness of St. John's Wort with traditional antidepressants and placebos is inconsistent at best. Recent analyses of large numbers of published studies (a meta-analysis) tend to conclude that St. John's Wort is effective for the short-term treatment of mild depression but not for the chronic treatment of severe depressive disorder. For instance, investigators have found St. John's Wort to be more effective than placebos and about as effective as traditional antidepressants (Kasper et al., 2006; Linde et al., 2005). Other research has suggested that St. John's Wort may be even more effective than traditional antidepressant medication. For instance, a recent study found that St. John's Wort was more effective than fluoxetine (Prozac), but not more effective than a placebo in decreasing symptoms of depression as measured by depression inventories (Fava et al., 2005). Knowing that the vast majority of studies find antidepressants to be more effective than placebos makes the interpretation of this study particularly difficult. And to further complicate this picture, evidence from long-term studies has found St. John's Wort to be ineffective for major depressive disorder when compared to traditional antidepressants (Gelenberg et al., 2004; Shelton et al., 2001). The National Institute for Health (NIH) also sponsored a large study of St. John's Wort by the *Hypericum Depression Trial Study Group* (Davidson, 2002). In this study, the effects of Hypericum, the SSRI sertraline, and an active placebo were compared. The results of this study are presented in Figure 3.10, which reveals that Hypericum was not as effective as sertraline when depression symptoms were measured by the Hamilton Rating Scale for Depression (a widely used inventory to measure depression severity). The results also reveal that all three groups improved over the eight-week treatment phase, including the placebo-treated patients. This observation is typical in studies of antidepressant effects, and it further illustrates the difficulty of separating placebo from treatment effects in clinical trials. These results are shown in Figure 3.10.

In animal studies, Hypericum appears to have effects similar to traditional antidepressants. That is, Hypericum decreases immobility time in forced swimming tasks and protects animals from the behavioral effects of acute stressors in learned helplessness and escape tasks (Butterweck, 2003; Sanchez-Mateo, 2007; Zanoli et al., 2002).

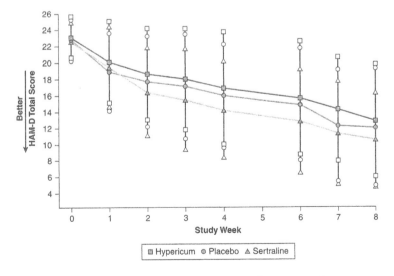

Figure 3.10 Hamilton Rating Scale for Depression (HAM-D) total mean score by treatment week. Higher scores indicate greater severity of symptoms.

Source: Davidson (2002).

Mechanisms of St. John's Wort Antidepressant Action

Evidence suggests that St. John's Wort increases serotonin and norepinephrine activity but not by acting on reuptake transporters, as do the SSRIs and SNRIs discussed previously. Rather, it appears to inhibit the reuptake and the vesicular storage of monoamine neurotransmitters, resulting in more being available in the synapse. Because the active ingredient of St. John's Wort, *Hyperforin*, does not appear to bind with either the reuptake transporters or the vesicular transporter proteins, its mechanism of action may be to increase intracellular sodium concentrations, which in turn interfere with reuptake and contribute to a Reserpine-like effect on storage vesicles (Müller, 2003; Roz & Rehavi, 2004). Hyperforin also increases the extra cellular concentrations of both GABA and glutamate by the same mechanisms. The putative antidepressant effects of St. John's Wort are believed to be mediated by its effects on both serotonin and norepinephrine availability (Müller, 2003; Roz et al., 2002; Zanoli, 2004).

In summary, St. John's Wort appears to be more effective than inert placebos for the short-term treatment of mild to moderately severe depression—an effect observed in numerous human and animal studies. Whether St. John's Wort is more effective than an active placebo for severe depression or for extended treatment durations is uncertain. Patients report fewer and less severe side effects with St. John's Wort compared to traditional antidepressants, the most common being gastrointestinal upset, sedation, restlessness, sexual dysfunction, and headache. The effects of St. John's Wort appear to be mediated by enhanced neurotransmitter release and reuptake inhibition. Because St. John's Wort also enhances the synthesis of the liver enzyme CYP3A4, which is involved in the metabolism of most drugs, it can decrease the duration of action and the effectiveness of other medication. Finally, St. John's Wort can contribute to serotonin syndrome when it is combined with other antidepressant medication (Boyer & Shannon, 2005; Izzo, 2004).

Bipolar Disorders

Rick was a completely normal high school kid. He was class president during his senior year and a member of the basketball team. He graduated as the only male valedictorian that year and was looking forward to attending a small, prestigious liberal arts college in the fall. Like most other kids his age, Rick experienced a full range of emotions, including a bout of depression after a year-long relationship with his girlfriend ended. This depression disappeared quickly, and he was seeing someone else within a few months. During the summer following graduation Rick experienced his first significant symptoms. While working for his father in a family-owned business, Rick made frequent trips for business purchases out of town. On this particular trip he failed to return from his three-hour drive and ended up staying in an out-of-town hotel. For the next few days he went on spending sprees, charging clothing and sports equipment on his father's business card. He returned a few days later after spending over $10,000. This first manic episode lasted a little over two weeks. During that time he slept very little, demonstrated bouts of anger and hostility, and talked enthusiastically about his new plans to open a clothing store of his own. This episode revealed behavior that was so uncharacteristic of Rick that his parents made arrangements for a psychiatric evaluation. He was not diagnosed with acute mania at that time, however. Rather, his psychiatrist reasoned that his behavior was completely normal—he was simply displaying some anxiety about attending college in a few months.

Midway through his first semester at college, Rick experienced his first severe depression. He stopped attending classes, slept for much of each day, rarely showered or changed clothes, and even attempted suicide by alcohol ingestion. On that occasion he consumed nearly a fifth of vodka before blacking out. Fortunately, he was taken to the hospital before respiratory depression killed him. Rick remained in a depressed mood for several more months and often self-medicated with marijuana. During Christmas break he was prescribed Prozac, and this appeared to help. Unfortunately, within a few months he experienced another manic episode. Throughout this episode he became so euphoric and enthusiastic about finding religion he did little else but publicly proclaim his religious faith and try to convince others of his special relationship with God. Rick could speak in the center of campus for hours at a time. After several days of exhibiting this behavior he was asked by the administration to leave college. His parents had him reevaluated and he was finally diagnosed with bipolar disorder. His medication was switched to lithium, which may have helped to terminate this second manic episode.

Rick stayed at his parents' home for the remainder of the year and worked intermittently at the family business. He stopped taking lithium after about six months and quickly returned to a severely depressed state. This episode of depression lasted about three months and was followed by about a month of relatively normal mood. Just about the time when his family thought they had seen the worst of his condition, Rick entered another manic state. As with his prior manic episode he began to have delusions about his special relationship with God and used every opportunity to demonstrate his newly found religiosity. Rick was convinced to go back on lithium and antidepressants. However, after several months of intermittent use he abandoned lithium for alcohol and marijuana. His life ended several months later in a fatal one-car accident.

Rick's case is not untypical. His first symptoms came as acute mania when he was 18 years old. This episode was followed within a few months by an episode of depression. The diagnosis of depression and its treatment with an SSRI may have actually hastened his second manic episode where he exhibited some psychosis. Non-compliance with lithium is also quite common and can lead to an even more severe depression with an increased risk of suicide.

Defining and Diagnosing Bipolar Disorders

Bipolar disorders are distinguished from other depressive disorders by the presence of either **manic** or **hypomanic episodes**. During a manic episode, a person experiences an excessive elevation in mood and euphoria often accompanied by extreme enthusiasm and energy. These manic episodes may also be characterized by psychotic features, such as delusional beliefs and hallucinations. Hypomanic episodes are similar but less severe than manic episodes. They are noticeable changes that impair social and occupational functioning, but do not include psychotic features or require hospitalization. These mood changes must be present for at least four days to be diagnostic. The depression associated with bipolar disorders is essentially indistinguishable from major depressive disorder and may be confused with it until a manic or hypomanic episode appears. Unfortunately, misdiagnosis and treatment with antidepressants may actually promote manic symptoms and therefore worsen a patient's condition. It has been estimated that as many as 30 percent of patients with bipolar disorders are inappropriately treated with antidepressants without mood-stabilizing medication.

Bipolar disorders occur with equal frequency in men and women and typically present in late adolescence or early adulthood. As many as six million people (about 2.5 percent of the population) in the United States are diagnosed with a bipolar disorder each year. The lifetime prevalence of these disorders may be as high as 4.4 percent of the population when we consider its various forms and severity (Merikangas et al., 2007; NIMH, 2021b).

The diagnostic criteria for bipolar disorders are complicated by the presence or absence of manic and depressive features as well as their appearance and severity upon diagnosis. The disorders include Bipolar I disorder, Bipolar II disorder, and **dysthymic disorder**. The *DSM-5* criteria for Bipolar I disorder require that a patient exhibit at least one manic or mixed episode. Often, but not required for Bipolar I diagnoses, are occurrences of major depressive episodes. If a patient has not yet presented a major depressive episode it is presumed that they eventually will. Most often the first manic episode immediately precedes or follows a period of major depression. The episodes of either mania or depression can vary in duration, but typically the depressive episodes are shorter than a bout of unipolar depression, lasting three to four months. Manic episodes typically last from a few days to several weeks. If an individual experiences four or more episodes of either depression or mania during the period of a year, the condition is referred to as **rapid cycling** bipolar disorder.

The distinctions between Bipolar I disorder, Bipolar II disorder, and dysthymia are more of symptom severity than of their presence. A diagnosis of Bipolar II disorder requires that at least one major depressive episode and one or more occurrences of hypomania have been presented. Bipolar II disorder does not require that a full-blown manic episode has occurred, and it is more prevalent than Bipolar I disorder. Between periods of depression and hypomania, individuals with Bipolar II disorder may function normally, whereas those with Bipolar I disorder are more likely to experience continued social and occupational difficulties. Dysthymia is characterized by the presence of hypomanic episodes intermixed with periods of mild to moderate depression, not meeting the criteria for a major depressive disorder. These bouts of depression and hypomania must be present for at least two years without remission. Dysthymia, and subthreshold bipolar disorder, may be the most prevalent, accounting for 2.4 percent of the 4.4 percent lifetime prevalence for these disorders (Merikangas et al., 2007; NIMH, 2021b).

Diagnostic Criteria for a Manic Episode

1. *A distinct period of abnormally elevated, expansive, or irritable mood lasting at least one week.* During these periods an individual may become more inspired and creative than normal. In fact, a large number of prominent scientists and writers claim much of their most productive work came during manic episodes. Compliance with medication schedules can become problematic, as some patients prefer these manic episodes to more normal and less creative periods. It is not uncommon for an individual to switch from an enthusiastic euphoric mood to irritability, particularly when their wishes are frustrated or denied.

2. *During the mood disturbance at least three of the following symptoms must have occurred:*

   a. *Inflated self-esteem or grandiosity.* Characterized by an inflated sense of self-confidence, individuals may embark on huge unrealistic projects, such as writing a novel, composing a symphony, or profess expertise in areas where they have no special knowledge. Grandiose delusions of identity are also common, including having a special relationship with God or some other religious figure.

   b. *Decreased need for sleep.* Individuals may either just wake much earlier than normal or go for days without sleep or feeling tired.

   c. *Excessive talking.* Manic speech is typically loud, rapid, erratic, and difficult to interrupt. The speech may be dramatic or jovial, with excessive gestures and movements. If in an irritable mood, the speech may be critical or even hostile.

   d. *Racing thoughts or ideas.* Along with excessive talking, an individual may describe their thoughts as racing and shifting among several simultaneous themes as if switching television channels rapidly. These racing and shifting thoughts contribute to the fast, erratic, and incoherent speech mentioned earlier.

   e. *Distractibility by irrelevant or unimportant stimuli.* For instance, an individual may become preoccupied with room furnishings or external noise, making concentration difficult. In some cases, it may be impossible to attend to relevant stimuli, further diminishing one's ability to converse and attend to work.

   f. *Increase in goal-directed social, work-related, or sexual activity.* Increases in sexual interest and activity are quite common. As well, individuals may become overly social with colleagues, friends, and family. Taking on considerably more work or obligation than normal is also characteristic of mania.

g. *Excessive involvement in pleasurable activities that have potentially painful consequences. This would include buying sprees, sexual promiscuity, or irrational business decisions.* Excessive self-confidence and grandiosity may lead to poor and irrational decisions about purchases and business decisions without appropriate consideration of their financial consequences. Additionally, an enhanced sexual drive may lead to promiscuous, frequent sexual activity with little regard for health or legal consequences.

3. *The mood disturbance is sufficient to cause marked impairment in occupational functioning or in usual social activities and relationships with others.* Most often bipolar disorders are only recognized by family, friends, and colleagues, and they may only be recognized after considerable damage to relationships has already occurred. In severe instances of mania, hospitalization may be required to prevent individuals from further harming others or themselves.

The symptoms of a full-blown manic episode and major depression may alternate every few months, or symptoms of both may be present together. Mixed episodes are being recognized with more frequency and are now considered to be a relatively common expression of bipolar disorder. In fact, many patients present symptoms of depression during manic episodes even if they are not severe enough to be considered a mixed episode or major depression.

Pathology of Bipolar Disorders

Of all the psychological disorders, perhaps the least is known about the pathology underlying bipolar disorders. Because of the nature of the disorders, cycling between manic and depressive episodes, the pathology must embody dynamic perturbations in neural structures and function. And, unlike the pathology of depression, which was largely revealed by an understanding of antidepressant drug action, relatively little has been learned about the pathology of bipolar disorders from mood-stabilizing drugs. Research continues to describe both genetic and structural correlations with bipolar disorders that may eventually reveal better clues to its evasive pathology.

Genetic Determinants of BPD

It has long been known that there are strong genetic contributions to bipolar disorders. These disorders occur much more frequently when there is a family history of the disease, and heritability studies suggest that the concordance rate among genetically identical (monozygotic) twins approaches 70 percent compared to a rate of approximately 12 percent for dizygotic twins. Genetic studies have found evidence for bipolar genes on a number of chromosomes, but as of yet there is no consensus about how many genes are involved or about their locations (Cassidy et al., 2007; Hamet & Tremblay, 2005). Recent attention has focused on the genes responsible for coding the serotonin transporter (5-HTT) and brain-derived neurotropic factor (BDNF) may be implicated in both major depression and bipolar disorders. Specifically, polymorphisms resulting in decreased expression of the serotonin transporter gene have been shown to be strongly correlated with both suicide ideation and the incidence of major depression in individuals experiencing major life stress (Canli et al., 2006; Caspi et al., 2003; Chen et al., 2014; Fears et al., 2014; Meier et al., 2013). A number of other studies have found strong correlations between the expression of the BDNF gene and bipolar disorders, suggesting that decreased BDNF synthesis may predispose individuals for these diseases (Lohoff et al., 2005; Müller et al., 2006; Nakata et al., 2003). However, not all studies have replicated these findings, suggesting that it may be too early to conclude that there is a causal association between genotypes for the expression of serotonin transporters, BDNF synthesis, and the susceptibility to bipolar disorders (Gonzalez-Castro et al., 2014; Kato, 2007; Wang et al., 2020).

Anatomical Determinants of BPD

Bipolar disorders are also associated with structural abnormalities in several brain regions. As shown in Figure 3.11, individuals who have had the disease for longer periods of time and have had recurrent episodes of mania have significantly enlarged lateral ventricles compared to those who have had only one episode or compared to healthy control subjects (Reite et al., 2010; Strakowski et al., 2002; Strakowski et al., 2005). Enlarged ventricles are believed to be indicative of the loss of neural tissue from surrounding brain structures. As neural degeneration occurs, ventricles gradually enlarge to occupy that space. Functional imaging studies suggest that the areas most afflicted in bipolar disorders include the prefrontal cortex, the amygdala, and the striatum (Figure 3.11).

The structural degeneration observed in bipolar patients is consistent with the abnormalities in BDNF synthesis described earlier in major depression. Decreases in BDNF levels have also been shown to be associated with the severe manic episodes in bipolar patients (Machado-Vieira et al., 2007). Furthermore, treatment with antidepressants as well as several mood stabilizers increases BDNF synthesis and contributes to **neurogenesis** in the hippocampus as well as in other brain structures implicated in depression (Baj et al., 2012; Castren et al., 2007; Duman et al., 2006; D'Sa & Duman, 2002; Laeng et al., 2004; Musazzi et al., 2009; Post, 2007; Wang et al., 2020).

In summary, genetic studies have strongly implicated several genes controlling the expression of the serotonin transporter and BDNF synthesis in both major depression and bipolar disorders. While it may be premature to link the expression of specific genes to predispositions for bipolar disorders, pharmacological evidence is mounting to support this argument. Antidepressants and mood-stabilizing drugs do contribute to the expression of serotonin transporters and to increased levels of BDNF in animals and humans. These adaptations have also been associated with neurogenesis in affected neural structures and to improvements in the symptoms of these diseases. In the following section we examine several drugs used in the treatment of bipolar disorders.

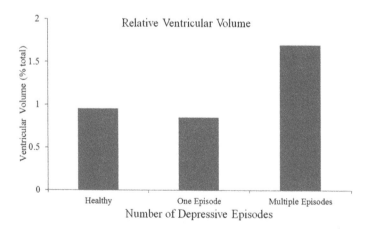

Figure 3.11 Ventricular volumes in bipolar disorder.

Source: Strakowski et al. (2002).

Pharmacological Treatment of Bipolar Disorders

Perhaps one of the most intriguing events in the history of psychopharmacology was John Cade's discovery of the **antimanic** properties of lithium in 1948. At that time, lithium was widely used as a substitute for salt in patients with high blood pressure and heart disease. Its medical use was quickly discontinued because it was toxic and occasionally lethal. Lithium was also found in several tonics used in Europe for a variety of ailments.

John Cade believed that mania was caused by an excessive amount of a normal byproduct of metabolism. To test this idea he collected urine from manic patients and injected it into guinea pigs. He reasoned the excess byproduct would be found in their urine. The urine from manic patients was certainly more toxic than that of normal people or from those suffering from other diseases, but it did not have manic effects. Cade isolated urea as the toxic compound in urine and continued to believe this to be the substance that caused mania, despite the fact that his animals did not exhibit any signs of it. To determine urea's toxic levels Cade needed to dissolve urea in different concentrations to test them for toxicity and manic-inducing properties. After many unsuccessful attempts to dissolve urea he found it was most soluble as lithium urate. Unfortunately, the lithium urate solutions did not cause manic responses in his guinea pigs either. Still not dissuaded by lack of evidence supporting his urea hypothesis, Cade persisted to believe that some substance excreted in the urine (most likely urea) caused manic episodes in his patients and the lithium subdued them. To evaluate the effects of lithium in his toxic compound he also injected animals with lithium carbonate. This compound caused his animals to become lethargic for several hours. In Cade's own words, "it may seem a long way from lethargy in guinea pigs to the control of manic excitement, but as these investigations had commenced in an attempt to demonstrate some possibly excreted toxin in the urine of manic patients, the association of ideas is explicable." Cade was now in a position to test the effects of lithium on his manic patients. One of his patients was described as "a little wizened man of 51 who had been in a state of chronic manic excitement for five years . . . amiably restless, dirty, destructive, mischievous, and interfering." Several days after lithium treatment commenced his patient was "more settled, tidier, less disinhibited, and less distractible." Other patients apparently responded similarly (Cade, 1949).

Although lithium carbonate treatment continued to gain support around the world, it was not approved by the FDA for the treatment of mania until 1970. One can wonder whether approval might have occurred much sooner had the simple compound been of any commercial value.

Lithium

Lithium (Li^+) is a light alkali metal with properties similar to those of sodium (Na^+), including its ability to substitute for sodium in ion exchange across neural membranes. Because it is highly reactive in air and water, sodium is rarely found in its elemental form. Lithium carbonate (Li_2CO_3) is one of the most common natural compounds of lithium, and this compound is also its pharmacologically active form. However, lithium citrate and lithium sulfate are also available pharmacologically. These compounds are sold under several brand names, but they all have the same pharmacological properties.

PHARMACOKINETICS OF LITHIUM

Lithium carbonate is easily absorbed into the bloodstream, but it crosses the blood–brain barrier relatively slowly. Lithium is not metabolized by liver enzymes, so it is excreted by the kidneys in compound form intact. It has an elimination half-life of approximately 18–30 hours.

The therapeutic dose of lithium falls within a very narrow index, and it is quite toxic and even lethal above these levels. Blood levels between 0.6 and 1.5 mEq/L (milliequivalents per liter of blood) are typically therapeutic. The higher range is typically used to treat acute mania, whereas blood levels between 0.6 and 1.0 mEq/L are used for maintenance.

Dosages causing blood levels to rise above 1.5mEq/L are often toxic and can produce severe side effects, including nausea and vomiting, abdominal pain, ataxia, tremors, slurred speech, and cognitive difficulties. Lithium toxicity can also occur if there is a sudden loss of salt either through excessive sweating or a decrease in dietary salt intake, as these may cause in an increase in the lithium/sodium ratio and hence blood levels of lithium. The long-term use of lithium may also contribute to significant weight gain, thyroid disease, skin rash, kidney dysfunction, and compromised immune function. Because of these troublesome side effects patients often discontinue taking their medication. Suddenly suspending medication can also have severe consequences by dramatically increasing one's risk of suicide or suicide attempts. Studies have reported a 16-fold increase in suicide attempts in patients who suddenly discontinued lithium therapy (Yerevanian et al., 2007). Recent reviews, however, continue to support the use of lithium for suicide prevention (Sarai et al., 2018).

PHARMACODYNAMICS OF LITHIUM

While lithium carbonate may be the simplest compound used to treat psychological disorders, its mechanisms of action remain paradoxically elusive. In normal individuals lithium taken in pharmacological doses has few discernible effects beyond some occasional abdominal discomfort. In patients with bipolar disorder it has remarkable effects on both the incidence and severity of manic and depressive episodes. It is also known to be an effective antidepressant and to decrease suicide ideation and attempts in patients with major depressive disorder (Guzzetta et al., 2007; Latalova et al., 2014).

Evidence accumulated over the past several years supports an argument that bipolar disorders, as well as major depressive disorder, result from downregulated BDNF synthesis and the resulting cascade of neurodegenerative effects occurring in the hippocampus and frontal cortex (Brunello & Tascedda, 2003; Einat et al., 2003; Hashimoto et al., 2004; Wang et al., 2020). Lithium has been shown to increase BDNF activity in these brain regions and to reverse degeneration by gene activation of protein synthesis (Brunello, 2004; Mai et al., 2002). Furthermore, lithium both reverses BDNF downregulation and a manic state induced in animals by d-amphetamine (Frey et al., 2006). Lithium also appears to increase serotonergic activity in the cortex and hippocampus by agonizing 5-HT_{1B} autoreceptors and 5-HT_{1B} heteroreceptors on dopaminergic neurons (Chenu & Bourin, 2006). This later effect is believed to mediate lithium's antimanic properties, perhaps by stabilizing the activity of central dopamine neurons. To summarize these effects, lithium treatment appears to reverse the neural degeneration in the hippocampus and frontal cortex caused by downregulated BDNF synthesis. Increases in BDNF contribute to gene activation and to cellular adaptations, leading to increased cortical serotonergic and dopaminergic activity during the depressive phase of bipolar disorder and a stabilization of dopamine activity during the manic phase (Berk et al., 2007; Liu et al., 2020). These alterations are currently believed to mediate the antidepressant and antimanic properties of lithium.

Lithium continues to be regarded as the "gold standard" for the treatment of bipolar disorders, despite its relative toxicity and high incidence of side effects. For these reasons, other drugs are replacing lithium as the principal drug for the management of bipolar disorders. Many of these newer drugs have also been utilized as **anticonvulsants** to treat seizure and anxiety disorders. These drugs may be used alone to treat acute mania or in combination with antidepressants to treat cycling bipolar disorders.

Valproic Acid (Valproate, Depakote)

Valproic acid was introduced in 1994 and approved as an anticonvulsant to treat seizure disorders, acute mania, and migraine headaches. While its mechanisms of action are not completely understood, valproic acid does stimulate BDNF synthesis and alter the activity of several neurotransmitters, including GABA and dopamine. In animal studies, valproic acid increases the number and synaptic growth of GABAergic neurons and it inhibits GABA reuptake, thereby elevating its inhibitory effects (Eckstein-Ludwig et al., 1999; Laeng et al., 2004). Valproic acid also increases dopamine release in the prefrontal cortex but apparently not in the nucleus accumbens (Ichikawa et al., 2005b). It may also protect and stimulate the neuronal growth of dopaminergic neurons through the neurotropic effects of BDNF (Chen et al., 2006; J. Wang et al., 2007). The anticonvulsant and antimanic actions of valproic acid may also be mediated by its inhibitory effects on the glutamate NMDA receptor. Excessive glutamate activity is believed to underlie both mania and seizures, and it can contribute to neuronal degeneration. Valproic acid inhibits NMDA receptor activity and may therefore protect against glutamate excitotoxicity (Chuang, 2005; Gobbi & Janiri, 2006).

Valproic acid is typically better tolerated than lithium and is often more effective for rapid cycling patients. Its most notable side effects include sedation, tremor, ataxia, nausea, and weight gain.

Gabapentin (Neurontin)

Gabapentin was approved in 1993 for the treatment of seizures, but it became a popular alternative to valproic acid and lithium for the *off label* (non–FDA approved) treatment of mania associated with bipolar disorders. It has also been used to treat anxiety, and it has been found to be effective in the management of neuropathic pain. Gabapentin was designed to both structurally and functionally mimic the neurotransmitter GABA. And, although gabapentin increases levels of GABA in the brain, its direct effects on GABA neurons remain unclear. Several presumed mechanisms of action have been suggested, and these may contribute to its antiseizure and antimanic effects.

Gabapentin decreases the influx of calcium into neurons by inhibiting a subset of voltage-dependent calcium channels (Cheng & Chiou, 2006; Rogawski & Loscher, 2004). As a result, glutaminergic activity, which is known to mediate seizure and manic episodes, is decreased in the cortex (Cunningham et al., 2004; Czapinski et al., 2005). Gabapentin also increases GABA-mediated inhibition at $GABA_A$ receptors in the hippocampus as well as in other brain regions (J. K. Cheng et al., 2006). It is unknown whether these diverse effects all share a common underlying mechanism. Gabapentin has a side effect profile that is similar to that of valproic acid. It may cause bothersome sedation, dizziness, ataxia, tremors, nausea, and weight gain.

A large number of antimanic and anticonvulsant drugs are currently available for treating bipolar disorders. Often these drugs are used in combination with other antimanic and antidepressant drugs. Most of these drugs are in the anticonvulsant category and are used to treat seizures, and not all are approved by the FDA for the treatment of bipolar disorders. The off-label use of these drugs for treating mania associated with bipolar disorders is often controversial because of a lack of research demonstrating their effectiveness (Mack, 2003). The newest drug approved by the FDA for bipolar disorder is aripiprazole (Abilify), which acts as a partial agonist at dopamine D_2 and serotonin 1_A receptors. Abilify is also approved for schizophrenia and acute mania. However, a recent study found it to be no more effective than a placebo, and that it contributed to rather severe side effects (Thase et al., 2008). At lower doses aripiprazole may also be used to augment antidepressant therapy (Philip

Table 3.7 Mood stabilizers and anticonvulsants.

Drug name	Brand name	Mechanism of action	Half-life hours	FDA-approved use
Lithium	Lithium carbonate	Serotonin agonist, dopamine agonist	18–30	acute mania
Valproic acid	Valproate, Depakote	Glutamate antagonist, dopamine agonist	9–16	acute mania, seizure disorders, migraine
Gabapentin	Neurontin	Glutamate antagonist, GABAa agonist	5–7	seizure disorders, neuralgia (pain)
Pregabin	Lyrica	GABAa agonist	5–7	neuralgia (pain)
Lamotrigine	Lamictal	Glutamate antagonist	33	bipolar disorders, seizure disorders
Oxcarbazepine	Trileptal	Glutamate antagonist	2–9	seizure disorders
Topiramate	Topamax	Glutamate antagonist, GABA agonist	21	seizure disorders, migraine
Quetiapine	Seroquel	Dopamine antagonist	6–7	acute mania, schizophrenia
Carbamazepine	Tegretol	Glutamate antagonist	12–17	acute mania, seizure disorders
Aripiprazole	Abilify	Dopamine D_2 agonist, serotonin 1_A agonist	75	schizophrenia, acute mania, bipolar maintenance
Zonisamide	Zonegran	Sodium and calcium channel blockade, dopamine agonist (?)	63	seizure disorders

et al., 2008). A number of drugs currently approved for bipolar disorder are presented in Table 3.7 with their common brand name, presumed mechanisms of action, half-life, and FDA-approved use.

Alternatives to Mood Stabilizers

Treating the often-severe depression in bipolar patients has been problematic. Mood stabilizers alone are often not adequate. Treating this depression with traditional antidepressants has always been controversial because of the high probability of making manic symptoms worse. Numerous studies have reported conflicting outcomes with antidepressants, including worsening the severity of depression and mania, even when used in conjunction with mood stabilizers (e.g., Zhang et al., 2013).

Lurasidone (Latuda)

In 2013 the FDA approved lurasidone, an atypical antipsychotic, for the treatment of bipolar disorders. In a large number of clinical trials, lurasidone was found to be effective in treating depression in bipolar patients when either used alone or with a mood stabilizer such as lithium (Alamo et al., 2014; Citrome et al., 2014; Loebel et al., 2014). Lurasidone acts as a potent antagonist at D_2 and 5-HT_7, 5-HT_{1A}, and 5-HT_{2A} receptors, in a manner similar to other atypical antipsychotics. Because of its relatively low affinity for histamine and cholinergic receptors, its adverse side effects are comparably lower.

Lumateperone (Caplyta)

The most recent addition to drugs used to treat bipolar depression is lumateperone (Caplyta) which was approved by the FDA in 2019. Lumateperone is also an atypical antipsychotic which has potent agonistic effects on 5-HT_{2A} receptors and relatively weak agonistic effects on dopamine D_2 postsynaptic receptors. While its mechanisms of action for bipolar disorder are not completely known, it is believed that lumateperone's agonist effects on both serotonin and dopamine contribute significantly to its antidepressant effects for both Bipolar I and Bipolar II disorders (Calabrese et al., 2021). Because the use of lumateperone in treating depression associated with bipolar disorders is quite recent, it may be several years before we understand its longer-term effectiveness.

Glossary

Active placebo a psychologically inactive drug that has some peripheral side effects that patients may recognize and thereby assume they are receiving actual treatment. For example, they may cause minor dry mouth, dizziness, or blurred vision.

Agoraphobia fear of being in open places where a panic attack may occur and from which it would be difficult to escape or help would be unavailable.

Anticonvulsant a drug used to treat seizure disorders. Occasionally used to treat symptoms of bipolar disorder.

Antimanic a drug used to treat bouts of mania or hypomania.

Atypical an atypical drug is a class of drug that differs significantly in its mechanism of action from other medication for a particular psychological disorder.

Bipolar disorder a severe mood disorder characterized depressive and manic episodes.

Brain-derived neurotropic factor (BDNF) a nerve growth factor essential for normal cell survival, receptor growth, and for the growth of new neurons.

CREB (cyclic adenosine monophosphate [or cAMP] response element binding protein) a second messenger activated by metabotropic receptors responsible for transcribing brain-derived neurotropic factor from a cell's DNA.

Deaminate an enzymatic reaction that deactivates a neurotransmitter by removing an essential amine chemical group from its molecular structure.

Downregulation a process that results in a decrease in synaptic activity caused by decreasing neurotransmitter synthesis, its release, and/or its receptor availability.

Dysthymic disorder a moderately severe mood disorder that is characterized by lengthy episodes of depression (at least two years).

First-generation drug the first class of drugs used to treat a particular psychological disorder.

Hypomanic episode a period of elevated, expansive, or irritable mood lasting at least four days. Less severe than a manic episode.

Lag time the delay of about 10–14 days between the onset of medication and observations of symptom relief in depression.

Major depressive disorder a severe mood disorder during which a person experiences depressive episodes without intermittent bouts of mania.

Manic episode a period of at least one week of excessively elevated mood, euphoria, or enthusiasm that may be interrupted by outbursts of anger or irritability.

Monoamine hypothesis the proposal that deficiencies in the monoamine neurotransmitters dopamine, norepinephrine, and/or serotonin cause depression.

Monoamine oxidase inhibitors (MAOIs) an antidepressant that blocks the activity of the degrading enzyme monoamine oxidase in the synaptic gap of monoamine neurotransmitters.

Neurogenesis the cellular process that contributes to neuronal growth.

Neuropathic pain associated with damage to, or overuse of, nerves. It may be associated with certain types of cancer, autoimmune disorders, or trauma.

Psychostimulant a drug that increase or stimulates cortical activity and arousal. Cocaine and amphetamines are psychostimulants.

Rapid cycling a condition where periods of depression and mania in bipolar disorder cycle at least four times in a year.

Reactive depression a period of depression associated with a significant life event, such as the loss of a spouse or significant other, loss of financial resources, or significant stress.

Second-generation drug a class of drugs that have supplemented or replaced first-generation drugs and differ significantly in their mechanism of action.

Serotonin syndrome a toxic reaction caused by excessive serotonin activity. Symptoms may include disorientation, confusion, visual disturbances, agitation, and mania.

Suicidality attempts, both successful and unsuccessful, at committing suicide.

Suicide ideation thoughts of suicide and/or planning suicide attempts.

Transcription a step in the process of expressing the activity of genes for the building of a specific protein.

Tricyclic antidepressant an antidepressant characterized by its three-ring molecular structure.

Upregulation a process that results in an increase in synaptic activity by increasing neurotransmitter synthesis, its release, and/or the availability of its receptors.

4 Anxiety and Stress-Related Disorders

Panic, Generalized Anxiety, Obsessive-Compulsive Disorder, and Post-traumatic Stress Disorder

Susan began her day as she always had. She rose early before her husband, started the coffee, and headed to the shower. She was rehearsing how she would conduct her sales meeting later in the morning when she began to feel as if someone, or something, had taken control of her body. Her heart rate jumped from a normal 65 to over 150 bpm in an instant. Her respiration was strained, and she could not get air into her lungs. She grabbed the bathroom counter as she began to lose balance in a spinning room. Her skin felt cold and clammy, but at the same time she felt as if she were burning alive. A terror like she had never experienced overwhelmed her as she realized she must have had a heart attack and was now dying. She tried to scream out to her husband but could not even make a sound. She was paralyzed with fear, knowing she was going to die in her bathroom. Susan felt as though an hour had passed when she realized that her breathing was now under her control. She took long deep breaths as her racing heart slowed back towards normal. Susan got up from the floor not even remembering the fall. At that moment her husband walked in carrying her morning coffee. She then realized this had all occurred in just a few minutes. What she didn't yet know was that this was only the first of many episodes to follow.

Susan had just experienced her first panic attack. Like over six million other Americans each year her attack was not preceded by warning or even noticeable anxiety. Another seven million people suffer from generalized anxiety, an additional eight million from post-traumatic stress disorder, over two million from obsessive-compulsive disorder (OCD), and many others from various debilitating phobias. In all, over 40 million persons in the United States alone currently suffer from some form of anxiety disorder, making them the most prevalent of all psychological disorders. In this chapter, we will examine the pathology and the pharmacological treatment of several of the most prevalent anxiety disorders. But first, let us begin by reviewing the neurobiology of normal fear and anxiety.

Biological Bases of Fear and Anxiety

Fear is an adaptive emotional response that involves changes in behavior, autonomic reactivity, hormonal activity, and in humans, the body sensations of these changes. These components of fear are integrated by several neural structures and glands, and they provide animals with the ability to adapt to potentially life-threatening circumstances. In addition, specific changes to these structures enable animals to learn about stimuli that are predictive of danger, thus providing them with the ability to avoid altogether situations that may be harmful. Several structures are critical to fear responses. These include the amygdala, the hypothalamus, the thalamus, and several areas within the cortex.

The amygdaloid nuclei are part of the limbic system and are located deep within the temporal lobes (Figure 4.1). They, or more specifically structures within the amygdaloid complex, receive sensory information about potentially threatening stimuli and initiate the various components of the fear response. The central nucleus of the amygdala sends information to a

DOI: 10.4324/9781003309017-4

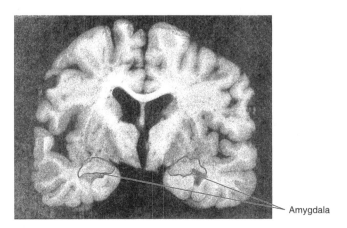

Amygdala

Figure 4.1 Coronal section of the human brain, revealing the amygdaloid nuclei located deep within the temporal lobes.

number of other brain structures, including the hypothalamus, which controls the hormonal component of the fear response, and to the pons and medulla, which control various fear responses, such as freezing, facial expression, and heart and respiration rates. Other brainstem structures receive neural input from the amygdala and control autonomic and cortical arousal. The amygdala, therefore, is the most important brain structure for the integration of sensory information and for the initiation of fear responses to it. Damage to the amygdala has long been known to disrupt emotional behavior. In fact, bilateral destruction of the amygdala was used early on to control psychiatric patients who did not respond to pharmacological treatment.

Several cortical areas are also important for fear as well as for other emotional responses. Two areas within the prefrontal cortex—the ventromedial prefrontal cortex and the orbitofrontal cortex—are particularly important (Figure 4.2). These prefrontal areas receive input from the thalamus, the ventral tegmentum, and the amygdala. They send output to the cingulate cortex, the hypothalamus, and inhibitory signals to the amygdala. These structures function to integrate emotional content from stimuli and to organize and guide our behavior in response to them. In humans, the prefrontal cortices additionally guide and control our emotional behavior in social contexts. Damage to these areas severely affects judgment in social situations and how an individual anticipates consequences of their behavior. The prefrontal areas would therefore be involved in interpreting fear-producing stimuli and in regulating or inhibiting fear responses in nonthreatening contexts.

The prefrontal cortices also send input to and receive output from the cingulate cortex, which is located deep within the central fissure, above the corpus callosum (Figure 4.3). The cingulate cortex also receives sensory information about body states during emotional responses. The emotion of fear, for example, is represented as a set of physiological and behavioral responses, including high heart rate, changes in respiration, posture, facial expression, muscle tension, and blood flow. These changes all contribute to the sensory information that is essentially mapped into the cingulate cortex and perceived as the feeling of fear. Damage to the cingulate does not disrupt the physiological state of an emotion, but it does disrupt our subjective feeling and our awareness of it.

When we experience fear, a cascade of physiological events results in changes in posture, facial expression, heart rate and blood flow, respiration, and cortical arousal. These changes allow animals to either flee from or confront the emotion-causing stimulus. When the emotional

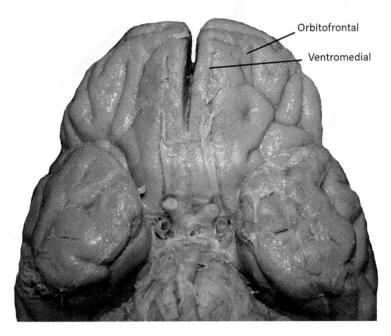

Figure 4.2 Ventral view of human brain. The ventromedial cortices lie adjacent to the midline on both halves of the brain. The orbitofrontal cortices lie above the eye orbits and adjacent to the ventromedial areas.

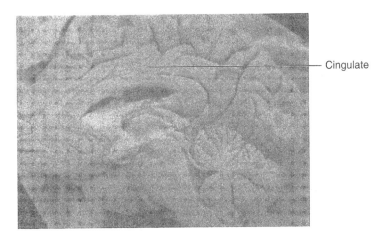

Figure 4.3 The cingulate cortex lies deep within the central fissure above the corpus callosum.

stimulus can be ignored, the prefrontal cortices send inhibitory signals to the amygdala, which in turn shuts off output to structures that cause these adaptive changes.

Anxiety differs from fear in that an emotion-causing stimulus does not need to be present to experience the emotion. Anxiety occurs when one perceives an expectation of a vague and uncertain threat as opposed to a specific danger. For instance, one may experience anxiety in preparation for an important exam. Anxiety also persists for extended durations once initiated and no specific pattern of behavior is motivated to terminate it. And, unlike fear, anxiety is not accompanied by specific postures or facial expressions. The physiological components of anxiety, however, are essentially identical to those of fear. Increases in autonomic activity lead to increased heart rate, blood pressure, muscle tension, and respiration. Additionally, anxiety is characterized by increased cortical arousal and vigilance. Anxiety makes it difficult to concentrate on other tasks and activities, and it contributes to disturbances in normal sleep patterns.

Both fear and anxiety are normal adaptive responses to specific and diffuse threats to our well-being. These emotional responses consist of physiological and behavioral changes that enable animals to more effectively deal with threat and uncertainty. When fear begins to occur to nonthreatening stimuli, or anxiety is excessive and persists for extended periods of time, however, these emotions can become debilitating, and they may contribute to cardiovascular diseases and to compromised immunity. As we will see, the distinctions between normal fear and anxiety, and pathological anxiety, are not always clear. In the following sections, we describe several of the most debilitating of the anxiety disorders.

Panic Disorder

The diagnosis of **panic disorder** requires the repeated and unexpected occurrence of panic attacks and at least one month of persistent worry about having other attacks or about the consequences of these attacks. Often the persistent worry is about whether an individual will actually die during an impending panic attack. According to the *DSM-5*, panic attacks are discrete periods of intense fear during which four or more of the following symptoms occur:

1. *Heart palpitations or accelerated heart rate.* Nearly everyone experiences the feeling of their heartbeat occasionally, but during a panic attack these palpitations are intense sensations of accelerated heart rate. These palpitations may contribute to other symptoms and a fear of an imminent heart attack.
2. *Sweating.* Sweating that occurs in the absence of exertion or excessively high temperatures.
3. *Trembling or shaking.* Feelings of trembling or shaking with fear. This may occur with the sensation of being immobile or frozen in place.
4. *Sensations of shortness of breath or breathing restriction.* Feeling as if one cannot get enough air in each breath. Respiration rate may increase to compensate for a lack of sufficient oxygen, and this can lead to dizziness and other symptoms of mild hypoxia.
5. *Feelings of choking.* The sensation of shortness of breath may also be related the sensations of choking or the feeling of tightening of the neck and airway.
6. *Chest pain.* Chest pains or abnormal chest sensations may be associated with higher-than-normal heart rates and palpitations. These sensations may also contribute to a fear of an imminent heart attack.
7. *Nausea or abdominal distress.*
8. *Dizziness, fainting, or lightheadedness.* Can be symptoms related to hypoxia caused by breathing difficulties.
9. *Derealization or depersonalization.* Feelings of unreality or being detached from oneself.
10. *Fear of losing control.* The inability to calm oneself or control the intensity of feeling. One may feel as if they are going crazy or mad.
11. *Fear of dying.* A common fear during panic attacks that can be exacerbated or confirmed by other symptoms such as high heart rate, palpitations, chest pains, and breathing difficulties.
12. *Paresthesia.* Numbness or tingling sensations typically of the limbs and face.
13. *Chills or hot flushes.*

Panic attacks can, and often do, happen without warning or without situational triggers, although after recurrence they may begin to occur in specific situations or places. For the diagnosis of panic disorder, however, the attacks must be unexpected or uncued, at least initially. Panic disorder may also be associated with a phobic avoidance that makes it difficult for people to be in crowded places, on public transportation, in theaters, or in places where escape might be difficult or embarrassing if and when a panic attack occurs. This phobia of experiencing a panic attack in inescapable situations is referred to as *agoraphobia*. Individuals with agoraphobia experience intense anxiety when they find themselves in, or even anticipate, situations where a panic attack might occur, and they often develop a phobic avoidance of these situations as a result. The phobic avoidance behavior may mitigate anxiety, but it often contributes significantly to other problems. In severe cases, agoraphobia can be so debilitating that an individual may find it impossible to leave the confines of their own home or room.

Generalized Anxiety Disorder

Mark is a first-year law student who has recently sought help for insomnia. He complains that on most nights he just cannot "shut off his brain." His mind shifts rapidly between assignments and projects he has not yet completed and the constant worry about his financial and medical conditions. Like many students, Mark has borrowed from several student loans, but his debt will not be unmanageable since he already holds the promise of a position at his father's law firm. This security, however, provides little respite from his fret about finances. Mark's medical concerns commenced when his father was diagnosed with prostate cancer several years earlier. Now Mark has noticed that he too has every symptom of an enlarged prostate. While lying awake much of the night he frequently makes bathroom visits that are pointless, and the assurances from his doctors that there are no signs of enlargement only convince Mark that they are missing something even more serious. Often, Mark's anxiety seems unrelated to anything explicit. In these cases, the feelings of anxiety and dread are just as intense, even though they have no particular focus.

While Mark had little trouble getting through college with his unrelenting worries, he is now having difficulty in law school. More and more frequently, he is finding that his anxiety interrupts his attention during class and his concentration while studying. On several occasions he has been embarrassed when professors called on him to comment and he had no idea what the preceding discussion was about. Pushing aside the incessant worrying during his study time is also getting much more difficult. Mark is now beginning to agonize about whether he will flunk out of law school and disappoint his parents even further.

It turns out that Mark has a much longer history of worrying about pleasing his parents than his latest academic concerns. While in high school, Mark was preoccupied with his athletic and academic competencies, even though he was a good student earning an athletic scholarship for track. He fought his less-than-perfect performances and his fear of competition with countless hours of training. During his high school years, Mark was diagnosed with depression and prescribed an antidepressant. After diligently following the prescription for almost a year he eventually discontinued it because it made him feel too lethargic. Mark claims he has never felt depressed, but only anxious and concerned about his future.

Generalized anxiety disorder (GAD) typically emerges in early adolescence or adulthood, as it did with Mark, but it can occur in children. The lifetime prevalence of GAD is about 5 percent of the population, and about seven million people suffer from it at any given time. It is not uncommon for GAD to disappear for several years and to reoccur during times of stress. The *DSM-5* criteria for a diagnosis of generalized anxiety disorder are as follows:

1. *Excessive anxiety and worry occurring for more days than not for at least six months.* The anxiety and worry are exaggerated far out of proportion for the perceived threat or peril. For instance, a child or adolescent may worry about their athletic or academic performance when they are in fact doing quite well. An adult may worry unnecessarily about an illness they or a family member may or may not actually have. During the

course of the disorder the focus of anxiety or worry often shifts from one concern to another, or there may be no specific focus at all.

2. *Difficulty in controlling the worry.* The worry and anxiety repeatedly interrupt their daily activities and work. These interruptions are difficult or impossible to quell and may persist for hours at a time.

3. *The anxiety and worry are associated with restlessness, fatigue, difficulty concentrating, irritability, muscle tension, and sleep disturbances.* Three or more of these symptoms must be present more often than not for at least six months.

4. *The anxiety, worry, or physical symptoms cause clinically significant distress or impairment in social or occupational functioning.* Anxiety and constant worry make normal social and occupational functioning difficult if not impossible. Normal activities and concentration are interrupted frequently. Headaches and gastrointestinal symptoms are also common.

Pathology of Generalized Anxiety Disorder

Generalized anxiety disorder does not appear to be heritable, and there is no identifiable gene linked with it. However, a number of studies have reported strong associations between responses to anxiety-provoking situations and the gene for monoamine oxidase A (MAOA) (Reif et al., 2014; Tadic et al., 2003). Evidence for associations between genes for the serotonin transporter (5-HTT) is mixed at best. Several researchers have found associations in humans (Gottschalk & Domschke, 2017; Stein et al., 2006) and in animal studies (Line et al., 2011), but others have been unable to confirm this relationship (Bortoluzzi et al., 2014). Therefore, conclusions about the role of specific genes in anxiety disorders are limited at the present.

It has also been suggested that GAD and major depression share a common etiology, with some individuals more prone to depression, some to anxiety, and others sharing features of both disorders. Researchers have found strong associations between the co-occurrences of major depression and generalized anxiety in large twin studies, suggesting a common genetic risk (Kendler, 1996; Kendler et al., 2007). Generalized anxiety disorder also co-occurs with other anxiety disorders—particularly social phobias, PTSD, and panic disorder.

Several neurotransmitter systems have also been implicated in GAD, with particular interest focused on the inhibitory neurotransmitter gamma amino butyric acid (GABA). A number of studies have found deficiencies in GABA receptor expression in patients with GAD. Researchers have further shown that messenger RNA (ribonucleic acid), which transcribes the GABA receptor, is also deficient and that these deficiencies can be restored following treatment with GABA agonist (Nasir et al., 2020; Rocca et al., 1998). Furthermore, GABA has long been known to exert inhibitory effects on nuclei within the amygdala and the hypothalamus. Both of these structures are implicated in the regulation of anxiety.

Studies with laboratory animals provide additional support for the role of GABA. One animal model of generalized anxiety utilizes an **elevated maze** with two enclosed and two exposed (open) arms. Researchers measure the latency to leave an enclosed arm and enter an exposed arm to receive food (inhibitory avoidance) as a measure of anxiety (cf. Graeff et al., 1998; Zangrossi & Graeff, 1997). Experimental animals tend to prefer maze arms that have protective sides over the exposed arms and leave to explore or retrieve food only after some hesitation. Drugs that are known to reduce anxiety in humans also decrease the latency to leave enclosed arms and increase time spent in exposed arms in the elevated maze. Microinjections of GABA agonists directly into hypothalamic structures which innervate the amygdala also decrease latencies to leave enclosed arms. This suggests that both GABA activity in the amygdala and anxiety are regulated by the hypothalamus (Bueno et al., 2007; Jie et al., 2018).

Animal models have also been useful in the identification and development of numerous anxiety-producing (**anxiogenic**) and antianxiety (**anxiolytic**) substances.

Dopamine appears to play a critical role in modulating stress and anxiety. During acute stress, dopamine activity is increased in several brain regions, including the nucleus accumbens and the frontal cortex (Abercrombie et al., 1989). Inhibitory dopamine projections from the ventral tegmental area (VTA) to the amygdala disinhibit stress responses that are normally suppressed by projections from the prefrontal cortex (see Figure 4.4). Further evidence of dopamine's role comes from studies using mice that have been genetically altered to not express the dopamine D3 receptor. These knockout mice fail to demonstrate stress-related responses to immobilization stress (Xing et al., 2013). Animals treated with dopamine antagonists appear to be protected from manipulations that typically induce fear and anxiety (de la Mora et al., 2010).

The neurotransmitters serotonin and norepinephrine have also been implicated in generalized anxiety. However, because generalized anxiety and depression can often be difficult to disassociate, the specific roles that these neurotransmitters play in anxiety has been difficult to corroborate, even though SSRIs are often prescribed to alleviate generalized anxiety. A common pathology underlying anxiety and depression seems to be the overexpression of $5\text{-}HT_{1A}$ autoreceptors, which are abundant in the prefrontal cortex, amygdala, and hippocampus (Albert et al., 2014). As we saw in Chapter 3, antidepressants can downregulate these receptors, allowing serotonin to more effectively modulate fear and anxiety. Results from several animal studies further suggest that serotonergic neurons in the dorsal raphe nucleus, which project to the forebrain, are involved in the regulation of anxiety (Pobbe et al., 2005; Sena et al., 2003). These ascending neurons receive inhibitory input from GABA neurons in this region of the brainstem.

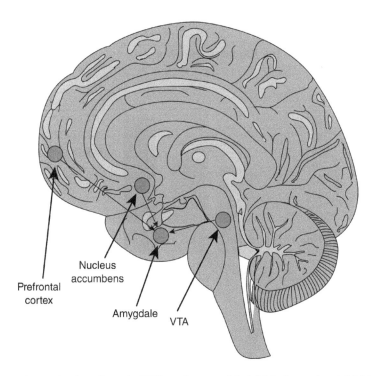

Prefrontal cortex

Nucleus accumbens

Amygdale   VTA

Figure 4.4 Dopamine projections from the VTA to the amygdala inhibit the anxiety-inhibiting projections from the prefrontal cortex to the amygdala. This disinhibition results in the expression of anxiety-related behaviors.

Using animal models such as the elevated maze (Figures 4.5 and 4.6) may be a useful way to clarify the interaction between serotonergic and GABAergic systems in anxiety. The elevated maze is believed to induce anxiety because of a conflict between an animal's natural tendency to explore novel environments and fear induced by heights. Anxiolytic drugs tend to increase exploratory time.

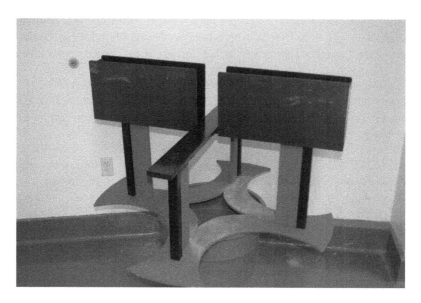

Figure 4.5 Elevated PLUS maze used to measure anxiety in laboratory animals. Latencies to leave enclosed arms and the amount of time spent exploring open arms are measures of anxiety.

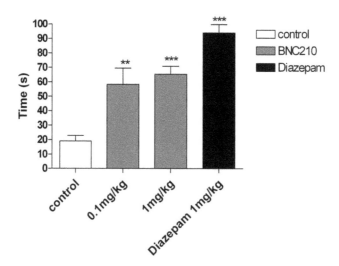

Figure 4.6 In an animal model of anxiety, GABA agonists increase time spent in exposed arms of an elevated maze. BNC210 is an experimental drug being developed as an anxiolytic. Diazapam is an anxiolytic and a GABA agonist.

Source: Reprinted with permission from Dr Sue O'Connor, Bionomics (2007).

To summarize, evidence from both human and animal studies suggests that GABA, dopamine, and serotonin dysfunction underlie generalized anxiety disorder. Several different mechanisms, including decreased GABA receptor expression and/or the overexpression of 5-HT$_{1A}$ receptors, may be involved. Drugs that enhance GABA activity are effective in alleviating the symptoms of generalized anxiety, and they decrease latencies to leave enclosed arms of an elevated maze. Serotonin 5-HT$_{1A}$ agonists are also prescribed for GAD, but whether they act specifically on anxiety-regulating mechanisms or whether they act indirectly by treating comorbid depression is unknown. Serotonin (5-HT$_{1A}$) agonists do decrease latencies to leave enclosed arms in elevated mazes.

Pharmacological Treatment of Panic and Generalized Anxiety Disorders

From the preceding discussion it should be no surprise that GABA agonists would be effective in alleviating many of the symptoms of both panic and generalized anxiety. In fact, long before the discovery of the neurotransmitter GABA, pharmacologists had discovered a class of drugs known for their anxiolytic and sedative effects. Only much later would they become known as GABA agonists. In 1903, several chemists working at the Bayer laboratories announced their discovery that barbital, a derivative of barbituric acid, had sedative properties in animals. This product was called barbital, and it was introduced a year later under the trade name Veronal. This was the first among a long list of barbiturate drugs, including Phenobarbital, that were widely used until the 1960s as antianxiety and sedation-inducing drugs.

Barbiturates

The barbiturate drugs are all powerful central nervous system depressants, and prior to their introduction only a few substances were known to induce sedation and quell anxiety. These substances included the narcotic opium and various preparations of alcohol. Much later, in the mid-1800s, bromide and chloral hydrate were introduced to bring on sleep and as anesthetics for surgery. With the discovery of barbiturates a new era of psychopharmacology began. Drugs could now be developed to produce profound changes in neural functioning and behavior.

The barbiturates all share a common molecular structure that contains the barbital nucleus shown in Figure 4.7. The main difference between these drugs is their half-life, which can range from several hours for Thiopental to over 100 hours with Phenobarbital. The short-acting,

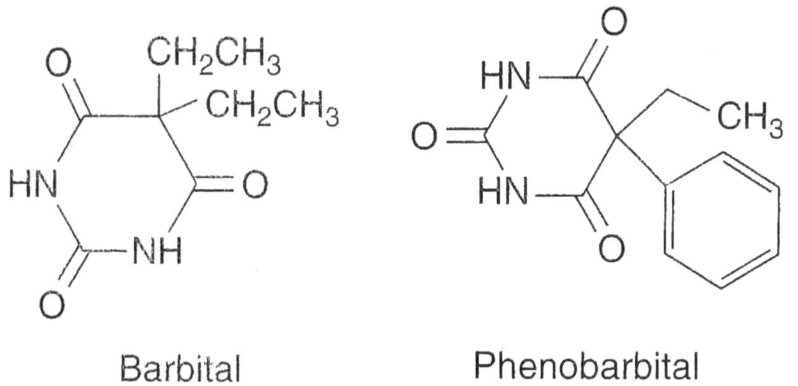

Barbital

Phenobarbital

Figure 4.7 All barbiturates share a common barbital nucleus.

Table 4.1 Barbiturates and their half-lives.

Drug name	Trade name	Half-life hours	Present use
Amobarbital	Amytal	10–40	Anesthesia, sedation
Butabarbital	Butisol	30–40	Sedation, seizures
Methohexital	Brevital	1–2	Short duration anesthesia
Pentobarbital	Nembutal	20–50	Anesthesia, sedation
Phenobarbital	Luminal	25–120	Sedation, seizures
Secobarbital	Seconal	20–40	Anesthesia, sedation
Thiopental	Pentothal	2–5	Short duration anesthesia

highly fat-soluble barbiturates like Thiopental can induce sleep or anesthesia within 20–30 seconds when administered intravenously. The longer-acting drugs have much lower fat solubility and may take up to an hour to produce an effect. The duration of action of the lower fat-soluble barbiturates such as Phenobarbital can be as long as 12 hours. Several common barbiturates and their half-lives are presented in Table 4.1. Over 50 different barbiturates have been marketed; many are no longer available in the United States.

The barbiturates produce behavioral effects that can be indistinguishable from alcohol intoxication. At lower doses they cause drowsiness and sedation in addition to disruptions in motor and cognitive abilities. At higher doses, or with barbiturates that are highly fat soluble, they induce sleep or a state of anesthesia. The anxiolytic effects of barbiturates cannot be separated from these effects, thus limiting their usefulness during most daytime activities. Because barbiturates disrupt REM (rapid eye movement or dream) sleep, their use in treating insomnia is also limited.

Barbiturates have a very narrow therapeutic index, and when combined with other GABA agonists, such as alcohol, they can suppress respiratory centers in the brainstem and have lethal consequences. Suicide by barbiturate and alcohol consumption was not at all uncommon prior to their largely discontinued used in the late 1960s. In spite of these disadvantages, barbiturates were extensively used to treat anxiety disorders, insomnia, muscle spasms, convulsions, and induce anesthesia before other safer drugs became available. The barbiturate sodium Amytal (amobarbital) was used in psychiatry to induce a hypotonic state during psychoanalysis called an **Amytal interview**. It was presumed that Amytal would increase a patient's ability to recall and verbalize repressed memories, making psychotherapy more effective. And, in forensic science it has a long history of use as a "truth serum" to elicit confessions from crime suspects. This use became disputed when it was recognized that false memories could easily be coerced from drugged suspects. Nonetheless, amobarbital has allegedly been used on al-Qaeda prisoners detained in Afghanistan and Cuba. Evidence obtained with the use of drugs is not allowed in US courts, however (*People v. Cox,* 271 N.W.2d 216 [1978]).

Mechanisms of Barbiturate Action

The barbiturates bind effectively to a specific subtype of receptor on the $GABA_A$ receptor complex called the barbiturate site. The $GABA_A$ receptor is an ionotropic receptor that controls the influx of Cl^- ions. This receptor has five membrane-spanning regions, which include subunits: two α, two β, and one γ, with other configurations possible. These subunits make up the Cl^- ion channel illustrated in Figure 4.8. In addition to a site for the neurotransmitter GABA there are four distinct receptor sites distributed on these subunits that selectively bind to GABA agonists: a barbiturate site, a benzodiazepine site, an alcohol site, and a steroid site.

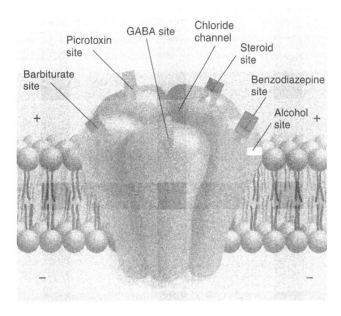

Figure 4.8 GABA receptor complex. Several drugs, including the barbiturates, benzodiazepines, and alcohol, act to facilitate GABA binding and chlorine influx.

When any of these receptors are bound to a specific agonist, the neurotransmitter GABA binds to its receptor more effectively and for longer durations, producing greater hyperpolarization of postsynaptic membranes. Hyperpolarization reduces the likelihood of postsynaptic cells producing an action potential, thus reducing the firing rate of receiving neurons. GABA antagonists (e.g., picrotoxin) bind effectively to other receptor sites and produce **convulsant** effects by inhibiting the binding of GABA. All barbiturates, however, are presumed to act by binding to the barbiturate site on the $GABA_A$ receptor complex. Unlike other GABA agonists, however, barbiturates can open the Cl^- channel and hyperpolarize postsynaptic membranes in the absence of GABA.

One of many mysteries of psychopharmacology is why these receptor subtypes have evolved on the $GABA_A$ receptor. Although they were named after the drugs that have high affinities for them it would certainly be presumptuous, if not mistaken, to assume they were waiting for these drugs to be discovered. The identification of a natural ligand called diazepam binding inhibitor (DBI), which prevents benzodiazepine binding and produces anxiety-like effects, has only partially resolved this mystery. To date, other natural ligands for these receptors have not been identified.

Side Effects of Barbiturates

The use of barbiturates to treat anxiety and insomnia has largely been discontinued because of severe side effects. At anxiolytic doses barbiturates cause confusion, impaired judgment, retarded reflexes, loss of muscle coordination, and impaired speech—effects similar to alcohol intoxication. Because of these intoxicating effects, most normal activities, including driving, work, and study are greatly impaired. When prescribed as a sedative to treat insomnia the barbiturates disrupt normal sleep cycles, including REM sleep. A few nights of REM deprivation may produce symptoms including irritability, aggressiveness, and poor concentration. After a week or more of REM deprivation, symptoms may escalate to delusions, hallucinations, and other symptoms of psychosis. When barbiturates are suddenly discontinued for sleep, REM rebound occurs, resulting in significantly increased durations of REM sleep.

Tolerance and dependence also occur rapidly to barbiturate use. Tolerance is mainly a result of increased liver metabolism and GABA receptor downregulation. Both of these mechanisms also decrease the effectiveness of other GABA agonist drugs—a phenomenon referred to as **cross tolerance**. In addition, tolerance to a barbiturate's sedating and antiseizure effects occurs more rapidly than to its respiratory-suppressing effects. This difference in the rate of tolerance acquisition decreases the therapeutic index, making a barbiturate overdose more likely. Physical dependence on barbiturates makes discontinuation difficult for most long-term users and can lead to seizures caused by an excitable rebound of CNS activity.

The barbiturates have also been linked to fetal abnormalities and cognitive impairments that are similar to those seen with **Fetal Alcohol Syndrome** (FAS). Female patients using barbiturates to control seizures or other disorders should be advised to suspend medication early in their pregnancy. Other drugs with a lower risk of adverse fetal effects may be more appropriate. Finally, combining barbiturates with other GABA agonists, such as alcohol, can accidentally cause respiratory depression and death. The CO_2-sensitive respiratory center located in the medulla contains $GABA_A$ receptors that regulate respiration in response to increased CO_2 levels. Excessive GABA inhibition decreases medulla responsiveness to CO_2 and depresses respiration.

Benzodiazepines

The introduction of barbiturates in the early 1900s ushered a promise that drugs could be developed to alleviate symptoms of behavioral disorders by altering brain chemistry. Epileptic seizures, severe anxiety, debilitating insomnia, muscle spasms, and a variety of other ailments were for the first time treated effectively and humanely. Surgical anesthesia, which to this point was induced by vapors of ether or chloroform, was also dramatically improved with the introduction of barbiturates. For nearly 50 years the barbiturates were the choice of treatment for these disorders and for surgical anesthesia.

In the 1960s, however, the treatment of anxiety disorders was revolutionized by the introduction of the benzodiazepines that were discovered in 1954 in laboratories at the pharmaceutical company Hoffman-LaRoche. In 1960, the first benzodiazepine was released as Librium, which was quickly followed by Valium. Since then, over 2,000 benzodiazepines have been synthesized, and approximately 30 have been marketed for their anxiolytic and hypnotic properties. Not all of these are currently available for use in the United States. Once the benzodiazepines became available they rapidly replaced the older barbiturates and became the most widely prescribed psychoactive drugs in the world.

The benzodiazepines all share a common three-ring molecular structure that largely determines their activity. The main differences are the specific molecules that are attached at the methyl (CH_3) sites and the Cl site on the rings shown in Figure 4.9. Substitutions on the CH_3 sites are typically with hydrogen molecules (H or H_2) and at the Cl sites typically nitrogen dioxide (NO_2). All the benzodiazepines have the same mechanism of action regardless of their specific molecular structures. The major differences are their half-lives and their fat solubility, which determines how quickly they enter the brain.

The half-lives of benzodiazepines can range from less than an hour with the ultra short-acting anesthetic Diprivan (propofol) to several days with the longer-acting anxiolytic Valium (diazepam). The effective half-lives of Valium and most other longer-acting drugs are extended by their active metabolite nordiazepam. Several common benzodiazepines and their respective half-lives are presented in Table 4.2. The longer and intermediate-acting benzodiazepines are

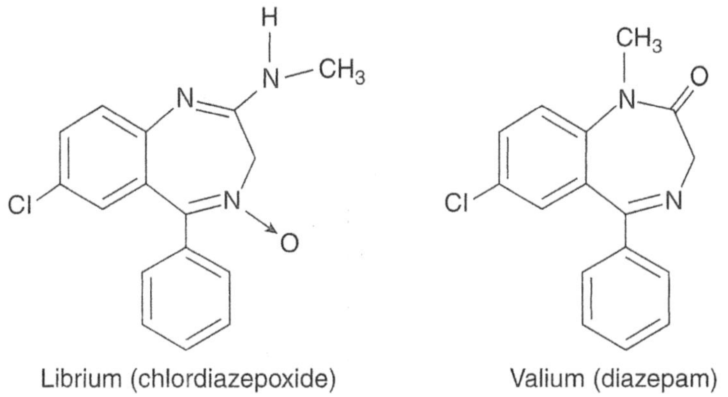

Librium (chlordiazepoxide)   Valium (diazepam)

Figure 4.9 The molecular structure of several common benzodiazepines. All the pharmacologically active benzodiazepines share a common three-ring nucleus. Substitutions with hydrogen molecules at the CH_3 sites and nitrogen dioxide (NO_2) at the Cl site are common structural arrangements for many of the benzodiazepines.

Table 4.2 Several common benzodiazepines and their half-lives.

Drug name	Trade name	Half-life hours	FDA-approved uses
Long-acting			
Diazepam	Valium	20–50	Anxiety, seizures, muscle spasms
Chlordiazepoxide	Librium	24–48	Anxiety, alcohol withdrawal
Flunitrazepam	Rohypnol	16–35	Insomnia, but not approved in the US
Clonazepam	Klonopin	30–40	Panic disorder, seizures
Intermediate			
Lorazepam	Ativan	10–20	Anxiety, seizures
Alprazolam	Xanax	12–15	Generalized anxiety, panic disorder
Short-acting			
Midazolam	Versed	2–4	Sedation, pre-operative anxiety
Oxazepam	Serax	3–21	Anxiety, alcohol withdrawal
Triazolam	Halcion	2–5	Insomnia
Propofol	Diprivan	1	Anesthesia
Antagonists			
Flumazenil	Romazicon	1–2	Overdose–reverses benzodiazepine effects

typically prescribed for anxiety and seizure disorders, while the shorter-acting drugs are most often used for insomnia and for surgical anesthesia.

Mechanisms of Benzodiazepine Action

Benzodiazepines all bind to the benzodiazepine site on the $GABA_A$ receptor complex illustrated in Figure 4.8. As with the barbiturates, benzodiazepines alter the shape of the $GABA_A$ receptor protein so GABA has a greater affinity for its site. When the inhibitory neurotransmitter GABA binds to its receptor the chlorine channel opens and allows for the influx of Cl^- ions, thereby hyperpolarizing the cell and making it less likely to fire. The anxiolytic and sedative effects of the benzodiazepines are mediated by $GABA_A$ receptors in the frontal cortex, the hippocampus, and several limbic structures, including the amygdala. Because the benzodiazepines

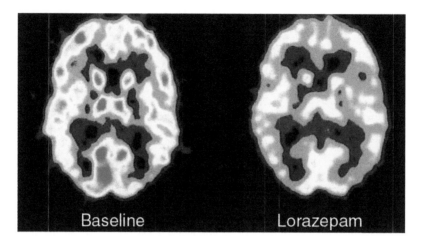

Figure 4.10 PET image showing decreased neural activity throughout the brain after benzodiazepine treatment. Red and orange colors indicate more neural activity than the yellow, green, and blue colors.

Source: © American Psychiatric Publishing. Inc.

do not open chlorine channels on their own, as do the barbiturates, the amount of neural inhibition they can produce depends on the availability of GABA (see Figure 4.10).

Not all benzodiazepines function as agonists on the GABA$_A$ receptor complex. The benzodiazepine flumazenil is a potent antagonist of benzodiazepines by competitively binding to the benzodiazepine site. In cases of suspected benzodiazepine overdose flumazenil effectively competes with and displaces other benzodiazepines at the receptor site. As a result, flumazenil reverses the anxiolytic, sedating, and motor effects caused by benzodiazepines. In large doses, flumazenil can produce anxiety, increases in muscle tone, and convulsions—effects opposite to those produced by other benzodiazepines.

Side Effects of Benzodiazepines

Because the benzodiazepines cannot open Cl⁻ channels on their own, as do the barbiturates, they are less likely to contribute to respiratory depression. Lethal overdose by benzodiazepines is therefore quite rare unless combined with alcohol or another GABA agonist. In combination with alcohol the benzodiazepines can cause a serious and sometimes fatal interaction by enhancing GABA neurotransmission. Other side effects of these drugs include marked sedation, cognitive impairments, retarded motor movements, and slurred speech—all effects observed with barbiturates and alcohol.

When combined with alcohol the benzodiazepine Rohypnol (flunitrazepam) produces euphoria, sedation, and amnesia. Because of these effects, Rohypnol has allegedly been used to facilitate date rape in a number of sexual assault cases. Prior to 1998, the drug Rohypnol, which is used in England and Mexico for the short-term treatment of insomnia, was colorless, tasteless, and could rapidly be dissolved in drinks. Consuming this cocktail would bring about sedating and amnesiac effects within about 15–20 minutes. Since 1998, a blue dye has been added to alert one to the presence of this drug in spiked beverages. Nevertheless, the FDA has not approved Rohypnol for use in the United States.

When used for the extended treatment of insomnia, the benzodiazepines disrupt normal sleep cycles and REM sleep, and discontinuation may cause rebounds in REM sleep, insomnia, and in anxiety. These effects are mediated by benzodiazepine receptor downregulation. Tolerance and dependence, also mediated by the downregulation of benzodiazepine receptor sites, occurs rapidly and may make discontinuation difficult for many patients. Although long-term use may cause physical dependence, there is little evidence from either human or animal studies that the benzodiazepines are addictive. This conclusion may be somewhat surprising since both benzodiazepines and alcohol share similar mechanisms of action. Perhaps the addictive potential of GABAergic drugs depends on how rapidly they enter the brain and on their ability to significantly increase dopamine activity in the mesolimbic system. The benzodiazepines are absorbed relatively slowly when compared with alcohol. In support of this hypothesis, the self-administration of benzodiazepines by laboratory animals is both variable and non-robust when compared to other abused drugs (Griffiths et al., 1991). A high rate of drug self-administration by animals is considered to be a reliable method of determining a drug's addictive potential.

In summary, the benzodiazepines represent a significant advance in the pharmacological treatment of anxiety disorders, seizures, muscle spasms, and insomnia compared with their predecessors, the barbiturates. All benzodiazepines agonize GABA neurotransmission by their activity on specific sites on the benzodiazepine receptor complex. Increases in inhibitory GABAergic activity decrease the firing rate of neurons in the frontal cortex, the hippocampus, and limbic structures assumed to underlie anxiety disorders. The benzodiazepines are safer than their predecessors and are rarely lethal by themselves in overdose. Their side effects are essentially the same as alcohol intoxication and the barbiturates, including sedation, cognitive impairment, retarded motor activity, and slurred speech. Although the benzodiazepines can cause physical dependence with long-term use, they have little or no addictive potential.

Third-Generation Anxiolytics

Partial GABA Agonists

In attempts to minimize the side effects of sedation and cognitive impairment associated with the benzodiazepines, a number of partial GABA$_A$ agonists have been investigated. A **partial agonist** has a high affinity for the GABA$_A$ receptor but has much less of an effect on the ability of GABA to bind than do full GABA$_A$ agonists. As you may recall, GABA$_A$ agonists alter the configuration of the GABA$_A$ receptor slightly, thus making it more structurally compatible for GABA. Partial agonists appear to produce even more subtle structural changes than do full agonists, such as the barbiturates and benzodiazepines. Several partial GABA$_A$ agonists have been investigated but are no longer being pursued for use in the United States. These include etizolam, which is available in Europe, imidazenil, pazinaclone, and bretazenil. In both human and animal studies these drugs appear to have similar anxiolytic effects but lower sedative and cognitive impairing effects than do the benzodiazepines. In addition, they appear less likely to induce tolerance and dependence (Mirza & Nielsen, 2006; Pinna et al., 2006; Sanna et al., 2005). The reasons for pharmaceutical companies not pursuing these alternatives aggressively may be due in part to the increased interest in SSRIs for treating anxiety disorders. However, interest in partial GABA agonists has continued with the development of several drugs used to treat insomnia.

Serotonin 5-HT$_{1A}$ Agonists

Because serotonin receptors are located through the brain regions known to be involved in anxiety, it should not be surprising to learn that serotonin agonists have anxiolytic properties. Genetically engineered 5-HT$_{1A}$ knockout mice lacking 5-HT$_{1A}$ receptors in the hippocampus, the amygdala, and the frontal cortex demonstrate exaggerated fear and anxiety compared to normal mice when tested in an elevated maze (Overstreet et al., 2003). In addition to increased behavioral anxiety, these mice have elevated autonomic activity, including increased heart rate and body temperature analogous to that observed in anxious humans. Injections of diazepam do not eliminate these stress responses, suggesting that interactions between GABAergic and serotonin 5-HT$_{1A}$ receptors are involved in anxiolysis (Albert et al., 2014; Celada et al., 2013; Pattij et al., 2002). Although several 5-HT$_{1A}$ agonists have been shown to have anxiolytic effects, buspirone is the only one approved for anxiety at this time. However, the off-label use of other serotonin uptake inhibitors, such as Prozac or Paxil, are commonly used to treat anxiety.

Buspirone (BuSpar)

Buspirone is a member of the azapirone group of 5-HT$_{1A}$ partial agonist drugs that were originally developed for their potential as antidepressants. And, although buspirone is used occasionally for the treatment of depression, it has not been approved by the FDA for this use. Buspirone is an effective anxiolytic, however, which has been established in numerous human and animal studies. In an extensive review of 36 clinical trials involving nearly 6,000 participants, buspirone was shown to be more effective than a placebo and as effective as benzodiazepines in treating generalized anxiety disorder (Chessick et al., 2006).

The agonistic effects of buspirone on 5-HT$_{1A}$ receptors result in downregulation or desensitization of these presynaptic autoreceptors and a corresponding increase in serotonin synthesis and release (Hensler, 2003). Typically it takes two or three weeks for buspirone to become effective—a time course similar to the adaptive changes observed in serotonin receptors. Because of the delay in its therapeutic effects, buspirone is not as useful as the benzodiazepines for treating acute anxiety. Buspirone is typically better tolerated than benzodiazepines and causes less sedation and fewer cognitive and motor-inhibiting effects. Additionally, buspirone does not cause dependence and there is no evidence for an abuse potential.

GABA$_B$ and GBH Receptor Agonists

Gamma-hydroxybutric acid (GBH) is only discussed here because of its historical significance and the recent discovery of a GBH receptor, not because it is currently used as an anxiolytic drug. In the 1960s, GBH was used in general anesthesia, as an anxiolytic, and as a sedative for the treatment of insomnia. More recently, GBH has been used recreationally and in athletics to enhance muscle growth through increased synthesis of growth hormone. In some cases, GBH has been reportedly used as a potent hypnotic to facilitate rape. Because GBH is odorless and colorless it is difficult to detect, and it could easily be dissolved in beverages and consumed without detection. GBH is also difficult to detect in urine samples, so the incidence of its use as a date rape drug remains largely unknown. Because it is now restricted, GBH use to facilitate rape is presumed to be quite rare.

GBH is a naturally occurring metabolite of GABA found in small amounts in both plant and animal tissues. Until quite recently GBH was believed to exert its sedating effects solely through the GABA$_B$ metabotropic receptor—a less common form of the GABA receptor distributed throughout the brain and spinal cord. It is now known that GBH also binds to a separate and specific presynaptic G protein-coupled receptor (GBH$_R$) that regulates adenyl cyclase activity and ultimately neurotransmitter release (Carter et al., 2009; Snead, 2000; Ticku & Mehta, 2008). At present there is no consensus about whether the behavioral effects of GBH are mediated by GABA$_B$ receptor agonism, the newly identified GBH receptor, or a combination of both.

Alternatives to Drug Therapy for Anxiety Disorders

The treatment of anxiety disorders with non-traditional pharmacotherapy has a long and controversial history. Although dozens of herbal remedies for anxiety have been utilized, only valerian and inositol are discussed here because there is some scientific evidence for their effectiveness.

Valerian (Valeriana Officinalis)

The herb **valerian**, which is extracted from the root of the valerian plant, shown in Figure 4.11, has a history dating back to Hippocrates, who may have been the first to describe its sedating and anxiolytic properties. Controversy about the evidence for these effects continues to the present. This controversy will continue until research on valerian is replicated by well-controlled clinical trials. The majority of the literature on the effectiveness of valerian has been either promoted by the herbal supplement industry or has been based on poorly designed studies or anecdotal evidence.

In a recent review of the research on the anxiolytic effects of valerian, researchers Miyasaka et al. (2007) found that only one study utilized random assignment of subjects into treatment conditions and included a placebo control. In this particular study, patients were randomly assigned to one of three treatment groups receiving valerian, diazepam, or a placebo. After four weeks of treatment the groups receiving valerian and diazepam scored lower on a subset of questions allegedly measuring the psychic symptoms of anxiety as measured by the Hamilton Anxiety Scale compared to the placebo group (Questions 1–6 in Figure 4.12). These results were confounded, however, by the fact that overall Hamilton Anxiety scores decreased in all three treatment groups (Andreatini et al., 2002), suggesting that both valerian and benzodiazepines were no more effective than a placebo, at least in these patients. The relative lack

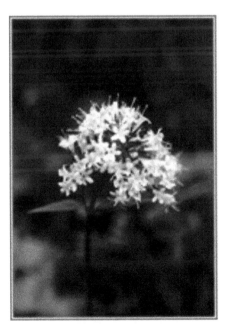

Figure 4.11 Valeriana officinalis.

HAMILTON ANXIETY RATING SCALE (HAM-A)

Classification of symptoms: 0 - absent; 1 - mild; 2 - moderate; 3 - severe; 4 - incapacitating

HAM-A score level of anxiety: < 17 mild; 18–24 mild to moderate; 25–30 moderate to severe

Symptoms   Date:_____

1. Anxious Mood   0 2 3 4
   - worries
   - anticipates worst
2. Tension   0 2 3 4
   - startles
   - cries easily
   - restless
   - trembling
3. Fears   0 2 3 4
   - fear of the dark
   - fear of strangers
   - fear of being alone
   - fear of animal
4. Insomnia   0 2 3 4
   - difficulty falling asleep or staying asleep
   - difficulty with nightmares
5. Intellectual   0 1 2 3 4
   - poor concentration
   - memory impairment
6. Depressed Mood   0 2 3 4
   - decreased interest in activities
   - anhedonia
   - insomnia
7. Somatic complaints - Muscular   0 2 3 4
   - muscle aches or pains
   - bruxism
8. Somatic complaints - Sensory   0 1 2 3 4
   - tinnitus
   - blurred vision
9. Cardiovascular Symptoms   0 1 2 3 4
   - tachycardia
   - palpitations
   - chest pain
   - sensory of feeling faint

10. Respiratory Symptoms   0 2 3 4
    - chest pressure
    - choking sensation
    - shortness of breath
11. Gastrointestinal Symptoms   0 2 3 4
    - dysphagia
    - nausea or vomiting
    - constipation
    - weight loss
12. Genitourinary Symptoms   0 2 3 4
    - urinary frequency or urgency
    - dysmenorrhea
    - impotence
13. Autonomic Symptoms   0 2 3 4
    - dry mouth
    - flushing
    - pallor
    - sweating
14. Behavior at Interview   0 2 3 4
    - fidgets
    - tremor
    - paces

TOTAL SCORE

Rater's signature _____

Figure 4.12 Hamilton Rating Scale. According to Hamilton, questions 1–6 address psychotic anxiety, while questions 7–14 address somatic anxiety.

Source: Hamilton (1959).

of well-designed clinical trials, as well as reliable measures of anxiety in humans, continues to make conclusions about valerian's effectiveness difficult at best. Additionally, there are few objective studies that examine valerian's effects on inhibitory avoidance or forced swimming in experimental animals. As we saw earlier, animal studies are particularly useful in corroborating human studies when outcome measures are largely subjective.

In the author's laboratory we isolated several active compounds in the valerian root extract, including GABA and valerenic acid. We compared the effectiveness of valerian with the known anxiolytic diazepam and samples of the active compounds extracted from valerian root using the elevated plus maze. In this study, female rats were randomly assigned to receive either an injection containing valerian root extract, diazepam, or saline. Additional groups received either valerenic acid or valerenic acid and GABA in the concentrations titrated from the valerian root

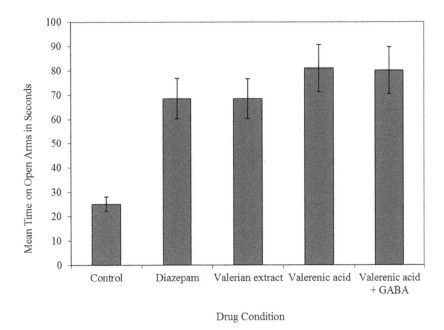

Figure 4.13 A comparison of the anxiolytic effects of valerian root extract, diazepam, valerenic acid, and valerenic acid with GABA in female rats using the elevated plus maze.

Source: Murphy et al. (2010).

extract. After 30 minutes, these animals were placed in the center of the plus maze suspended four feet above the floor. The time these animals spent exploring open arms of the maze is shown in Figure 4.13. In this experiment, valerian extract was as effective as diazepam in increasing exploration—a measure of a drug's anxiolytic effects (Murphy et al., 2010).

Mechanisms of Valerian Action

Despite the fact that research on valerian's anxiolytic properties is fragile, evidence that the herb acts as a GABA$_A$ receptor agonist suggests that valerian at least has anxiolytic potential. Specifically, valerian, and its main constituent valerenic acid, were both shown to induce neuronal inhibition in experimental animals in a manner similar to, but slightly less potent than, the GABA$_A$ agonist muscimol (see Figure 4.14). Valerian apparently potentiates the inhibitory effects of GABA by binding to specific subunits on the GABA$_A$ receptor complex (Khom et al., 2007; Yuan et al., 2004). Whether the neuronal inhibiting effects of valerian are sufficient to produce an anxiolytic effect in people remains to be demonstrated in clinical studies.

Inositol

Inositol is a natural isomer (a molecule made up of the same elements as another but in a different structural arrangement) of glucose, and it is a precursor to several of the phosphate-based second messengers (shown in Figure 4.15). Found in a variety of foods, including bran cereals, nuts, and fruits, including oranges and melons, inositol (*myo*-inositol) is also synthesized by the body and is a member of the vitamin B complex. Inositol has been reputed to treat

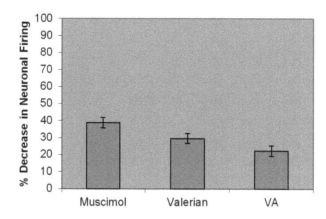

Figure 4.14 Percentage decrease in neuronal activity in rat brainstem following treatment with the $GABA_A$ agonist muscimol, valerian, or valerenic acid (VA).

Source: Yuan et al. (2004).

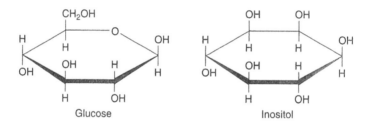

Figure 4.15 Inositol $(C_6H_{12}O_6)$ is a structural isomer of glucose $(C_6H_{12}O_6)$.

panic disorders, generalized anxiety, OCD, and depression. Evidence for these effects is sparse relative to the abundance of research supporting the effectiveness of traditional anxiolytic drugs for these disorders.

A few studies have shown inositol to be more effective than a placebo and as effective as fluoxamine (an SSRI) in treating panic disorder and in reducing the severity of anxiety as measured by the Hamilton Rating Scale (Benjamin et al., 1995; Palatnik et al., 2001). Why the researchers did not compare inositol with either barbiturates or benzodiazepines is unclear. As with valerian, inositol research often lacks the kinds of scientific rigor that makes conclusions about its effectiveness speculative. Furthermore, the mechanisms of action that underlie the putative effects of inositol have yet to be described, although inositol is involved in second messenger systems in many neural pathways, including serotonin.

In summary, alternatives to drug therapy for anxiety disorders have been proposed and some experimental evidence supports their use. Evidence described earlier using animal studies suggests that valerian may be effective, and the mechanism of action of valerian on $GABA_A$ receptors is at least consistent with its alleged anxiolytic effects. However, the glucose isomer inositol has limited experimental support for treating anxiety (Mukai et al., 2014), and its mechanism of action remains elusive, although inositol does function in the second messenger systems of most neurons, including neurons that are known to underlie anxiety. Because neither of these substances cause significant side effects, or interact measurably with other anxiolytic or antidepressant drugs, their sensible use is not discouraged. In fact, as a first treatment attempt they might not only be effective but are better tolerated and cause appreciably fewer side effects than prescription antianxiety medication.

Obsessive-Compulsive Disorder (OCD)

Obsessive-compulsive disorder is a disorder characterized by recurrent, unwanted thoughts (obsessions) and repetitive behaviors (compulsions). Obsessions may consist of thoughts of contamination or infection, repeated self-doubt, a need for order, aggressive impulses to hurt someone or shout out an obscenity, or sexual imagery. Compulsions, which may include hand washing, counting, checking, cleaning, or hoarding miscellaneous items, are often performed with the anticipation of preventing obsessive thoughts or making them go away. Performing these repetitive behaviors appears to only provide temporary, if any, relief. Not performing these behaviors, however, tends to increase one's anxiety and obsessive thoughts. Patients with OCD recognize that their obsessions and compulsions are excessive and unreasonable, but this recognition does little to subdue their anxiety.

OCD typically emerges in early adolescents or adulthood, but it can occur in children. The lifetime prevalence of OCD is about 2.5 percent of the population, and over two million people suffer from it at any given time. The prevalence of OCD is about equal for males and females but may be more prevalent among males in the child population. The majority of patients with OCD experience cycling periods with and without symptoms and experience the most debilitating symptoms during times of stress.

The *DSM-5* criteria for a diagnosis of OCD are as follows:

1. *The presence of obsessions, compulsions, or both.* Obsessions are recurrent and persistent thoughts, impulses, or images that mark anxiety or distress. In addition, these obsessions are not simply worries about real-life problems and the patient realizes that the obsessive thoughts are a product of their own mind and not imposed by another. Compulsions are repetitive behaviors that the person feels driven to perform and are aimed at preventing or reducing distress or some dreaded event.
2. *The obsessions and compulsions cause marked distress, are time consuming, and they significantly disrupt a person's normal routine, occupational functioning, and their social activities.*

Carl, a 24-year-old college student, began seeing a psychologist at his girlfriend's request because of his persistent checking behavior. Once they began living together she was shocked by his inability to sit through a television show, a complete dinner, or even a conversation without getting up to check to be sure the kitchen stove was off or to lock the door to their apartment. During the night, Carl would often get up to verify that everything was off and secure. Carl even insisted that they leave the theater in the middle of a movie because he was certain that the door to their apartment was left open. Reassuring him that she had checked was of little use once he began obsessing about it.

Carl's obsessions appear to have begun in high school when he became obsessed with arranging and rearranging things in his room. At first his parents encouraged his cleanliness and the order of his personal things. When he went off to college they assumed his behavior would change in the presence of roommates who would likely be much messier than he. While Carl wasn't obsessed with the disorder of their shared dorm room, his obsessions about his own possessions persisted. Carl was meticulous about the folding and the order of clothes in his small closet and drawers. He also became concerned about the shared sink in their room. He spent hours washing and disinfecting the shared area where his roommate shaved and brushed his teeth. Any amount of hair or toothbrush splatter in the sink or on the counter repulsed him.

After several months, Carl was granted a request to move into a single dorm room. In his single room Carl was aware that his excessive concern about order was unusual. He was even embarrassed when others commented about how clean and orderly everything was. At one point, prior to friends coming to visit, he actually disorganized everything to make his dorm look "normal." Carl found this to be so distressing that he spent their entire visit rearranging again rather than playing cards. Living in the shared space of dormitories was getting more and more difficult for Carl. His obsessions over the sanitary conditions of the showers, the many doorknobs, and the shared kitchen space distracted him much of the time. He was also concerned about leaving his dorm room door unlocked and needed to check it frequently throughout the day. By his senior year Carl had moved into a small but new apartment. Within a few months his girlfriend joined him, only to be stunned by his unusual behavior.

After two visits to the university psychologist Carl was referred to a psychiatrist at the university hospital for medication. Following a brief visit Carl was prescribed Zoloft, which he continues to take today. His obsessive symptoms of anxiety have improved, but his ritualistic checking has not. Carl's symptoms seem to come and go over time and are most severe when he is under stress.

Assessment of Obsessive-Compulsive Disorder

One of the most common assessment tools for diagnosing the severity of OCD is the Yale-Brown Obsessive Compulsive Scale (Y-BOCS) (Goodman et al., 1989). This ten-item scale is presumed to measure both obsessive and compulsive symptoms. It is mentioned here because it is often used to evaluate the effectiveness of treatment medication as well as the effectiveness of cognitive behavioral therapy. Researchers are also interested in developing animal models of OCD to study its underlying pathology, as well as to investigate drug effectiveness. Several animal models have been proposed that involve inducing OCD symptoms with drugs (e.g., quinpirole) which increase dopamine activity in the striatum and produce compulsive checking-like and hoarding behaviors in animals (e.g., Eagle et al., 2014; Fernandez-Guasti et al., 2003; Joel, 2006; Szechtman et al., 1998). Drugs that effectively decrease OCD symptoms in human patients appear to diminish OCD-like symptoms in animals as well.

Pathology of Obsessive-Compulsive Disorder

Of all the anxiety disorders, OCD has the clearest connection to abnormal neuroanatomy and function. The prevailing view of OCD argues that it is a biological disease involving neural dysfunction in circuitry between the orbitofrontal cortex, the cingulate gyrus, the caudate nucleus, the globus pallidus, and the thalamus. This neural circuit forms a loop where dopamine hyperactivity in the caudate nucleus inhibits the globus pallidus, which normally suppresses thalamic activity (illustrated in Figure 4.16). Excessive dopamine inhibition in the globus pallidus is presumed to disrupt the normal inhibitory control the globus pallidus has over the thalamus. Increased activity in the thalamus of OCD patients produces increased activity in the orbitofrontal cortex via the cingulate gyrus. This proposal is supported by several neuroimaging studies (Saxena et al., 1998) and volumetric studies of these structures (Atmaca et al., 2007; Chen et al., 2022). Furthermore, OCD patients who had been successfully treated with SSRI medication showed normalized functioning in the caudate nucleus compared to patients treated for depression (Saxena et al., 2003). A number of patients with severe OCD have benefited from surgically disrupting the excitatory input from the cingulate gyrus to the frontal cortex by a procedure known as a **cingulotomy**, which severs this connection. Surgical intervention is only an option when patients don't respond to medication (e.g., Sheth et al., 2013).

Pharmacological Treatment of Obsessive-Compulsive Disorder

The observation that symptoms of OCD are dissipated with serotonin agonists (SSRIs and SNRIs) has led to the hypothesis that serotonin dysfunction underlies this disorder. It is

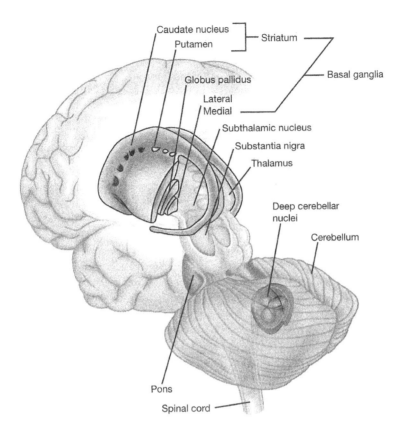

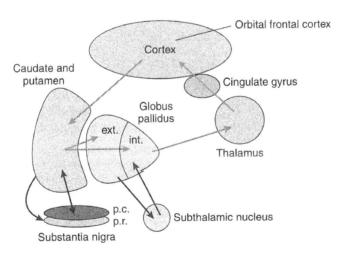

Figure 4.16 Neural structures implicated in OCD (top). Normally, thalamic activity suppresses activity in the orbitofrontal cortex via the cingulate gyrus. In OCD, hyperactivity in the caudate nucleus suppresses inhibitory input from the globus pallidus to the thalamus. This results in an increase in activity in the thalamus, cingulate gyrus, and orbitofrontal cortex (bottom).

Table 4.3 FDA-approved medication for the treatment of OCD. Other serotonin agonists may be equally effective but are used off label.

Drug name	Trade name	Class
Clomipramine	Anafranil	SNRI
Fluoxetine	Prozac	SSRI
Fluvoxamine	Luvox	SSRI
Paroxetine	Paxil	SSRI
Sertraline	Zoloft	SSRI

important to note, however, that there is little evidence for serotonin dysfunction in OCD (Westenberg et al., 2007). There is also little agreement about which serotonin receptors may be involved when symptoms are improved (Lin, 2007). It does appear, however, that it is serotonin reuptake inhibition that mediates the effectiveness of treatment, even with the dual serotonin-norepinephrine reuptake inhibitors. A number of these drugs are described in Table 4.3. There is a growing consensus that serotonin agonists are initially effective in 50–60 percent of OCD patients. Non-responders may eventually respond to another serotonin agonist or to combinations of drug and cognitive behavioral therapy (Simpson et al., 2013).

Patients who respond to treatment with serotonin agonists also reveal decreases in blood flow to the thalamus compared to patients who don't respond to drug treatment—a finding consistent with thalamic hyperactivity contributing to OCD symptoms (Ho Pian et al., 2005; Weeland et al., 2021). Treatment with the serotonin agonist fluvoxamine has also been shown to increase dopamine (D_2) receptor availability in the caudate nucleus. This secondary effect of serotoninergic activity is presumed to normalize hyperexcitability in the caudate nucleus and the thalamus (Moresco et al., 2007).

In conclusion, OCD is a serious and debilitating condition that affects a significant portion of the population. Disruptions in neural circuits between the caudate nucleus, globus pallidus, and the thalamus appear to cause increased activity in the cingulate gyrus and the orbitofrontal cortex. Evidence supporting this hypothesis comes from numerous imaging and surgical studies, as well as animal models of OCD. While there appears to be evidence for a genetic contribution to OCD, there is little agreement on the details of its underlying pathology or on the details of serotonin involvement. Drugs that increase serotonin activity, however, do effectively decrease symptoms in many patients and they appear to normalize hyperexcitability in the caudate nucleus and the thalamus.

Post-traumatic Stress Disorder

A significant number of individuals who experience severe stress associated with a disaster, an accident, military combat, rape, or who witness a horrific crime may continue to experience stress and anxiety through intrusive memories or dreams of these traumatic events. About 11 percent of the rescue and recovery workers after the 9/11 attacks on the World Trade Center in New York continue to be traumatized by their memories, and many of these individuals could not continue to live and work in New York City. About 9 percent of the population, over 24 million people, in the United States will experience post-traumatic stress disorder at some point during their lifetime. The *DSM-5* lists the following criteria for a diagnosis of post-traumatic stress disorder (PTSD):

1. Exposure to actual or threatened death, serious injury, or sexual violence by directly experiencing it or witnessing it as it occurred to others.

2. The traumatic event is persistently experienced as intrusive recollections, dreams, or flashbacks.
3. Persistent avoidance of stimuli associated with the trauma indicated by efforts to avoid thoughts, activities, places, or people associated with the event.
4. Negative alterations in cognitions and mood associated with the traumatic event.
5. Marked alterations in arousal and reactivity associated with the traumatic event.
6. These disturbances have occurred for at least one month and cause significant distress or impairment in social, occupational, or other areas of functioning.

Pathology of Post-traumatic Stress Disorder

Stress causes profound changes to structures in the brain that regulate fear and anxiety. Among these changes are significant decreases in both hippocampal and prefrontal cortex volumes and an increase in dendritic density and activity in the amygdala. The decreases in hippocampal volume, particularly in the region of the dentate gyrus, are a result of increased glucocorticoid and catecholamine release during the stress response. Decreases in the volume of the medial prefrontal cortex may also be related to increased glucocorticoid and catecholamine activity. As a result, stimuli associated with traumatic events cause enhanced amygdala responsiveness that is not suppressed by cortical inhibition (Chen et al., 2018). Recent functional neuroimaging studies confirm that the medial prefrontal cortex is hypoactive in PTSD patients. Additionally, PTSD patients demonstrate heightened responses in the amygdala following exposure to trauma-related stimuli (Karl et al., 2006; Miller et al., 2006; Shin et al., 2006). It is believed that heightened amygdala responsiveness to emotional stimuli and hypoactive inhibitory input from descending prefrontal cortical regions underlies post-traumatic stress disorders. Evidence for decreased GABA inhibitory activity in PTSD patients comes from a recent study comparing the ability of the GABA$_A$ antagonist flumazenil to bind to GABA receptors in PTSD patients with normal control subjects. Radioactively labeled (^{11}C) flumazenil was injected into both groups of subjects and measured using PET scans. Significantly, decreased densities of GABA$_A$ receptors were found in PTSD patients (see Figure 4.17).

Animal studies also confirm that stress hormones and the catecholamines contribute to neuronal atrophy and degeneration in the hippocampus, whereas stress manipulations cause enhanced dendritic branching and growth in the amygdala. These structural changes lead to

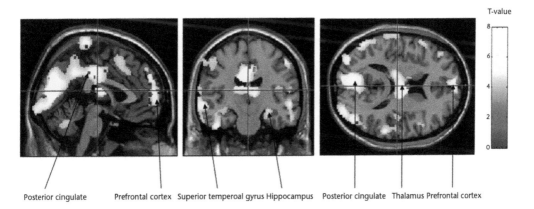

Figure 4.17 Areas with decreased GABA$_A$ receptor binding in PTSD patients are indicated in yellow.
Source: Geuze et al. (2008).

enhanced emotionality in laboratory animals and seem to parallel those changes observed in humans with PTSD (Bremner, 1999; Dannlowski et al., 2012; Vyas et al., 2002).

Glossary

Amytal interview an interrogation of a witness after the administration of sodium amytal (truth serum). Evidence obtained under the influence of such drugs is not admissible in court.

Anxiogenic a drug or substance that induces or exacerbates anxiety.

Anxiolytic a drug or substance that is used to treat anxiety.

Cingulotomy surgically disrupting the excitatory input from the cingulate gyrus to the frontal cortex. Occasionally used to treat drug-resistant obsessive-compulsive disorder.

Convulsant a drug or substance that can induce seizures or convulsions in subjects.

Cross tolerance tolerance developed to one drug may be expressed to other similar-acting drugs that the patient has not had before.

Elevated maze an apparatus used to evaluate the effects of drugs on anxiety responses in laboratory animals. Designed with two enclosed and two open arms and suspended about three feet above the ground. The proportion of time spent in open arms is a measure of a drug's anxiolytic effect.

Fetal alcohol syndrome a severe developmental disorder caused by fetal exposure to alcohol or other similar-acting drugs.

Generalized anxiety disorder chronic worry about events with no specific threat. Characterized by restlessness, fatigue, difficulty with concentration, and sleep disruptions.

Inositol a derivative of the glucose molecule with putative anxiolytic properties.

Obsessive-compulsive disorder (OCD) a severe psychological disorder characterized by the persistence of unwanted thoughts or disturbing images. Compulsive, often ritualistic, behaviors may also occur in attempts to mitigate the obsessive thoughts.

Panic disorder experiencing repeated and unexpected panic attacks as well as anxiety about impending attacks.

Partial agonist a drug that binds to and agonizes a receptor but with less intensity than a full agonist.

Post-traumatic stress disorder (PTSD) a severe stress disorder brought about by an extreme traumatic experience.

Valerian an herbal remedy promoted to treat insomnia and anxiety. Derived from the root of valerian plants.

5   Psychotic Disorders

Schizophrenia

David was first diagnosed with schizophrenia when he was 26 years old. At that time he was in his fourth year as an architect student at the University of Oregon. David's life prior to attending the university was not unusual. He had many high school friends, he was outgoing, and he was exceptionally bright. Any eccentricities in his behavior during these years were attributed to deep passion for everything he did, but particularly drawing. While in college, David began to withdraw socially during his freshman year. He started college as an art major, and he spent most of his time immersed in his drawings. At first his artwork earned him praise because of his obsession with detail, but later this fixation began to take over and he could never complete his assignments. He preferred spending time alone and would often be observed wandering aimlessly on campus failing to recognize or respond to those who knew him.

During his third year, David's advisor suggested he may do well in architecture since he seemed more intrigued with drawings of buildings. David's sketches were becoming increasingly complex and not well suited to his assignments. Discussions with his mentors were getting more and more frustrating as his elaborations began to reveal his psychosis. David would talk enthusiastically about his design concepts only to be met with an outright rejection of his increasingly bizarre ideas. By this point David was becoming convinced that his professors were concealing their real interest in plagiarizing his work by their rejection of it. Rather than continuing to work in the student lab in the architecture building, David found it necessary to do his work in secret because his professors were spying on him. Within a few months David was convinced that co-conspirators of the plagiarism scheme were tapping his phone and following him everywhere. By now he was having great difficulty sleeping and was spending his time altering his drawings to conceal the innovations he had made.

After seeing and discussing his recent work, David's parents realized that their son needed professional help. Several appointments later he was diagnosed with paranoid schizophrenia and given a prescription for clozapine. David's psychiatrist encouraged him to schedule monthly appointments and to return to school to finish his architecture degree. David remained on the medication for several months and was showing signs of improvement, but he felt the medication dampened his creativity and made it difficult to draw. His paranoia quickly returned when he discontinued medication, forcing him to leave school altogether. During our initial visit, David's enthusiasm for architecture was easy to draw out—so too was his paranoia of members of the department at the university who were conspiring to steal his creations. It wasn't at all unusual for David to hear voices threatening him if he didn't reveal his work. One familiar voice threatened "We know where you live, David" on numerous occasions.

While David could respond sensibly to questions about his past, he would lapse into an incoherent speech where sentences were only loosely connected when we discussed his plans about his future. His thoughts also seemed to shift unpredictably, making it difficult to follow. If one didn't know of his medical condition they might be easily convinced of his architectural genius during a rant about building design.

Of all the psychological disorders, schizophrenia is perhaps the most serious and debilitating. It typically emerges in early adulthood, and although there may be periods of remission, schizophrenia is a chronic life-long illness for most patients. The lifetime prevalence of schizophrenia

DOI: 10.4324/9781003309017-5

worldwide is about 1 percent (1 in every 100 individuals during their lifetime), but it may be higher in some ethnic groups than others. For instance, there appears to be a greater incidence among African-Caribbeans living in England than any other group. Schizophrenia is also known to run in families. Sons and daughters of parents with schizophrenia have a tenfold increase in risk of developing the disease than others. And, although the concordance rates among monozygotic twins are significantly greater than dizygotic twins, there is no consensus on which gene or genes are involved. Schizophrenia does appear to have a strong genetic contribution, but environmental factors seem to play an even greater role in its etiology. Schizophrenia is a complex collection of diseases that affect all aspects of human functioning. It causes disturbances in affect, cognitive functions, speech and language, perception, and even movement. The most distinctive, and diagnostic, features of schizophrenia, however, are the presence of psychotic delusions and hallucinations.

This chapter discusses psychotic disorders with an emphasis on schizophrenia. We will examine its diagnostic criteria, its pathology, and the pharmacological approaches to its treatment. Other psychotic disorders, including schizoaffective disorder, delusional disorder, and schizophreniform disorder are not discussed separately here because their pathology and treatment do not differ significantly from that of schizophrenia.

Defining and Diagnosing Schizophrenia

The *DSM-5* diagnostic criteria for schizophrenia require that two or more of the following symptoms be present for a significant portion of the time during the month preceding its diagnosis:

1. *Delusions.* Delusions are strongly held beliefs that are quite clearly contradictory to external evidence. They often consist of misinterpretations of perceptions and everyday experiences. The most common theme in schizophrenia seems to be delusions of persecution, where the individual feels as if they are being watched, followed, or ridiculed behind their back. Another common theme is delusions of reference that might include feelings that comments by others, song lyrics, television personalities, news reports, or passages from books are purposely directed at them. Delusions may also be bizarre in that they are clearly impossible and not understandable by others who share the same religious and cultural experiences. For example, a bizarre delusion may be that one inhabits the body of another or that parts of one's body have been exchanged with another person. Sometimes bizarre delusions include themes of control where one's thoughts or behaviors are being manipulated by others, even aliens.

2. *Hallucinations.* Hallucinations are perceptual experiences that are not consistent with, or happen in the absence of, external stimuli. Schizophrenic hallucinations may occur in any sensory modality (visual, olfactory, auditory, gustatory, or tactile) but auditory hallucinations are the most frequent. The most common theme for auditory hallucinations is familiar voices that are quite critical and judgmental. For example, a patient may hear, upon passing a woman on the sidewalk, "you raped her" or "you hurt that woman." Voices from God, the Devil, or any other supreme being can also occur, but these are less frequent. Rarely do patients with schizophrenia act on commands from auditory hallucinations. Magnetic imaging studies conducted while patients are experiencing an auditory hallucination suggests that they represent misattributed subvocal speech, since they activate the same auditory structures as external speech not structures associated with hearing speech (Plaze et al., 2006).

3. *Disorganized speech.* Often the speech of a schizophrenic is so disorganized, fragmented, and incoherent it can be difficult to converse with them. Switching topics frequently,

excessive detailed elaboration, and grandiose ideas are common. This author spent four hours on a flight from Washington, DC, to Portland listening to a patient with schizophrenia describe the origins of matter and the universe. Frequently, he made up words to describe strange forces that have yet to be identified. Challenges to his theory only fueled his conviction and led to even greater fabrication. Occasionally, speech can be so disjointed it is referred to as *word salad*. In these cases, individual words are clearly spoken, but there is no coherent sentence structure or meaning to utterances.

4. *Grossly disorganized or catatonic behavior.* The ability of patients with schizophrenia to conduct normal activities can also be severely disrupted. Goal-directed behavior is often thwarted by distractions and changes in plan. Maintaining appropriate hygiene, dress, and manners in social settings may also deteriorate over time. In extreme examples, motor stereotypes and catatonia begin to emerge. Catatonia is a state of waxy flexibility where posture can be molded into or held in uncomfortable positions for extended periods of time.

5. *Negative symptoms.* Schizophrenia symptoms are often described as either *positive* (excessive or distorted) or *negative* (in absence or deficit). The symptoms described in the previous examples are **positive symptoms** since they represent exaggerations or distortions of behavior. Examples of negative symptoms might include a flat or muted expression, lack of speech, avolition, and long periods of non-reactive immobility. A preponderance of **negative symptoms** tends to occur in later stages of the disease and may be associated with greater neural damage. The prognosis of patients displaying predominantly negative symptoms is typically not good.

Prior to the discovery of **antipsychotic** drugs in the 1950s, patients with schizophrenia were, for the majority, housed in mental institutions with few treatment options. Physical restraint was used for severely agitated patients, as was insulin administration to dramatically lower blood glucose levels and induce a state of **insulin shock**—a comatose state that was maintained for about an hour. **Electric shock therapy** (electro convulsive therapy or ECT) is still used to treat drug-resistant depression, but it is only rarely used on patients with schizophrenia who do not respond to drug treatment or need immediate management. The rationale behind electroconvulsive shock therapy originally was that seizures were never observed during acute states of schizophrenia. The induction of a seizure may, therefore, prevent the occurrence of psychosis. None of these treatments affected the course of schizophrenia, and all were essentially replaced as pharmacotherapy gained prominence in the late 1950s.

The most widely used surgical procedure was a **frontal lobotomy**, which was introduced as a treatment in the late 1930s by the Portuguese physician António Moniz. Moniz received the Nobel Prize in 1949 for refining this procedure at a time when there were no treatment options for severe schizophrenia. The lobotomy (or leucotomy) procedure involved either separating the prefrontal areas from the remainder of the frontal cortex by knife cuts, or by destroying these areas with ice picks inserted behind the eyes (Figures 5.1 and 5.2). About 40,000 lobotomies are believed to have been performed in the United States before it was finally banned in all states. The last lobotomies performed in the United States were conducted in the late 1980s.

Pathology of Schizophrenia: Dopamine Hypothesis

The **dopamine hypothesis** of schizophrenia can be traced back to early research on the effects of antipsychotic drugs on animals (Carlsson & Lindqvist, 1963; Randrup & Munkvad, 1965) and to the discovery of the mechanism of action of the first effective antipsychotic drugs (van Rossum, 1966). This hypothesis proposes that schizophrenia is caused by excessive dopamine activity in the striatum and mesolimbic pathways, and perhaps a decrease in dopaminergic activity in the prefrontal cortex. A number of observations provided early support for this hypothesis, including evidence that dopamine agonists such as cocaine and amphetamine induced psychotic symptoms. Large doses or prolonged use of these drugs can cause positive psychotic symptoms that appear indistinguishable from schizophrenia symptoms—a state referred to as amphetamine psychosis. Additionally, the psychoses induced by amphetamine, methamphetamine, or cocaine are treated with traditional antipsychotic medication that block dopamine (D_2) receptors. Finally, a number of postmortem studies revealed that psychotic patients had increased numbers of dopamine (D_2) receptors, which may have contributed to hyperactive dopamine activity in the striatum and mesolimbic areas. It is important to point out, however, that not all studies have found increased numbers of D_2 receptors, particularly studies involving patients who have had schizophrenia for long periods of time.

Perhaps the most compelling support for the dopamine hypothesis comes from **amphetamine challenge** and **receptor competition** studies. Amphetamine challenge estimates

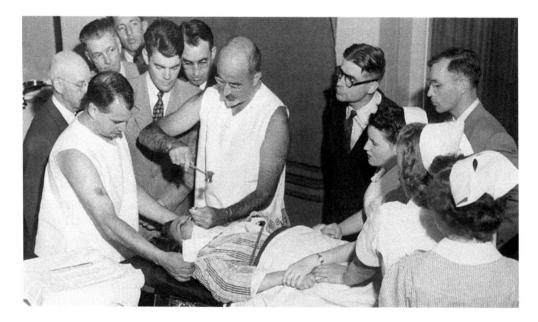

Figure 5.1 Dr. Walter Freeman performing a prefrontal lobotomy in the United States.

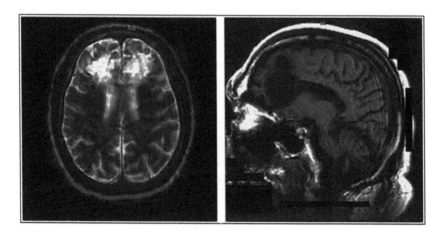

Figure 5.2 Brain section revealing the damaged frontal lobes after lobotomy.

Source: Lapidus et al. (2013).

dopamine release by scanning for radioactive markers of dopamine receptor occupancy following the administration of amphetamine. Amphetamine increases synaptic dopamine by blocking dopamine reuptake and vesicular transporters. When compared to matched controls, patients with schizophrenia exhibit significantly greater dopamine release following amphetamine administration (Abi-Dargham et al., 2000; Laruelle, 1998). Patients with schizophrenia also show greater D_2 receptor density than do normal control subjects. Both of these findings are consistent with the dopamine hypothesis. In addition, the only predictor of a drug's antipsychotic efficacy is its ability to block dopamine receptors. The ability of a drug to compete with dopamine for D_2 receptors is measured by its capacity to displace a radioactive dopamine ligand. Clinically effective doses of antipsychotic drugs are highly correlated with their ability to compete for and block D_2 receptors, as shown in Figure 5.3. Similar correlations are not observed for other receptor types even though additional neurotransmitters (e.g., serotonin) have been implicated in schizophrenia.

According to the dopamine hypothesis, the positive symptoms of the disease are associated with hyperdopamine activity in the striatum and the mesolimbic system, while negative symptoms and cognitive impairment result from hypodopaminergic activity in mesocortical pathways to the prefrontal cortex. There appears to be a reciprocal relationship between mesocortical and mesolimbic dopaminergic activity, such that hypodopaminergic functioning in the prefrontal cortex may lead to the disinhibition of, and therefore increased, mesolimbic dopamine activity (Abi-Dargham & Moore, 2003; Joyce, 1993). Evidence from neuroimaging

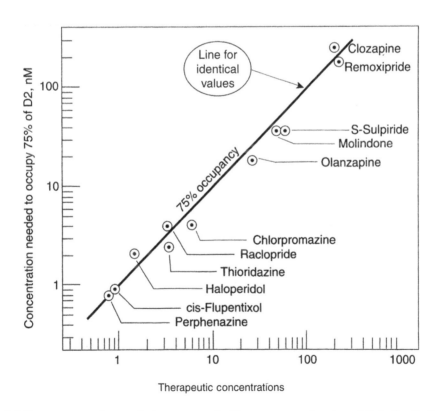

Figure 5.3 Drug concentration required to compete for D_2 receptors as a function of clinically effective dose. An antipsychotic's therapeutic dose is nearly identical to its concentration needed to occupy 75 percent of D_2 receptors. Drugs lower along the diagonal line bind more tightly than dopamine on D_2 receptors, while those higher along the line bind more loosely than dopamine.

Source: Seeman and Tallerico (1998).

studies also suggests that schizophrenia is associated with hypoactive prefrontal cortices. There is a marked reduction in frontal lobe activity in patients with schizophrenia when compared to normal controls. This reduction in activity, seen in Figure 5.4, is believed to be associated with hypodopaminergic activity in these regions.

Beyond the Dopamine Hypothesis: NMDA and GABA Dysfunction

While the dopamine hypothesis continues to be the most prominent theoretical explanation for schizophrenia, there is also evidence that GABAergic and glutaminergic systems are involved. This evidence comes from several observations: First, the drugs phenylcyclidine and ketamine, both glutamate NMDA receptor antagonists, produce effects that mimic schizophrenia, including hallucinations, delusions, thought disorders, and, perhaps most interestingly, negative symptoms. Repeated administration of these NMDA antagonists also produces structural changes that resemble those observed in schizophrenia. It has been proposed that the psychotic symptoms and neural degeneration seen following phenylcyclidine and ketamine administration result from a disruption of glutaminergic innervation of GABA neurons in the thalamus and basal forebrain. The effect of NMDA receptor blockade, as shown in Figure 5.3, would be disinhibition of GABA and an increase in cortical glutamate and acetylcholine activity. Neural degeneration, and the negative symptoms of schizophrenia, may result from cortical glutamate excitotoxicity (Olney et al., 1999; Stone et al., 2007; Uno & Coyle, 2019). Excitotoxicity is a process whereby neurons are destroyed when glutamate neurons become depolarized for long durations. Prolonged depolarization leads to an excessive influx of Ca^{++}, which activates several cell-damaging enzymes.

Secondly, patients with schizophrenia have depressed numbers of NMDA receptors in the thalamus and the hippocampus. It is presumed that glutamate dysfunction in these subcortical regions leads to excitotoxic glutamate activity in the cortex and the development of negative symptoms in later stages of schizophrenia. We will review several antipsychotic

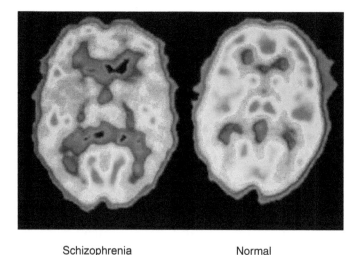

Schizophrenia   Normal

Figure 5.4 PET images of a schizophrenia brain (left) and a normal brain (right). The frontal lobes are at the top of each image. These images reveal decreases in frontal lobe activity in schizophrenia (top of each image) as well as enlarged ventricles (blue areas in the center).

Source: Buchsbaum and Hazlett (1998).

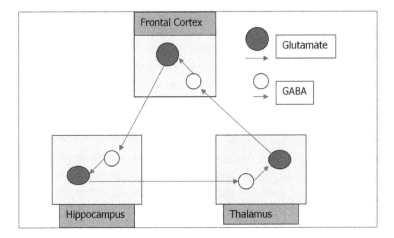

Figure 5.5 A simplified model for glutamate excitotoxicity. Hypoactive glutamate in the thalamus leads to decreased GABA inhibitory control over glutamate in the frontal cortex. Glutamate excitotoxicity causes damage to neurons receiving glutamate in the frontal cortex and to GABA neurons in the hippocampus.

Source: After Stone et al. (2007).

drugs that may be utilized during early stages of schizophrenia to diminish cortical and hippocampal excitotoxicity and to decrease the development of negative symptoms of schizophrenia (Figure 5.5).

In summary, the dopamine hypothesis has received considerable support during the 40 years since its inception. Evidence from the pharmacodynamics of antipsychotics drugs, amphetamine-induced psychosis, amphetamine challenge, and receptor competition studies are all consistent with this hypothesis as an account for the positive symptoms of schizophrenia. Glutamate dysfunction arising from subcortical regions may lead to excitotoxic effects of elevated cortical and hippocampal glutamate neurons and contribute to the development of negative symptoms often observed during later stages of the disease. In the following sections we discuss the evolution of drug therapy for schizophrenia and other psychotic disorders.

Abnormalities in Brain Structure

Patients with schizophrenia may also display abnormalities in cell densities and organization in the hippocampus and the amygdala. Normally cells in the hippocampus arrange in columnar fashion, much like cortical cells do. However, in schizophrenia hippocampal cells are arranged in a disorganized manner (see Figure 5.6). There is also a loss of cell volume in the frontal lobes, the hippocampus, and the amygdala in schizophrenia. It has long been known that patients with schizophrenia have significant memory impairments, specifically in verbal and visual memories. It is believed that these impairments are associated with hippocampal dysfunction rather than a general decrease in global functioning (Nelson et al., 1998).

While it is possible that some or all of these abnormalities could be the consequence of long-term use of medication or caused by the progression of the illness itself, many researchers believe that they begin during early development. Support for this comes from studies revealing strong correlations between the duration of schizophrenia symptoms, but not the duration of time on medication.

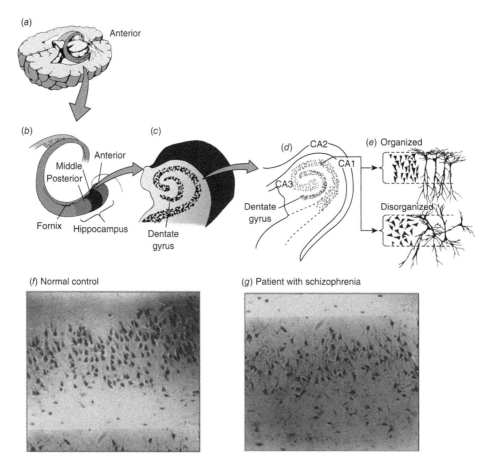

Figure 5.6 Hippocampal cells are less dense and arranged in a disorganized manner in schizophrenia.

Pharmacological Treatment of Schizophrenia and Psychotic Disorders

Phenothiazines

By the 1950s, it is estimated that over half a million patients were hospitalized in mental institutions in the United States for schizophrenia. These patients had few non-surgical treatment options and they typically remained in these institutions for much of their adult lives. The serendipitous discovery of the antipsychotic effects of a class of drugs called phenothiazines in the mid-1950s literally changed the lives of most patients with schizophrenia. The phenothiazine, chlorpromazine (Thorazine), was originally used as an antiemetic (antinausea) agent, but it was quickly observed to have remarkable sedative properties. Chlorpromazine was used to sedate patients with severe burns or trauma as well as to sedate agitated patients prior to surgery. Its first use to treat psychotic patients may have occurred in France in 1952, where 38 patients were treated with daily injections (Turner, 2007). Chlorpromazine appeared to relieve the symptoms of psychosis in these patients without producing heavy sedation. Within a few years of its approval for treating psychosis, the number of hospitalized patients in the United States was reduced by at least one half. Chlorpromazine is credited with liberating hundreds of thousands of patients from the harsh and often cruel conditions of mental institutions, but it may also have contributed to the simultaneous increase in the homeless population wandering the streets of our bigger cities. Patients often discontinued the use of their medication as they developed troubling and often serious side effects from it. Once they discontinued medication most of these patients found that they were unable to function outside of an institution. Many of these patients were unmonitored and simply faded into the streets.

The mechanisms of action of chlorpromazine were not understood when it was first approved by the FDA in 1954; in fact it was alleged to have predominantly sedative and antihistamine properties. It was becoming clear, however, that its antipsychotic effects were not related to its sedative effects. In other words, patients were not merely sedated out of their psychotic symptoms. Since the discovery of the antipsychotic effects of chlorpromazine a number of other phenothiazines were introduced. All phenothiazines have similar mechanisms of action, but differ to some extent in their side effect profiles.

Mechanisms of Phenothiazine Action

The antipsychotic effects of the phenothiazines are mediated by their antagonism of dopamine D_2 receptors, although they do have partial affinity for other dopamine receptor subtypes. Phenothiazines compete effectively with dopamine at these sites, thereby decreasing dopamine neural transmission. It is estimated that the phenothiazine dose required to obtain a therapeutic effect must be sufficient to occupy between 70 and 80 percent of D_2 receptors (Seeman & Tallerico, 1998). Dopamine D_2 receptors are found both postsynaptically and as presynaptic autoreceptors in the basal ganglia, the mesolimbic system, the hippocampus, the amygdala, and throughout the cortex. The initial response to phenothiazine treatment is an increase in dopamine synthesis and release because of autoreceptor antagonism. Chronic blockade of the inhibitory D_2 autoreceptors leads to upregulation and a greater sensitivity to the inhibitory effects of the autoreceptors on dopamine synthesis and release. The time course of these neuronal adaptations corresponds with the lag time to the onset of their antipsychotic effects.

The phenothiazines also block norepinephrine α_1 and α_2 receptors, acetylcholine muscarinic receptors, and histamine H_1 receptors to different extents, and many of the undesirable side effects of the phenothiazines are mediated by these receptors.

Side Effects of Phenothiazines

The side effects caused by phenothiazines vary depending upon the extent of receptor involvement. Blockade of norepinephrine α_1 and α_2 receptors results in hypotension, tachycardia, and sedation. Blocking muscarinic receptors causes dry mouth and eyes, dilated pupils, blurred vision, decreased sweating, and memory impairment. Competing with histamine at H_1 receptors contributes to its sedative effects.

The phenothiazines also cause serious and often debilitating motor effects by blocking D_2 receptors in the basal ganglia. These symptoms, referred to as **extrapyramidal symptoms**, resemble the motor impairments seen in Parkinson's disease. Extrapyramidal suggests that these symptoms are caused by disruptions to neurons outside of the major pyramidal tracks descending from the medulla. Long-term treatment with phenothiazines can lead to a more serious motor disorder called **tardive dyskinesia**. Dyskinesia refers to the involuntary movements and motor tics often of the mouth and tongue, and tardive, meaning slow or delayed, comes from the observation that these dyskinesias often continue long after the drug has been discontinued. Unfortunately there is no treatment for tardive dyskinesia other than terminating the use of antipsychotic medication, and even then these disorders may persist. Because of the serious motor disorders caused by long-term treatment with phenothiazines, other drugs have been developed in an attempt to minimize these effects. However, given that the antipsychotic effects and the extrapyramidal effects are both mediated by D_2 receptors, these efforts have been largely frustrated.

Non-Phenothiazine Antipsychotics

Haloperidol (Haldol) was the first non-phenothiazine used for the treatment of psychotic disorders. Although introduced as an antipsychotic in the late 1960s, it wasn't actually approved for this use by the FDA until 1988. The pharmacodynamics of haloperidol are essentially identical to the phenothiazines even though they are not structurally related to them. Haloperidol competes for and blocks dopamine D_2 receptors as effectively as most phenothiazines, so it is an effective antipsychotic, but it also produces the severe extrapyramidal side effects mediated by its effects on dopamine D_2 receptors in the basal ganglia described earlier. Haloperidol's effects on norepinephrine α_1 and α_2 and acetylcholine muscarinic receptors contribute to its autonomic effects, including blurred vision, dizziness, dry mouth and eyes, constipation, and hypotension. Haloperidol has less affinity for histamine H_1 receptors, so sedation is not as problematic as with the phenothiazines.

Several other non-phenothiazines were developed as alternatives to the phenothiazines and to haloperidol in the 1970s, including loxapine, molindone, and pimozide. These drugs are not discussed in detail here, as their mechanisms of antipsychotic action are essentially the same as haloperidol, with the exception that loxapine also competes for and antagonizes serotonin 5-HT_2 receptors. Whether this contributes to its antipsychotic effects is unknown. Because their side effect profiles are also similar to the phenothiazines and haloperidol, they have remained relatively obscure.

New Generation (Atypical) Antipsychotics

The 1990s were celebrated as the *decade of the brain* because of rapid advances in the neurosciences and psychopharmacology. During this decade, a number of novel drugs were developed to treat psychotic disorders without causing serious extrapyramidal side effects. The mechanisms of action of these newer drugs also differed from their predecessors, and for this reason they are referred to as **atypical antipsychotics**. The first atypical antipsychotic introduced in 1990 was clozapine; this was quickly followed by the introduction of several others listed in Table 5.1. The atypical antipsychotics all differ somewhat in their mechanisms of action, but most antagonize dopamine D_2 and serotonin 5-HT_{2A} receptors to varying extents. We will examine several atypical drugs in some detail. Several of the most common antipsychotic drugs are described in Table 5.1.

Clozapine (Clozaril)

Clozapine was the first antipsychotic that appeared to improve the symptoms of schizophrenia without causing severe extrapyramidal (Parkinsonian-like) effects. In addition, clozapine is effective in many patients that don't respond to phenothiazines, and it is known to alleviate the negative symptoms and cognitive deficits that are often observed in schizophrenia.

PHARMACODYNAMICS OF CLOZAPINE

Antipsychotic drugs all differ in their affinities for dopamine receptors, and dopamine D_2 receptors specifically. Drugs that bind more competitively than dopamine itself are not displaced when dopamine is present, while drugs that bind more loosely can be displaced by

Table 5.1 Three major classifications of antipsychotic drugs.

Drug name	Trade name	Half-life hours	Receptor effects
Phenothiazines			
Chlorpromazine	Thorazine	8–33	D_2 antagonism
Fluphenazine	Prolixin	15	D_2 antagonism
Mesoridazine	Serentil	2–9	D_2 antagonism
Perphenazine	Trilafon	9	D_2 antagonism
Prochlorperazine	Compazine	4–6	D_2 antagonism
Thioridazine	Mellaril	7–13	D_2 antagonism
Trifluoperazine	Stelazine	12	D_2 antagonism
Triflupromazine	Vesprin	5	D_2 antagonism
Non-Phenothiazines			
Haloperidol	Haldol	12–38	D_2 antagonism
Loxapine	Loxitane	4	D_2, 5-HT_2 antagonism
Molindone	Moban	1.5	D_2 antagonism
Pimozide	Orap	55	D_2 antagonism
New Generation (Atypical)			
Amisulpride	Solian	12	D_2 antagonism
Aripiprazole	Abilify	75	D_2 partial agonism, 5-HT_{1A} agonism
Clozapine	Clozaril	5–16	D_2, 5-HT_2 antagonism
Paliperidone palmitate	Invega Hafyera	24–49 days	D_2, 5-HT_{2A} antagonism
Olanzapine	Zeprexa	21–54	D_2, 5-HT_2 antagonism
Quetiapine	Seroquel	6–7	D_2, 5-HT_2 antagonism
Risperidone	Risperdal	20–24	D_2, 5-HT_2 antagonism
Ziprasidone	Geodon	6–7	D_2, 5-HT_2 antagonism, 5-HT_{1A} agonist

available dopamine. Furthermore, drugs that bind tightly are all associated with a greater incidence of extrapyramidal side effects than drugs that are less competitive. It appears that when drugs bind tightly to D_2 receptors they disrupt dopamine transmission in the basal ganglia, causing these side effects. Drugs that are less competitive than dopamine in the basal ganglia cause far less disruption to dopamine neurotransmission and cause fewer motor side effects. Because there is relatively less dopamine present in the mesolimbic system, when compared to the basal ganglia, drugs that only bind weakly to D_2 receptors can effectively antagonize dopamine in these structures and induce their antipsychotic effects (Seeman & Tallerico, 1998; Seeman et al., 2006).

Clozapine only competes weakly with dopamine receptors even though it occupies 75–80 percent of D_2 receptors, at least transiently—a level comparable to the phenothiazines and haloperidol, and illustrated in Figure 5.3. Therefore, clozapine can be an effective antipsychotic without causing extrapyramidal side effects (Seeman & Tallerico, 1998). In addition to antagonizing D_2 receptors, clozapine also antagonizes serotonin 5-HT_{2A} receptors. How antagonism at these receptors mediates its antipsychotic effects, if at all, remains unclear. What is known, however, is that dopamine neurons originating in the ventral tegmental area are regulated by excitatory serotonergic activity. Antagonizing these excitatory influences does decrease downstream release of dopamine in the nucleus accumbens (Broderick, 1992). In addition to weak competition with dopamine at dopamine receptors, clozapine may also contribute to decreased dopamine release, thereby enhancing its dopamine antagonistic effects.

SIDE EFFECTS ASSOCIATED WITH CLOZAPINE

Although clozapine remains one of the most widely prescribed antipsychotics, it is not without significant side effects, one of which can be fatal. Clozapine produces considerable sedation in a large proportion of patients. This effect is most likely a result of high occupancy of histamine receptors. In addition, dizziness, hypotension, high heart rate, dry mouth and eyes, and constipation are all common. These effects are also common with phenothiazines and haliperdol and are mediated by activity at noradrenergic α_1 and α_2, acetylcholine muscarinic, and histamine H_1 receptors. Clozapine is also associated with an increased risk of hyperglycemia and diabetes.

The most serious, but rare side effect of clozapine is a condition known as agranulocytosis, which is a life-threatening deficiency of white blood cells. Agranulocytosis occurs in approximately 0.8 percent of patients taking clozapine. It appears to be caused by an intermediate metabolite of clozapine, which causes excessive oxidative stress to white blood cells (Fehsel et al., 2005). Careful monitoring of white cell counts during the first year of treatment is an effective way to detect this condition early enough to avoid serious consequences to immune system function.

Risperidone (Risperdal)

Risperidone was approved by the FDA in 1993 for the treatment of schizophrenia and more recently in 2007 for the treatment of schizophrenia and bipolar disorders in children and adolescents aged 10–18. It has also been approved to treat autism and disruptive behaviors in children. It has been used off label (non-FDA approved uses) to treat depression, obsessive-compulsive disorder, eating disorders, and anxiety disorders.

PHARMACODYNAMICS OF RESPERIDONE

Resperidone, as with clozapine, competitively blocks both dopamine D_2 and serotonin 5-HT_{2A} receptors. In addition, it competes with noradrenergic α_1 and α_2 receptors. At relatively low therapeutic doses, resperidone competes weakly with dopamine and has a low risk of extrapyramidal side effects. However, at higher therapeutic doses, resperidone binds tightly with dopamine D_2 receptors and can cause Parkinsonian motor symptoms (thus its low position on Figure 5.3). For this reason, resperidone may be a first choice for treatment at lower doses or it may be used in combination with clozapine for treatment-resistant patients.

In addition to extrapyramidal side effects, resperidone can cause dizziness, sedation, headache, hypotension, and high heart rate, which are mediated by its noradrenergic effects. Weight gain, hyperglycemia, and an increased risk of diabetes are also side effects. The mechanisms responsible for these later effects remain unknown.

Amisulpride (Solian)

While not yet approved by the FDA, amisulpride has been used in Europe and Australia to treat schizophrenia. Amisulpride has been shown to be as effective as other atypical antipsychotics, such as clozapine and olanzapine; it isn't associated with hyperglycemia and other metabolic side effects, as are the other atypical drugs. In addition, amisulpride has been demonstrated to be more effective in treating depression associated with psychotic symptoms than other atypical agents (S. Kim et al., 2007; Vanelle et al., 2006).

Pharmacodynamics of Amisulpride

Amisulpride is discussed here because its mechanisms of action are unusual when compared to other atypical antipsychotics. Amisulpride is a potent blocker of both D_2 and

D_3 dopamine receptors, but it appears to act preferentially, in low doses, on presynaptic autoreceptors. Unlike other atypical antipsychotics it does not block serotonin $5\text{-}HT_{2A}$ receptors. Blockade of D_2 autoreceptors causes an increase in dopamine synthesis and release in these neurons. Consequently, its antidepressant effects are believed to be mediated by increased dopamine activity, similar to bupropion (Wellbutrin). Amisulpride at low doses is also more effective than other antipsychotic drugs in alleviating negative symptoms (Olié et al., 2006). Amisulpride binds relatively weakly with dopamine receptors in the basal ganglia, and it therefore produces fewer extrapyramidal side effects than traditional antipsychotics (Seeman, 2002). In addition to fewer and less severe extrapyramidal side effects, amisulpride causes less of the weight gain that is problematic with all other atypical antipsychotics.

Because amisulpride is as effective as other atypical antipsychotic drugs without antagonizing serotonin $5\text{-}HT_{2A}$ receptors, the role of serotonin in atypical antipsychotics remains elusive. In animal and human studies, there is no clear relationship between a drug's affinity for serotonin $5\text{-}HT_{2A}$ receptors and extrapyramidal symptoms. In fact, resperidone has a high affinity for serotonin $5\text{-}HT_{2A}$ receptors and is known to produce these symptoms (Nyberg et al., 1999). The most predictive feature of an antipsychotic's propensity to cause extrapyramidal symptoms is how tightly it competes for dopamine D_2 receptors (shown in Figure 5.7) in the basal ganglia (Kapur et al., 2000; Seeman & Tallerico, 1998; Seeman, 2002), not for its affinity for serotonergic or cholinergic receptors.

Pharmacodynamics of Aripiprazole (Abilify)

Aripiprazole (Abilify) is also a unique antipsychotic, in that it has both agonizing and antagonizing effects on dopamine, depending on existing dopamine activity. Aripiprazole was approved by the FDA in 1996 for the treatment of schizophrenia in adults, and in 2007 for adolescents. As we discussed earlier, positive symptoms of schizophrenia are believed to be caused by excessive dopamine activity in the mesolimbic pathway. Traditional

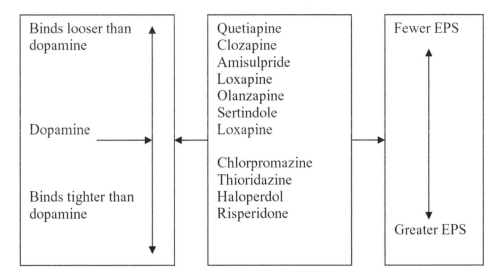

Figure 5.7 Antipsychotic drugs that bind more tightly to dopamine D_2 receptors tend to produce more severe extrapyramidal side effects (EPS) than do drugs that bind more loosely and for shorter durations.

Source: Seeman and Tallerico (1998); Seeman (2002).

antipsychotics decrease this activity by antagonizing, or blocking, most DA_2 receptors. Aripiprazole has dual effects. When dopamine activity is high in schizophrenia it acts to only moderately reduce it, thereby minimizing the motor side effects of traditional antipsychotics. It has this action because although it has high affinity for dopamine receptors it only competes weakly with dopamine, thereby only partially agonizing dopamine receptors. In addition, dopamine activity in the mesocortical system is low in patients with schizophrenia displaying negative symptoms, and Aripiprazole increases DA_2 activity there, again by agonizing DA receptors. A drug with these unique effects is called a **partial agonist**. A partial agonist exerts agonizing effects at receptors, but not as powerfully as the natural ligand. So, with high dopamine concentrations it decreases dopamine activity and at low dopamine concentrations it increases it. Aripiprazole also acts as a 5-HT_{1A} receptor agonist increasing serotonin activity in limbic structures related to mood. Because of this antidepressant action, Aripiprazole may be used in patients who do not respond to traditional antidepressants.

PHARMACODYNAMICS OF PALIPERIDONE PALMITATE (INVEGA HAFYERA)

Paliperidone palmitate (Invega Hafyera) received FDA approval for adults with schizophrenia in 2021. While its mechanisms of action are not completely known, it is believed to act as a D_2 and 5-HT_{2A} receptor antagonist, much like the antipsychotics discussed earlier. Paliperidone palmitate is quickly metabolized into paliperidone, the principal metabolite of risperidone. In clinical trials paliperidone palmitate was found to be equally as effective as risperidone. The principal difference is that paliperidone palmitate has a much longer half-life (24–49 days) compared to risperidone's half-life of about one day. Because of its long half-life paliperidone palmitate is administered by injection only four times per year (Daghistani & Rey, 2016).

Glutamate and Glycine Agonists

A large number of studies have reported that patients with schizophrenia have depressed numbers of NMDA receptors in the thalamus and the hippocampus. It is alleged that glutamate dysfunction in these subcortical regions leads to excitotoxic glutamate activity in the cortex and to the development of negative symptoms in later stages of schizophrenia. Drugs that enhance glutamate activity might therefore be more effective in alleviating negative symptoms and cognitive impairment than dopamine antagonists by themselves (Javitt & Coyle, 2004).

There are several ways to increase glutaminergic NMDA activity. One way would be to directly increase NMDA activity with glutamate agonists. Although a number of these agonists are available for research, increasing glutamate activity generally would likely increase the rate of glutamate excitotoxicity by activating other glutamate receptors. Research has therefore focused on specific NMDA receptor agonists and on glycine, which modulates glutamate effects on NMDA receptors. Both of these pharmacological approaches are being investigated as potential treatments to improve negative symptoms with mixed results. In a review of recent research Tuominen et al. (2006) reported that the NMDA receptor agonist D–cycloserine seemed ineffective in treating negative symptoms, but the glycine receptor agonists glycine and D–serine were just marginally effective. These conclusions were confirmed in the large *Cognitive and Negative Symptoms in Schizophrenia* study recently sponsored by the NIH. In this trial neither glycine nor D–cycloserine were consistently more effective than a placebo in improving negative symptoms in the 157 patients studied (Buchanan et al., 2007).

How Are the Effects of Antipsychotic Drugs Measured?

Animal Research

In animal studies, several models of psychosis have been utilized to investigate the effectiveness of antipsychotic drugs. One of the earliest animal models, **amphetamine-induced psychosis**, was based on the observations of psychotic behavior in amphetamine users. The most prominent symptoms are those that mimic paranoid schizophrenia, and they are typically treated in emergency rooms with phenothiazines. In animal studies, rats or mice are given repeated doses of amphetamine, which causes an increase in the incidence of stereotyped behaviors (repetitive motor movements). At high doses, catatonic states (a waxy flexibility) can be observed, where animals will hold unusual postures for extended periods of time. Both of these behaviors are easily observed and measured in experimental animals. Drugs suspected of having antipsychotic properties can be administered to animals in amphetamine psychosis to test for their effects. All known antipsychotic drugs alleviate amphetamine-induced psychosis in laboratory animals to some extent.

Another animal model, referred to as **prepulse inhibition** (PPI), is also based on abnormalities in the reactions of schizophrenic patients. In this case, however, the observation is that psychotic patients don't appear to filter extraneous stimuli as do normal subjects. This

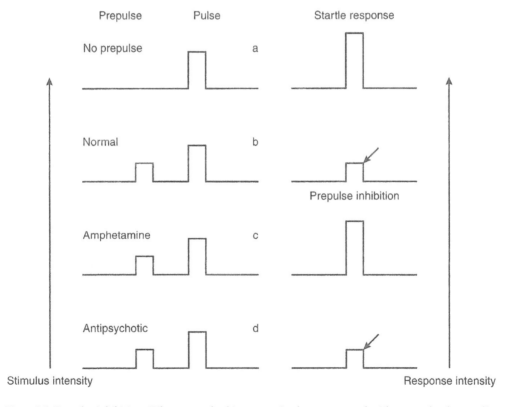

Figure 5.8 Prepulse inhibition. When normal subjects or animals are presented with a prepulse that predicts the pulse stimulus the startle response is inhibited (a–b). Dopamine agonists such as amphetamine disrupt prepulse inhibition, resulting in a larger startle response (c). Antipsychotic medication reinstates prepulse inhibition (d).

may reflect a deficit in sensorimotor gating, which is considered to be the brain's ability to close the gate on irrelevant sensory information. In a prepulse inhibition experiment a subject is presented with a warning stimulus (a prepulse, typically a loud sound) for several milliseconds before being presented with a much more intense stimulus (the pulse). Presentation of the prepulse inhibits the startle response to the pulse in normal subjects, as shown in Figure 5.8. In animal studies, prepulse inhibition can be disrupted by drugs that agonize dopamine, such as amphetamine or cocaine. Disruptions in prepulse inhibition are reversible with antipsychotic medication, making this a useful animal model for drug investigation.

Human Research

Measuring the effects of antipsychotic medication in human experiments is typically done with clinical evaluation scales. For example, the Clinical Global Improvement (CGI) scale requires clinicians to rate the changes observed from a baseline phase to a treatment follow-up stage in three categories: severity of illness, global improvement, and efficacy. Each of these indices is rated by the clinician to obtain a total CGI score. Average CGI scores for different groups of treated patients are then compared to determine relative effectiveness of different treatment protocols. To avoid biases in both patient responses and clinician ratings these studies are often conducted in a double-blind manner where neither the patient nor the clinician knows which medication (or placebo) a patient has received. A number of other scales—including the Positive and Negative Schizophrenia Syndrome Scale for Schizophrenia (PANSS), and the Brief Psychiatric Rating Scale (BPRS)—are also used in a similar manner. Each of these evaluation scales require clinicians to rate the severity of positive and negative symptoms, as well as side effects before and after treatment. Often researchers employ several of these evaluation scales as well as personal observations in their assessment of drug effectiveness.

Although most clinical research utilizes evaluation scales to rate changes in schizophrenia behavior, some studies are beginning to employ more objective measures, including startle responses and sensorimotor gating measured by the prepulse inhibition (PPI) test mentioned earlier. In several recent studies involving patients with schizophrenia, PPI deficits were found to be correlated with symptom severity. That is, patients with more severe symptoms or greater cognitive deficits also had greater deficits in sensorimotor gating (Hazlett et al., 2007; Swerdlow et al., 2006). Other studies are using PPI to compare the effectiveness of antipsychotic medication in patients with schizophrenia (e.g., Kumari et al., 2002, 2007; Mena et al., 2016; Sato, 2020); Wynn et al., 2007). In many of these studies, atypical antipsychotics seem to be more effective than the phenothiazines or haloperidol in reinstating prepulse inhibition. Figure 5.9 shows the results of a carefully conducted study that compared subjects who were taking phenothiazine antipsychotics (e.g., chlorpromazine) with subjects who were matched for age, duration of illness, and rating scores for the severity of negative symptoms who were taking risperidone. The treated groups were also compared to an age-matched group of healthy control subjects. In this study, risperidone (an atypical antipsychotic) was more effective than phenothiazine treatment in restoring PPI to near-normal values. Researchers speculate that PPI restoration is a good predictor of cognitive improvements and decreases in the severity of negative symptoms and might therefore be a valuable test of the effectiveness of newly developed antipsychotic drugs.

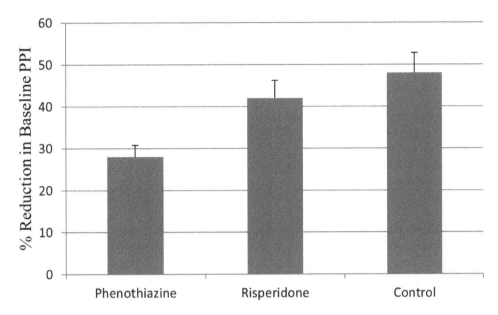

Figure 5.9 Comparison of the effects of risperidone and phenothiazine antipsychotic medication on prepulse inhibition (PPI) in patients with schizophrenia. The bars represent the percentage reduction in eyeblink startle responses over baseline. Larger percent PPI values represent greater prepulse inhibition. Risperidone restores PPI to levels observed in healthy control subjects.

Source: Kumari et al. (2002).

How Effective Is Pharmacological Treatment?

There is little doubt that the majority of patients with schizophrenia improve with medication, particularly with the newer-generation antipsychotics, or combinations of them, that have minimized the serious motor side effects and the sedation caused by the older phenothiazines. Nevertheless, a significant proportion of these patients do not receive additional psychological counseling and psychosocial intervention, as recommended in the *Practice Guideline for the Treatment of Patients with Schizophrenia*, second edition, published by the American Psychiatric Association in 2004. Schizophrenia is a chronic, degenerative brain disease that at the present can only be managed by the careful selection of medication and psychosocial training. While there is no cure for schizophrenia, early detection and pharmacological treatment may slow or even suspend its progression in many patients.

Drug therapy does not work for all patients with schizophrenia, however. Estimates of the proportion of patients who will respond to pharmacological treatment vary between 60 and 85 percent, depending on which drugs were initially prescribed, the duration of illness, and whether additional medication was tried after an initial non-response to treatment. Eventually, between 75 and 85 percent of patients with schizophrenia do respond, at least partially, to medication.

Few viable alternatives to drug treatment for schizophrenia are currently available. Patients who do not respond to pharmacological treatment, or who need immediate intervention, may respond to electroconvulsive therapy (ECT), either alone or in combination with antipsychotic medication. Electroconvulsive therapy remains controversial, but it has been demonstrated to be effective, at least for the short term, for refractory or non-responding patients (Braga & Petrides, 2005; Grover et al., 2019).

Glossary

Amphetamine challenge scanning for radioactive markers of dopamine receptor occupancy following the administration of amphetamine. A measure of dopamine activity in the brain.

Amphetamine-induced psychosis a psychotic state similar to schizophrenia, induced by amphetamine overdose.

Antipsychotic a drug that is used to treat symptoms of schizophrenia and other psychotic disorders.

Atypical antipsychotics antipsychotic drugs that differed in their mechanism of action from their predecessors, the phenothiazines. Clozapine was the first atypical antipsychotic to be widely used.

Dopamine hypothesis excessive dopamine activity in the mesolimbic-cortical systems of the brain underlie schizophrenia and its symptoms.

Electroconvulsive therapy the induction of a severe seizure in a patient by delivering electric shocks to the head. Used as a treatment for drug-resistant schizophrenia and depression.

Extrapyramidal symptoms severe motor impairment following disruptions to neurons outside of the major pyramidal tracks descending from the medulla. These symptoms are often caused by the long-term use of phenothiazine drugs.

Frontal lobotomy separating the prefrontal areas from the remainder of the frontal cortex by knife cuts or by destroying these areas with ice picks inserted behind the eyes. Used as an early treatment for severe psychosis.

Insulin shock a comatose state induced by severe hypoglycemia following an injection of insulin. Used as an early treatment for schizophrenia.

Negative symptoms symptoms of schizophrenia characterized by features removed from normal behavior and functioning. They include lack of affect, social withdrawal, cognitive impairment, and muscle rigidity.

Positive symptoms symptoms of schizophrenia that are characterized by features that are added to normal behavior and functioning. They include delusions, hallucinations, motor symptoms, and emotional turmoil.

Prepulse inhibition the ability to inhibit a startle response to a strong stimulus if given a warning signal or prepulse stimulus. Patients with schizophrenia show deficits in prepulse inhibition.

Receptor competition the ability of a drug to compete with a neurotransmitter for receptor binding is measured by its capacity to displace a radioactive ligand. Used to predict drug effectiveness against schizophrenia symptoms.

Tardive dyskinesia involuntary movements and motor tics, often of the mouth and tongue, observed after long-term phenothiazine use.

6   Attention and Developmental Disorders

Attention-Deficit/Hyperactivity Disorder
and Autism Spectrum Disorder

The attention and neurodevelopmental disorders cover a wide range of conditions that typically emerge during early childhood and in many cases continue through adolescence and adulthood. These disorders include attention-deficit/hyperactivity disorder and autism spectrum disorder, which are discussed in this chapter because many of their symptoms are managed with medication. A number of other psychological disorders discussed in this text (including depression, anxiety, and schizophrenia) may appear during childhood, but they are not generally classified as attention or neurodevelopmental disorders. Other neurodevelopmental disorders, including intellectual disability, language disorder, and social communication disorder, are not discussed in this text.

Attention-Deficit/Hyperactivity Disorder

Attention-deficit/hyperactivity disorders (ADHD) are characterized by a pervasive inability to attend to tasks and are often associated with disruptive and excessive motor activity and impulsivity. Children with ADHD have difficulties maintaining attention, following instructions, or completing tasks. Often they will begin one task, only to be quickly distracted by another, making it difficult to complete or follow through with any. Approximately 8 percent of the child population between the ages of 4 and 17 is diagnosed with ADHD at any given time. Attention disorders affect over 4.5 million children of whom a substantial proportion (over 2.5 million) are taking medication to alleviate their symptoms. Attention disorders are typically first observed in young children as they begin to develop independent locomotion. A diagnosis of ADHD, however, usually occurs in elementary school, where its symptoms begin to interfere with normal functioning. In many cases, ADHD symptoms dissipate in late adolescence or early adulthood. Symptoms of inattentiveness may persist, however, in as many as 50 percent of all cases well into adulthood. Adulthood ADHD frequently co-occurs with other behavioral disorders, including depression, anxiety, conduct disorder, drug abuse, and/or antisocial behavior. Attention disorders may also co-occur with other developmental disorders, including autism and Asperger's disorder. In this chapter, we focus on ADHD but include the diagnostic criteria and pharmacological treatment of these developmental disorders as well.

Josh's parents suspected their child was hyperactive when he was first learning to walk at two years of age. Compared with other children his age, Josh was in constant motion and was little deterred by his numerous falls and altercations with furniture. Like other children, he liked toys, but rarely spent time with any particular one before moving on to the next. It was as if he were merely attempting to grab and relocate a toy rather than actually play with it. Josh was easily irritated with other children and rarely played with them. In the first grade Josh had difficulty attending to reading materials presented by his teacher and he appeared easily frustrated by the experience. He was passed on to second grade without knowing how to read, with the assumption that he was merely slow. At home Josh was getting increasingly demanding of attention from his parents. He couldn't entertain himself and he needed constant supervision to complete

DOI: 10.4324/9781003309017-6

his schoolwork. And even though he was beginning to read in second grade, he would not do it on his own. Josh displayed both behavioral problems and learning difficulties throughout his elementary school years. He ignored the demands of his teachers and behaved aggressively towards other students. His parents assumed he was acting out frustration and insecurity from his family relocating three times during these years.

The diagnosis of ADHD occurred midway through seventh grade when Josh's teacher recommended a psychological evaluation. His school psychologist referred him to a psychiatrist who, after a 20-minute visit, diagnosed him with ADHD and prescribed Ritalin. Josh has been on and off ADHD medication since then. Now in high school, Josh finds little relief from medication. It contributed significantly to insomnia, which only seemed to exacerbate his inattentiveness and ability to concentrate. Josh now worries about whether he will earn good enough grades to attend college. He acts out frustration with his poor performance; he remains disorganized both at home and at school, is easily distracted, and has few friends.

For a diagnosis of an attention disorder using the *DSM-5*, symptoms of either inattention or hyperactivity-impulsivity must be present for a period of at least six months prior to the diagnosis:

A. At least six of the following symptoms of inattention have been present to a point that they are disruptive and inappropriate for the child's developmental level:

1. Often does not give close attention to details or makes careless mistakes in school-work, work, or other activities.
2. Often has trouble keeping attention on tasks or play activities.
3. Often does not seem to listen when spoken to directly.
4. Often does not follow instructions and fails to finish schoolwork, chores, or duties in the workplace (not due to oppositional behavior or failure to understand instructions).
5. Often has trouble organizing activities.
6. Often avoids, dislikes, or doesn't want to do things that take a lot of mental effort for a long period of time (such as schoolwork or homework).
7. Often loses things needed for tasks and activities (e.g., toys, school assignments, pencils, books, or tools).
8. Is often easily distracted.
9. Is often forgetful in daily activities.

B. At least six of the following symptoms of hyperactivity-impulsivity have been present to an extent that they are disruptive and inappropriate for the child's developmental level:

1. Often fidgets with hands or feet, or squirms in seat.
2. Often gets up from seat when remaining in seat is expected.
3. Often runs about or climbs when and where it is not appropriate (adolescents or adults may feel very restless).
4. Often has trouble playing or enjoying leisure activities quietly.
5. Is often "on the go" or often acts as if "driven by a motor."
6. Often talks excessively.
7. Often blurts out answers before questions have been finished.
8. Often has trouble waiting one's turn.
9. Often interrupts or intrudes on others (e.g., butts into conversations or games).
10. Some symptoms that cause impairment were present before age seven.
11. Some impairment from the symptoms is present in two or more settings (e.g., at school/work and at home).
12. There must be clear evidence of significant impairment in social, school, or work functioning.

Pathology of ADHD

While causes of attention-deficit/hyperactivity disorder remain elusive, there appears to be a consistent pattern of cortical **hypoarousal** and an increase in **theta activity** in ADHD patients when compared to normal children and adolescents. Electroencephalagraph (EEG) studies, such as the one shown in Figure 6.1, typically find a higher theta/**beta activity** ratio among ADHD subjects than in normal subjects, which is consistent with cortical hypoarousal, particularly in the frontal and cingulate cortices (Dickstein et al., 2006; Martella et al., 2020; Rowe et al., 2005; Snyder & Hall, 2006; Zang et al., 2007). Cortical hypoarousal would account for poor attentiveness and concentration as well as behavioral hyperactivity.

Imaging studies (fMRI) also find decreases in thalamic sensory activity, suggesting abnormalities in the **reticular activating system**. Decreases in cholinergic input to the **sensory thalamus** and to the **thalamic reticular nucleus** may contribute to cortical hypoarousal and an EEG pattern that is uncharacteristic of the normal beta-predominant pattern observed during wakefulness (see Figure 6.2). Corticothalamic projections from the frontal cortex back to the TRN are believed to underlie **attentional regulation** (Zikopoulos & Barbas, 2006) and may also be hypoactive in ADHD. These findings may account for the difficulties ADHD patients have in attending to objects or tasks for extended periods of time. Stimuli or tasks that would normally arouse the cortex via the thalamocortical pathway are apparently inhibited by the thalamic reticular nucleus (TRN). During normal wakefulness, cholinergic input to the TRN disinhibits the **attentional gate** allowing for cortical arousal. In ADHD the attentional gate is essentially closed and the cortex remains under aroused (see Figure 6.2).

Research also indicates that children with ADHD may express delayed cortical maturation when compared to age-matched controls. In a large study conducted at the National Institute of Mental Health, researchers using magnetic resonance imaging compared cortical thickness in 223 children with ADHD with 223 normal controls. While these groups showed similar developmental patterns in their primary sensory cortices, there were significant differences

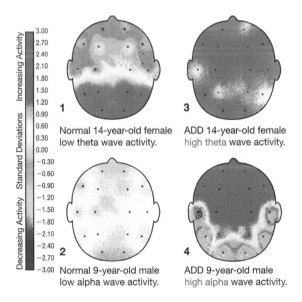

Figure 6.1 Quantitative EEG (Q-EEG) patterns from normal and ADHD-affected children. Excessive slow wave activity (alpha and theta activity) is characteristic of ADHD.

Source: Reproduced with permission from Jay Gunkelman (2014).

in cortical thickness in remaining cerebral areas. These deficits were most pronounced in the prefrontal regions of ADHD patients (Shaw et al., 2007). What is presently unknown is whether delayed cortical maturation is a result of cortical hypoarousal or the cause of it.

Stimulant drugs appear to normalize cortical activity by increasing beta activity and decreasing slower wave **alpha** and theta activity in the frontal cortices (Loo et al., 2004; Pliszka, 2007; Song et al., 2005). These effects are most evident in ADHD subjects who respond well to stimulant medication. Stimulant drugs may act directly on catecholamine pathways within the frontal and cingulate cortices, by facilitating ascending cholinergic activity to the thalamus, or by both of these mechanisms.

Decreased activity in the brain's arousal systems and their targets in cortical areas often appear contradictory to the hyperactive and impulsive symptoms observed with ADHD. That is, how could an individual with hyperactivity be under aroused? While it has been suggested that cortical hypoarousal is causally related to inattention and distractibility, hyperactivity and impulsivity, on the other hand, may be attempts by patients to increase neural arousal by engaging in ADHD-typical behaviors, including self-stimulation and attention-seeking (Antrop et al., 2000; White, 1999). The excessive appearance of these behaviors typifies ADHD.

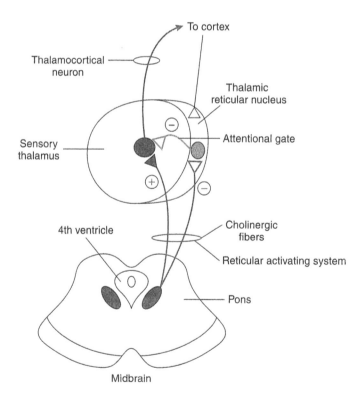

Figure 6.2 Cholinergic neurons originating in the pons project to both the sensory thalamus and to the thalamic reticular nucleus (TRN). During normal wakefulness, projections to the sensory thalamus facilitate thalamocortical activity, while projections to the TRN disinhibit the inhibitory influence the TRN has over the sensory thalamus (inhibition of inhibition = facilitation). The effect is to open the "attentional gate," allowing sensory input to reach and arouse the cortex. In ADHD, the reticular activating system is hypoactive, resulting in the inhibition of the sensory thalamus. Projections from the thalamus to the cortex are therefore inhibited, contributing to cortical hypoarousal and a more synchronized EEG pattern characterized by abnormal theta activity.

Dopamine Deficit Theory of ADHD

The **dopamine deficit theory** of ADHD proposes that depressed dopamine activity in the caudate nucleus and frontal cortices may contribute to cortical hypoarousal. Research from a variety of studies provides evidence for an increased expression of the dopamine transporter in ADHD patients (Chun et al., 2019; Swanson et al., 2007; Volkow et al., 2007). Specifically, studies using radioactive ligands for the dopamine transporter have found increased DAT numbers in ADHD patients in the caudate nucleus when compared to matched control subjects. As illustrated in Figure 6.3, these differences were not observed in the putamen, however (Spencer et al., 2007). The **dopamine transporter (DAT)** plays a key role in regulating dopamine activity throughout the brain by determining synaptic dopamine availability. An increase in DAT expression in the caudate nucleus and frontal cortices is believed to diminish dopamine availability and receptor activity in ADHD. Depressed dopamine activity is presumed to contribute to cortical hypoarousal and inattention.

Measuring ADHD Severity and Improvement

Like other psychological disorders, ADHD cannot be objectively measured, so clinicians and researchers need to rely on psychological evaluation to determine its severity and whether treatments are effective. It is important for students and researchers alike to understand just how this research is conducted to better evaluate treatment effectiveness.

Perhaps one of the most widely used assessment scales for measuring treatment outcomes for ADHD is the Connor's Global Index (CGI) scale. The Connor's scale comes in several different forms, including assessments to be used by parents and teachers. A subscale of the Global Index (CGI-ADHD) is typically used to assess changes in ADHD specifically and is based on the *DSM-IV* diagnostic criteria. Like psychological evaluations discussed in previous chapters, the CGI requires raters to judge the severity or frequency of an assortment of symptoms and behaviors. Figure 6.4 shows a representative comparison of treatment outcomes as measured by the Connor's ADHD subscale. In this study, 128 patients aged 6–14 participated. These subjects were randomly assigned to receive either Ritalin or a placebo for two weeks. Baseline

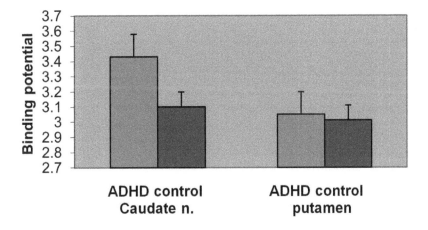

Figure 6.3 Dopamine transporter (DAT) binding. Increased dopamine transporter (DAT) expression (means and SE) in the caudate nucleus but not in the putamen in 21 ADHD patients compared to 26 matched control subjects.

Source: Data derived from Spencer et al. (2007).

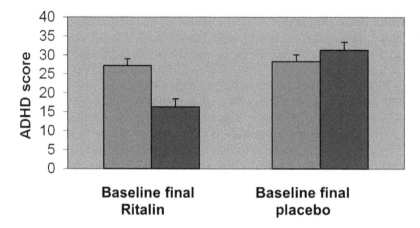

Figure 6.4 The effects of Ritalin vs. placebo on Connor's ADHD rating scores (means and standard errors). Ritalin significantly reduced symptom severity from a pretreatment baseline to the final treatment at 14 days. Scores slightly worsened for the placebo group.

Source: Data summarized from Biederman et al. (2003).

ADHD scores were assessed by the Connor's ADHD scale before treatment commenced and again after the final treatment at 14 days. In this comparison Ritalin significantly reduced symptom severity, while the placebo had no discernable effect. Other psychological assessment scales are used to evaluate ADHD, and they tend to reveal similar results.

A more objective assessment involves either fMRI or EEG to measure changes in cortical activity following treatment. The costs and limited availability of these methods, however, often restrict their use to smaller research studies at major research institutions.

Pharmacological Treatment of ADHD

Amphetamines and Methylphenidate

In 1999, the National Institute of Mental Health (NIMH) published its findings from a 14-month study of treatment options for ADHD. A major conclusion from this study was that treatments that included stimulant medication were far superior to intensive behavioral treatment or community-based treatment alone. In addition, children treated with medication (either alone or in combination with intensive behavioral therapy) showed greater improvements in academic performance and social skills than children in the non-medicated comparison groups. The use of stimulant medication is now widely considered to be vital to an effective treatment program, even in younger children. Concerns about the potential risks of stimulant abuse and increases in substance abuse appear to be unwarranted. In fact, drug abuse risk appears to decrease among stimulant-treated ADHD patients compared to their non-treated cohorts (Faraone et al., 2007). Because an increase in substance abuse risk is associated with ADHD, these findings are particularly noteworthy, since they reveal stimulant medication may actually protect against later drug abuse.

Amphetamines have been used for the treatment of ADHD since the early 1930s. These stimulant drugs include dextro-amphetamine (Dexadrine), dextro/levo-amphetamine (Adderall), and the most recently approved amphetamine for ADHD, lisdexamfetamine (Vyvanse).

The dextro-amphetamine isomer is the main compound and active ingredient in Adderall and Vyvanse, which contain other amphetamine structural isomers.

Methylphenidate (Ritalin) and dexmethylphenidate (Focalin) are also stimulant drugs that are virtually indistinguishable in their effects from the amphetamines. Daytrana, a methylphenidate, is only available as a skin patch to provide slower, extended release, as well as to reduce abuse potential. Research comparing the effectiveness of amphetamines and methylphenidates reveal little differences in their effectiveness or side effect profiles. Both of these classes of drugs are available in rapid and extended-release formulations. At the time of writing, methylphenidate and other amphetamine compounds accounted for over 90 percent of the prescription medication for ADHD.

MECHANISMS OF AMPHETAMINE AND METHYLPHENIDATE ACTION

Amphetamines (including methamphetamine to be discussed later) have perhaps some of the most complex and wide-ranging synaptic effects of any psychoactive drug (see Figure 6.5). They increase synaptic concentrations of both norepinephrine and dopamine by several distinct mechanisms. First of all, amphetamines block **reuptake transporters** for norepinephrine as well as increase the amount of NE released into the synapse. Both of these effects contribute to enhanced NE activity in both the brain and the peripheral nervous system.

Amphetamines also contribute to increased dopamine activity by several different mechanisms. Amphetamines bind to the vesicular transporter and cause dopamine to be released from its storage vesicles into the cytoplasm of the terminal button. This "free" dopamine is then transported into the synaptic cleft by amphetamine-induced reversal of the dopamine transporter (DAT). Amphetamines also increase the amount of dopamine released from synaptic vesicles during neuronal signaling. These combined mechanisms enhance extra cellular concentrations of dopamine significantly.

The mechanisms by which amphetamines contribute to cortical arousal in ADHD appear to be complex as well. Dopamine contributes to cortical arousal via the mesocortical pathway originating in the nucleus accumbens (see Figure 6.6). Increased NE activity contributes to cortical arousal via the reticular activating system originating in the **locus coeruleus** (see Figure 6.7). The relative contributions of these systems to ADHD remain unknown; however, as discussed in the previous section, depressed dopamine activity in the caudate nucleus and the prefrontal cortices are presumed to play important roles in ADHD symptoms. Amphetamines may act to increase and stabilize this activity.

SIDE EFFECTS OF AMPHETAMINE AND METHYLPHENIDATE

While the amphetamines remain the treatment of choice for ADHD and narcolepsy, they are not without significant side effects. The most noticeable effects are insomnia, nervousness, irritability, weight loss, and dizziness. Because amphetamines enhance noradrenergic activity peripherally as well as centrally, they may also cause hypertension, tachycardia, and cardiac arrhythmias. In excessive doses or overdose amphetamines are known to induce psychotic states, seizures, and cardiac failure. While these effects may seem extreme, the most common side effects with prescribed doses are well managed by dosing early in the day and by using slower release formulations or transdermal patches.

In 2003–2005, several studies were released suggesting that methylphenidate (Ritalin) might be associated with an increase in cancer (El-Zein et al., 2005). However, larger follow-up studies conducted in Germany found no such association (Walitza et al., 2007). Methylphenidate was also implicated in delayed growth in children, but again, researchers investigating this alleged side effect monitored 229 children for two years and found no evidence for delayed

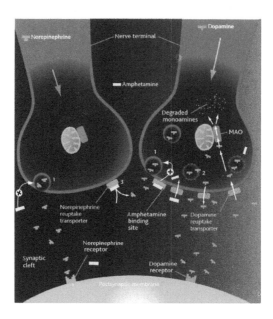

Figure 6.5 Amphetamines (including methamphetamine) increase the availability of dopamine in several distinct ways, including (1) by binding to the presynaptic membrane of dopaminergic and noradrenergic neurons, which increases the release of both norepinephrine and dopamine from synaptic vesicles; (2) by causing the transporters for dopamine to act in reverse, transporting vesicular dopamine back into the terminal and to transport this "free" dopamine into the synaptic cleft; and (3) by blocking the reuptake transporter for norepinephrine.

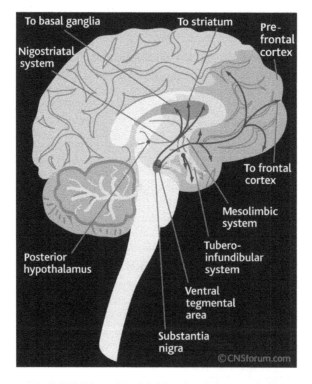

Figure 6.6 Dopamine pathways originate in the substantia nigra and ventral tegmental area of the pons. The nigrostriatal system innervates the basal ganglia while the mesolimbic-cortical system projects to the nucleus accumbens and to the frontal cortex.

growth or maturation (Wilens et al., 2005). Methylphenidate continues to be the most widely prescribed drug for ADHD, but because of the stigma associated with stimulant use, and its alleged potential for abuse, physicians and parents are seeking alternatives.

Alternatives to Amphetamine and Methylphenidate for ADHD

Several effective alternatives to amphetamines are now available for treating ADHD, including atomoxetine (Strattera) and modafinil (Provigil). While both of these drugs are promoted as non-stimulants, they do resemble the amphetamines in that they block reuptake transporters for norepinephrine and dopamine, and they do promote wakefulness and increases in activity (Madras et al., 2006). Specifically, modafinil (Provigil) appears to increase norepinephrine and dopamine activity in the brainstem and forebrain areas that regulate sleep and promote wakefulness (Wisor & Eriksson, 2005). Recent research suggests that modafinil may activate hypothalamic centers that regulate sleep–wake cycles by inducing orexin release (Kim et al., 2007b; Rao et al., 2007). Orexin is an excitatory neuromodulator that regulates the activity of catecholamine brainstem nuclei involved in arousal. Modafinil appears to promote alertness by increasing histamine release in the **tuberomammillary nucleus** of the hypothalamus. His- tamine activity in the hypothalamus is known to regulate sleep and wakefulness by activating hypothalamic nuclei involved in arousal. Increasing histamine activity contributes to wakeful- ness, while histamine blockade causes drowsiness and sedation. The potent sleep-promoting effect of antihistamines is well known.

Modafinil is approved for narcolepsy and excessive sleepiness associated with sleep apnea and shift-work sleep disruptions. Its off-label use for ADHD is supported by several studies,

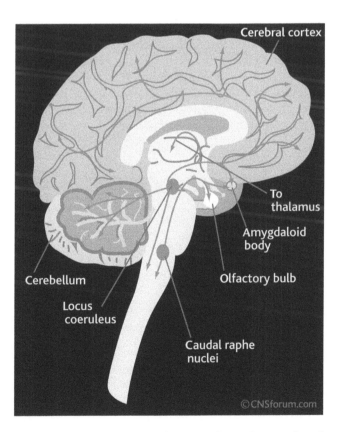

Figure 6.7 Norepinephrine pathways originate in the locus coeruleus and project along the reticular activating system to the frontal cortex.

including comparison studies with methylphenidate. For example, Amiri et al. (2008) found modafinil to be as effective as methylphenidate in reducing ADHD symptoms with fewer side effects. Subjects taking modafinil reported better appetites and fewer sleep difficulties than those taking methylphenidate. Other side effects associated with modafinil included headache, nervousness, agitation, dry mouth, and hypertension—all similar to the amphetamines and methylphenidate.

Atomoxetine (Strattera) is a catecholamine agonist that selectively blocks reuptake transporters for norepinephrine. It may also increase dopamine activity in the frontal cortex indirectly. Originally developed as an antidepressant, atomoxetine was tested for efficacy in ADHD patients because of its effects on norepinephrine transporters. A number of studies have found atomoxetine to be as effective as methylphenidate or more effective than placebos in well-designed studies. Meta-analyses of research also conclude that atomoxetine is effective in treating ADHD (Cheng et al., 2007; Fu et al., 2022). While atomoxetine is promoted as a non-stimulant, its agonizing effects on norepinephrine activity, as well as its side effect profile, resemble amphetamine and methylphenidate. Its most notable side effects include gastrointestinal discomfort, decreased appetite, insomnia, agitation, increased heart rate, and hypertension. A comparison of 120 atomoxetine- and 114 placebo-treated patients using the Connor's ADHD rating scale is presented in Figure 6.8. As shown, atomoxetine significantly reduced ADHD symptoms after 14 days of treatment. Several commonly prescribed drugs for ADHD are described in Table 6.1.

Autism Spectrum Disorder

Autism spectrum disorder described in *DSM-5* now includes Asperger's disorder and Rett disorder—a rare genetic condition that only occurs in females. Individuals previously (pre-*DSM-5*) diagnosed with Asperger's disorder would now be diagnosed with autism spectrum disorder without language or intellectual impairment. Considerable debate continues among clinicians and researchers about whether these are distinct conditions with different underlying pathology or whether they represent an autism continuum with Asperger's disorder, being a less severe and more functional appearance of autism. It now appears that together the autism disorders may affect as many as 90–110 in every 10,000 children (Kogan et al., 2009). Autism spectrum disorder occurs about four times more frequently in males than in females. The reason for the wide variation in prevalence estimates appears to be related to inconsistencies

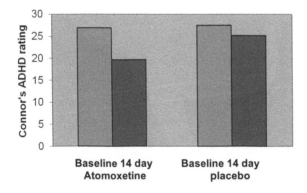

Figure 6.8 Changes in ADHD symptoms. Comparison of atomoxetine and placebo treatment on Connor's ADHD evaluation scores. Atomoxetine significantly reduced ADHD symptoms relative to placebo controls.

Source: Data from Spencer et al. (2002).

Table 6.1 Commonly prescribed drugs for treating ADHD.

Drug name	Trade names	Mechanisms of action
Amphetamine	Dexadrine, Adderall, Vyvanse	Increases both NE and DA availability in synapse by multiple mechanisms
Methylphenidate	Ritalin, Metadate, Concerta, Daytrana	Increases both NE and DA availability in synapse by blocking reuptake transporters
Dexmethylphenidate	Focalin	Increases both NE and DA availability in synapse by blocking reuptake transporters
Atomoxetine	Strattera	Increases NE activity by selectively blocking NE reuptake transporters
Modafinil	Provigil	Increases NE activity in hypothalamus by blocking reuptake transporter; increases orexin release in hypothalamus; increases histamine release in tuberomammillary neurons
Premoline	Cylert	(Discontinued in 2005 because of liver toxicity)

Note: Other drugs may be used in addition to those mentioned here to address specific symptoms that may co-occur with ADHD. These may include antidepressants, anxiolytics, and in some cases antipsychotics.

in survey methods, the use of different diagnostic criteria, and whether children with low IQ are included in the estimate.

Autism disorder was first named in 1943 by Leo Kramer, who identified a group of 11 children with the condition **early infantile autism**. At about the same time, Hans Asperger, an Austrian physician, used the term **autistic psychopath** in his description of what was known as Asperger's disorder. Prior to the use of these terms, autism and Asperger's disorders fell into categories of mental retardation and **infantile schizophrenia**.

The first symptoms of these disorders are most often observed by parents who notice a marked lack of responsiveness to others or objects, a tendency to withdraw from social interaction, and a lack of verbal and nonverbal communication. In many cases, these children engage in repetitive and self-abusive behaviors. While autistism spectrum disorder may co-occur with other developmental disorders, including mental retardation and growth abnormalities, these conditions are not required for a diagnosis.

According to the diagnostic criteria (*DSM-5*) the following indicators must be present for a diagnosis of autistism spectrum disorder:

A. Persistent deficits in social communication and social interaction as manifested by the following:

   1. Deficits in social-emotional reciprocity, exemplified by failures in back-and-forth communication, or failures to respond to social interactions.
   2. Deficits in nonverbal communicative behaviors used for social interaction. For example, abnormalities in eye contact, lack of appropriate facial expression, and misunderstanding of body language.
   3. Deficits in developing and maintaining relationships. This could be exemplified by an absence of interest in peers or making friends.

B. Restricted, repetitive patterns of behavior, activities, or interests:

   1. Stereotyped or repetitive motor movements.
   2. Insistence on sameness, inflexible routines, and ritualized patterns of behavior.

3. Highly restricted, fixated interests that are abnormal in intensity or focus.
4. Hyper- or hyporeactivity to sensory input or unusual interest in sensory aspects of the environment.

Jeffery appeared to be perfectly normal in every way until he was about two and a half years old. While other children his age were learning to speak, he was becoming more and more withdrawn. His parents assumed he was having hearing problems because he reacted very little to their commands or attempts to engage him verbally. By three years of age Jeffery's behavior was becoming more and more concerning. He would clutch a toy, showing no interest in others given to him and he rarely responded to attempts by his parents to play. Attempts by his brother, who was a year and a half older, to engage in play were also rejected by withdrawal or outburst of anger. While his older brother could be entertained by television, Jeffery didn't even appear to realize that it was on. He could sit for long periods, content to manipulate a moving part on a small toy while rocking back and forth. Abrupt noises or appearances of others would often cause Jeffery to react strongly, as if he were suddenly surprised anyone else was present. Tests of his hearing were conducted with great difficulty and followed by a referral to a child psychiatrist. Jeffery was determined to have normal hearing, but was diagnosed with autism spectrum disorder at the age of four.

Jeffery displays several characteristic abnormalities of autism disorder. He shows a total lack of verbal communication, a deficit in emotionality, no ability to interact or connect with his peers, and stereotypy in his motor movements. The prognosis for Jeffery is poor, as he will likely present abnormalities in language usage and emotionality for much of his life. Treatment will include various attempts at behavior modification to teach him personal hygiene and minimal social skills. Medication for his agitation and bouts of depression will also be used. As Jeffery enters his teenage years he will become increasingly aware of his condition and just how different he is from other kids his age. The painful recognition that he is socially awkward as well as his developing sexuality will likely lead to a deterioration of his condition. Outbursts of aggression will increase to express his increasing frustration and to combat the hurtful comments and gestures offered by his classmates.

Pathology of Autism Spectrum Disorder

While the causes of autism spectrum disorder remain elusive, perhaps some of the most consistent pathological correlates of this disorder are **cortical underconnectivity** and deficits in both functioning and volume of the anterior cingulate cortex. The theory of cortical underconnectivity proposes that autism is a result of deficits in **white matter** that makes up the cortical circuits that integrate intrahemispheric connections. These integrative circuits are essential for normal cognitive and social functioning, which require the integration of activity from a variety of cortical structures involved in social, language, problem solving, and decision-making functions (Barnea-Goraly et al., 2004; Just et al., 2012; McAlonan et al., 2004; Silk et al., 2006; Verly et al., 2014). For instance, a number of studies comparing individuals with autism with normal subjects have reported less connectivity and synchronized activity in left temporal areas involved in language comprehension in autism. Using fMRI, Just et al. (2004, 2012) found that patients with autism showed less activity in the left inferior frontal gyrus (Broca's area) but more activity in the left posterior superior temporal gyrus (Wernicke's area) while engaged in sentence-comprehension tasks (Figure 6.9). For example, subjects were asked to read a sentence displayed on a computer monitor and then were asked to respond by identifying the recipient of action.

Example of sentence-comprehension task:

The cook thanked the father.
Who was thanked? Cook or father?

A Autism group

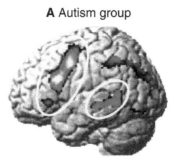

B Control group

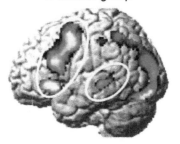

Sentence Comprehension

Figure 6.9 Brain activity measured by fMRI in autism and normal control subjects during a sentence-comprehension task. Subjects with autism (A) showed less activity in the left inferior frontal gyrus but
more activation in the left superior temporal gyrus (circled areas) than control subjects (B).

Source: Image from Just et al. (2004).

Additionally, these authors found that activation between these language areas was less
temporally synchronized in individuals with autism during comprehension tasks. That is,
there was a significant delay in cortical activation during the comprehension tasks when
compared to subjects without autism. Functional underconnectivity is presumed to account
for that wide range of deficits observed in autism—including language comprehension,
judgment, and social cognition—which require the integration and temporal synchronization of activity from several cortical areas. Deficits in the development of myelination
throughout the corpus callosum and the cortex are presumed to underlie autism disorder
(Chen et al., 2022)

In addition to underconnectivity, autism disorders are also associated with abnormalities in
the corpus callosum, which connects the left and right cortical hemispheres. The **corpus callosum** is a band of approximately 200 million interconnecting myelinated axons that unite left
and right cortical areas, as well as intrahemispheric regions. A number of studies have reported
reductions in corpus callosum size, particularly in the anterior (genu) and posterior (splenium)
regions (see Figure 6.10), in autism (Barnea-Goraly et al., 2004; Hardan et al., 2000; Hughes,
2007; Just et al., 2007, 2014). It has been proposed that this reduction constrains functional
connectivity within and across cortical regions. A moderate correlation between genu area
and functional connectivity between frontal and parietal areas supports this hypothesis (see
Figure 6.11).

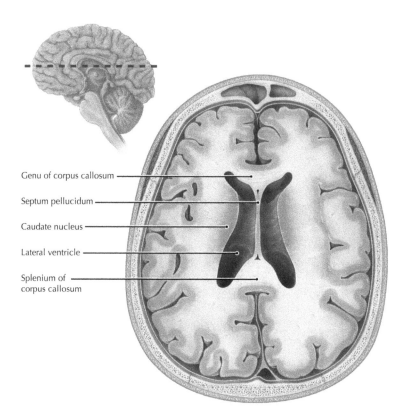

Figure 6.10 Horizontal section through the human brain revealing the corpus callosum. The anterior genu and posterior splenium are significantly reduced in size in individuals with autism.

Underconnectivity may be linked to a deficit in the protein **neuregulin**, which signals Schwann cells to myelinate axons. Myelination is critical for normal signaling within the brain and is a major determinant of signal velocity. Throughout the nervous system myelin maintains a constant thickness ratio to axon diameter (Michailov et al., 2004). The timing and duration of neuregulin signaling is therefore critical for normal myelination. It has been proposed that deficits in neuregulin signaling may lead to under-myelination in autism (Yoo et al., 2015).

Pharmacological Treatment of Autism Spectrum Disorders

Unlike other disorders discussed in this text, autism disorder is not believed to be a consequence of abnormal synaptic activity or neuronal communication. Therefore, the development of pharmacological interventions has been frustrated. However, there has been a recent interest in a number of clinical studies suggesting that pure **cannabidiol** (CBD-a non-intoxicating cannabinoid found in marijuana) may be effective in treating autism as well as co-occurring symptoms, including anxiety, hyperactivity, seizures, and/or severe behavioral agitation (Bilge & Ekici, 2021; Fleury-Teixeira et al., 2019; Fusar-Poli et al., 2020). At the time of this writing researchers had not yet identified the mechanisms of CBD action which improve autism symptoms and the FDA had not approved the use of CBD for autism. Cannabinoids are discussed in more detail in Chapter 9.

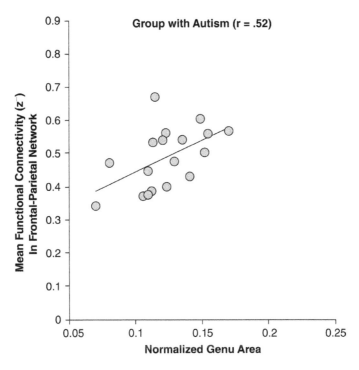

Figure 6.11 Moderate positive correlation between the size of the genu of the corpus callosum and functional connectivity between the frontal and parietal areas.

Source: Just et al. (2007).

Table 6.2 Drugs used off label to treat symptoms accompanying autism spectrum disorder.

Drug name	Trade name	Behavioral symptoms	Classification
Methylphenidate	Ritalin	inattention, hyperactivity	stimulant
Lorazepam	Ativan	hyperactivity, anxiety	anxiolytic, hypnotic
Diazepam	Valium	hyperactivity, anxiety	anxiolytic, hypnotic
Fluoxetine	Prozac	pediatric depression, anxiety, OCD	antidepressant
Fluoxamine	Luvox	depression, anxiety, OCD	antidepressant
Sertraline	Zoloft	depression, anxiety, OCD	antidepressant
Clomipramine	Anafranil	depression, anxiety, OCD	antidepressant
Haloperidol	Haldol	psychosis, behavioral agitation, tics	antipsychotic
Risperidone	Risperdal	psychosis, behavioral agitation, mania	antipsychotic
Olanzapine	Zyprex	psychosis, behavioral agitation, mania	antipsychotic
Carbamazepine	Tegretol	bipolar depression, seizures, mania	antimanic, antiseizure
Lamotrigine	Lamictal	bipolar depression, seizures, mania	antimanic, antiseizure
Topiramate	Topamax	pediatric seizures, migraine	antiseizure
Valproate	Depakote	seizures, migraine	antiseizure

The co-occurring conditions often associated with autism are typically managed with drugs that have been approved for other psychological disorders and are therefore used off label (a non-FDA-approved use) for autism disorder. A list of drugs that are commonly prescribed along with the behavioral symptoms they effectively manage is presented in Table 6.2. All of these drugs are described in some detail in other chapters, so their mechanisms of action will not be discussed here.

Glossary

Alpha activity defined as EEG activity between 8 and 12 Hz characteristic of a relaxed or meditative state.

Attention-deficit/hyperactivity disorder a disorder characterized by difficulties in attention to tasks, excessive motor activity, and impulsivity. Often diagnosed in early childhood but may persist into adulthood.

Attentional gate the inhibitory influence of the thalamic reticular nucleus to regulate sensory information along the thalamocortical pathway.

Attentional regulation the process whereby cortical input to the thalamus filters and allows attention to specific sensory information.

Autistic psychopath term first used by Hans Asperger to describe what is now known as Asperger's disorder.

Autism spectrum disorders these include autism disorder, Asperger's disorder, and Rett's disorder.

Beta activity desynchronized EEG activity ranging between 13 and 30 Hz typical of the normal aroused state.

Cannabidiol (CBD) a non-intoxicating cannabinoid found in marijuana

Corpus callosum a band of approximately 200 million interconnecting myelinated axons that unite left and right cortical areas as well as intrahemispheric regions.

Cortical underconnectivity deficits in white matter that make up the cortical circuits that integrate inter and intrahemispheric connections.

Dopamine deficit theory depressed dopamine activity in the caudate nucleus and frontal cortices may contribute to cortical hypoarousal in ADHD.

Dopamine transporter (DAT) proteins on the presynaptic membrane that selectively transport extracellular dopamine back into the terminal button. Responsible for dopamine reuptake.

Early infantile autism term first used by Leo Kramer in 1943 to describe what is now known as autism.

Hypoarousal a decrease in cortical arousal characterized by an increase in slow wave alpha and theta activity observed with an electroencephalograph (EEG).

Infantile schizophrenia a term used under the original classification scheme proposed by Eugen Bleuler to characterize autism.

Locus coeruleus a nucleus of noradrenergic cell bodies located in the pons near the fourth ventricle.

Neuregulin a protein that signals Schwann cells for axon myelination.

Reticular activating system a system of neurons originating in the reticular formation of the brainstem projecting to the thalamus and cortex. The reticular activating system is involved in attention and cortical arousal.

Reuptake transporters proteins on the presynaptic membrane that transfer neurotransmitter substances in the synaptic gap back into the terminal button.

Sensory thalamus regions of the thalamus that receive sensory information and project it to the cortex via the thalamocortical pathway.

Thalamic reticular nucleus outer cortex of the thalamus that regulates the sensory thalamus and activity along the thalamocortical pathway. Functions as an "attentional gate" by allowing or inhibiting sensory input to the cortex.

Theta activity cortical EEG activity in the range of 3.5–7.5 Hz often observed during the early stages of sleep.

Tuberomammillary nucleus a nucleus of histaminergic cell bodies located in the ventral surface of the hypothalamus. Believed to be involved in cortical arousal.

White matter large groups of fast-conducting myelinated axons that interconnect regions of the brain. Often compared to gray matter, which consists of unmyelinated neurons. Inside of the brain the white myelinating matter consists of a kind of glial cell called an oligodendrocyte. Outside of the brain, in the spinal cord, this myelinating glia is called a Schwann cell.

7   The Pharmacology of Opiates and Analgesia

The Opiates: Opium, Morphine, Heroin, and Codeine

The use of **opium** (Figure 7.1) can be traced back at least to 4500 BC, when early Egyptian images and Sumerian texts depict its use both medicinally and for religious or ritualistic purposes. Its use as a potent analgesic is described in several early medical texts, including the original Egyptian text, the Papyrus, written in approximately 1600 BC. The use of unprocessed opium as an analgesic continued throughout the world through much of the nineteenth century.

Opium was largely discontinued only after **morphine**, its main active compound, was isolated in 1805 by the German chemist Friedrich Sertürner, who named it after Morpheus, the Greek god of dreams. With its isolation, and the invention of the hypodermic syringe in the mid-1800s, morphine quickly emerged as a popular and effective analgesic for surgical pain, as a cough suppressant, and to treat fevers and diarrhea. Even 150 years after its commercial introduction, morphine continues to be the most valuable postsurgical analgesic available, in spite of efforts to identify even more effective and less addictive compounds. One such attempt resulted in a compound known as diacetylmorphine, which was heavily marketed in 1898 by Bayer pharmaceuticals under the brand name **Heroin** (see Figures 7.2 and 7.3).

The availability of opium and heroin in the late 1800s and early 1900s led to a significant increase in opiate addiction worldwide. In 1914, the **Harrison Narcotic Act** was passed as one attempt to begin to regulate the manufacture and distribution of opiates and cocaine, which was mischaracterized as a narcotic by this legislation. The Harrison Narcotic Act effectively eliminated any legal source for opiates for all nonmedical uses. In fact, in its original interpretation, the Narcotic Act even prohibited prescribing controlled amounts of heroin to patients who were in treatment programs. Neither the Narcotic Act, nor its successor the **Controlled Substance Act**, however, has done much to curtail the illicit importation and distribution of heroin in the United States.

Pharmacology of the Opiates

The pharmacologically active compounds in opium are principally morphine, **codeine**, and thebaine alkaloids. **Alkaloids** are nitrogen-containing natural compounds that are produced by a variety of plants. In fact, most of the psychoactive compounds discussed in this chapter and the next are alkaloids or they are derived from them. The relationships between the natural alkaloids of opium are illustrated in Figure 7.4. In addition to natural opiate alkaloids, a number of synthetic opiate compounds have been produced as potent analgesics (see Table 7.1). The term **opiate** refers to any natural derivative of opium, as well as all

DOI: 10.4324/9781003309017-7

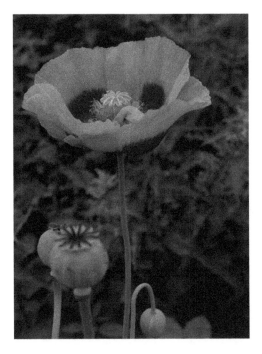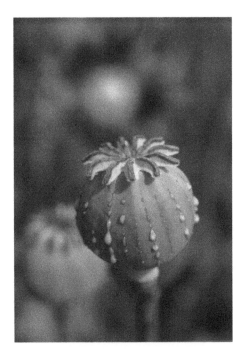

Figure 7.1 Pink flowers of the opium poppy Papaver somniferum, largely grown in Afghanistan, India, and Mexico. The milky latex sap (opium) extracted from immature seed pods contains morphine and codeine, which can easily be transformed into heroin.

endogenous compounds that bind to opiate receptors. **Opioids** are synthetic compounds that mimic the effects of opiates. Many useful analgesics are opioids. A common opioid is the synthetic fentanyl (Duragesic, Abstral, and Subsys are brand names). Fentanyl is about 50–100 times more potent than morphine and is used to treat severe cancer pain and pain following surgery. It has become popular as a street drug and has led to numerous deaths around the world. Of the more than 70,000 deaths caused by opiates and opioids in 2020, over 54,000 of these were attributed to fentanyl (CDC, 2022). Currently most of the illicit fentanyl originates in China.

Morphine and heroin are typically administered by intravenous injection, while codeine and the synthetic opiates are most often taken orally. Once administered, opiates readily cross the blood brain barrier and reach all bodily tissues fairly rapidly. The structural modification to heroin (see Figure 7.5) makes it much more lipid soluble, and it reaches the brain within seconds of an injection—a property that gives heroin the ability to produce an intense "rush" or "high." In addition, because morphine and codeine are also water soluble, only 20–30 percent of the administered dose is actually available to reach the brain. The rest is rapidly excreted. In the liver, morphine and heroin (heroin is converted into morphine during its metabolism) are metabolized into **morphine-6-glucuronide**, which is a potent active metabolite. Morphine and its metabolite both have half-lives of approximately one to three hours, so the duration of analgesia produced by morphine is extended significantly.

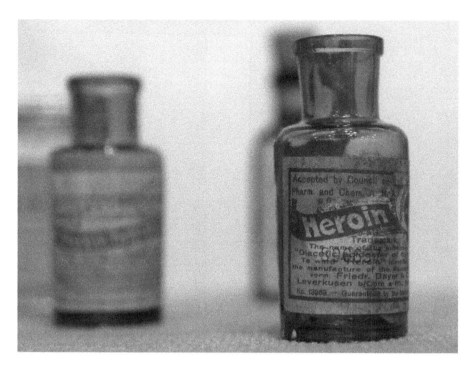

Figure 7.2 The Heroin brand name of diacetylmorphine marketed by the German pharmaceutical company Bayer.

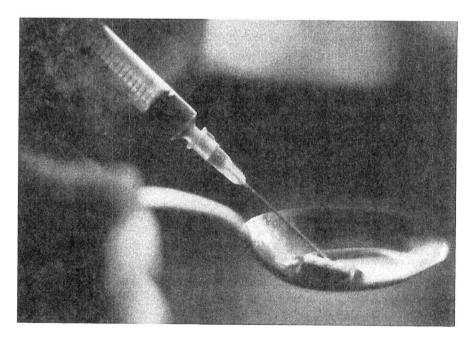

Figure 7.3 A small block (about 250 mg) of brown heroin is typically heated in a spoon with citric acid and water until it dissolves. Citric acid is commonly used as a buffering agent to increase heroin's water solubility. The liquid form of heroin can then be injected intravenously.

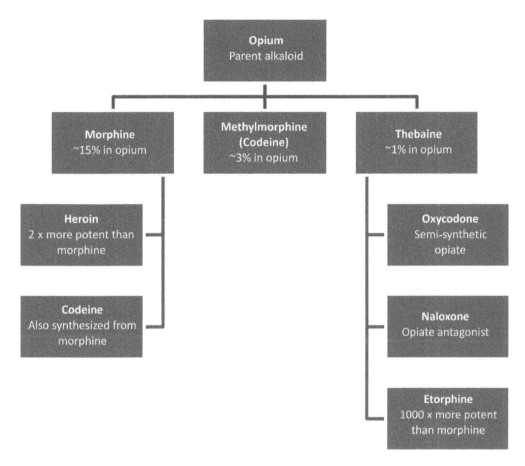

Figure 7.4 Relationships between common natural opiate derivatives.

Table 7.1 Several common natural and synthetic opiate/opioid compounds and their half-lives.

Drug name	Trade name	Origin	Half-life hours
Morphine	Morphine	opium	1–3*
Diacetylmorphine	Heroin	opium	10–20*
Methylmorphine	Codeine	morphine	2–3
Hydrocodone	Vicodin	codeine	1.5–3
Oxycodone	OxyContin	thebaine	2–3
Methadone	Dolophine	synthetic	15–22
Levomethadyl	Orlaam	synthetic	48–72**
Buprenophine	Suboxone	synthetic	36–73
Pethadine	Demerol	synthetic	3–4
Propoxyphene	Darvon	synthetic	6–12
Pentazocine	Talwin	synthetic	2–3
Fentanyl	Duragesic, Abstral, Subsys	synthetic	13–22

*active metabolite
**discontinued 2003

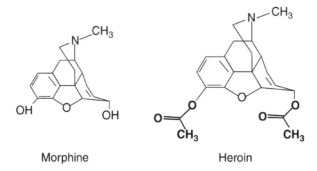

Figure 7.5 Molecular structures of morphine and heroin. The two acetyl groups (in bold) increase heroin's
lipid solubility and allow it to pass through the blood–brain barrier more rapidly than morphine.

Mechanisms of Opiate Analgesic Action: Brainstem

The opiates have a complex spectrum of effects on neural activity that include analgesia, euphoria, and respiratory depression. We will examine these mechanisms of action
separately in this chapter. First we will look at the neural pathways for pain sensation and
analgesia.

Pain sensations arise from several sources, including intense pressure, extremes in hot
or cold temperature, inflammation caused by tissue injury or infection, chemical irrita-
tion, and assaults or damage to skin or bone tissues. These sources of stimulation activate
pain receptors called **nociceptors**, which transduce stimulation into neural activity along
pain-transmitting neurons. Pain signals travel along myelinated Aδ fibers and unmyelinated
C fibers. Myelinated Aδ fibers transmit "fast" pain signals, which are perceived as sharp
localized pain, whereas unmyelinated C fibers transmit delayed or slow, dull pain. It is quite
common to experience dull or throbbing pain after the initial sharp piercing pain caused
by tissue damage. These distinct perceptions are transmitted and processed along different
neurons and pathways to the brain. The perception of pain is highly variable among people
and can be affected by psychological states as well as by drugs. For example, all of us are
familiar with the powerful analgesia caused by an extreme emotion or the excitation that
may occur after an accident. Depression, on the other hand, has long been known to increase
the perception of pain.

Nociceptors have their cell bodies in the dorsal root of the spinal cord called the dorsal root
ganglia (ganglia for cell bodies). These neurons terminate in the dorsal horn of the spinal cord
and release the excitatory neurotransmitter **substance P**. The origin of the name *substance P*
is unclear, but it was first isolated in powder form, it is a peptide, and it signals pain messages.
Its name could be derived from any or all of these anecdotes. From the dorsal horn, signals
ascend via the **spinothalamic pathway** to the thalamus, the somatosensory cortex, and to
the anterior cingulate cortex (Figure 7.6). The cingulate cortex is believed to be involved in
the feeling, or body representation, of the pain sensation. Damage to the anterior cingulate
does not eliminate pain signaling or the reflexive responses to pain, but it does disrupt our
feelings of pain.

Ascending information from the spinothalamic pathway and information originating in the
hypothalamus project to the periaqueductal gray area (PAG) of the pons, where the descending
pain pathway originates. The PAG projects to the locus coeruleus and to the raphe nucleus of

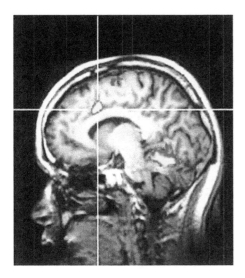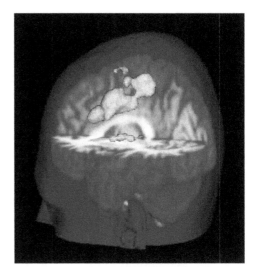

Figure 7.6 Pain caused by extreme heat is perceived in the anterior cingulate gyrus as well as the somatosensory cortex (left). Pain-induced activation of the thalamus, the somatosensory cortex, and the anterior cingulate cortex (right).

the medulla. Excitatory adrenergic neurons (yellow) from the locus coeruleus, and inhibitory serotonergic neurons (green) from the raphe nucleus, converge in the dorsal horn of the spinal cord where they inhibit the release of substance P (Figure 7.7). In addition, endogenous opiates and their receptors throughout the descending pathway modulate pain signaling. Endogenous opiates are involved in at least two ways within the spinal cord to modulate pain. First, opiates modulate the activity of the serotonergic and noradrenergic neurons in the medulla that project to the dorsal horn, and secondly, small interneurons within the dorsal horn release opiates that inhibit the release of substance P (Figure 7.8). These interneurons are activated by descending noradrenergic neurons. In addition to opiate receptors in the brainstem and spinal cord, opiate receptors in the cingulate cortex, the thalamus, the striatum, the **nucleus accumbens**, and the amygdala are also involved in modulating pain perception as well as the emotional components of pain.

Mechanisms of Opiate Analgesic Action: Cortex

While brainstem mechanisms clearly mediate pain signaling, several cortical structures are implicated in pain perception. As discussed earlier, patients with damage to their cingulate cortices respond to pain signals, but they are disassociated from them. That is, they don't perceive pain as their own. The insular and cingulate cortices and the body sensing areas of the sensory cortex are essential for the mapping of body states and the feelings of emotions, including pain (e.g., Bechara et al., 2003; Damasio et al., 2000).

Just how endogenous opiates and opiate drugs modulate pain perception has remained elusive. The observation that transcranial electrical stimulation of the prefrontal cortex induces analgesia in patients with either experimentally induced or chronic pain suggests that the prefrontal cortex is involved in analgesia, but its pharmacological mechanisms were only recently discovered. In an experiment conducted by Taylor et al. (2012), experimental

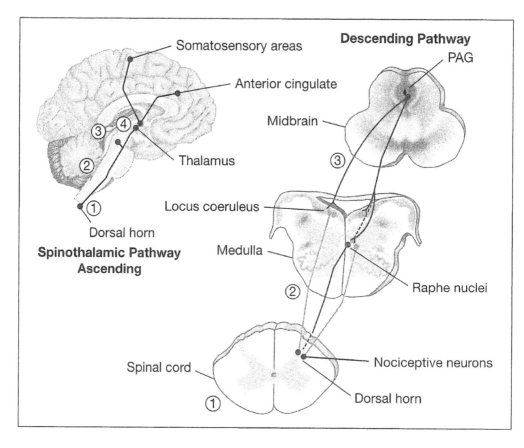

Figure 7.7 Ascending and descending pain pathways. Nociceptive pain neurons carry information from pain
and temperature receptors to the dorsal horn of the spinal cord to the thalamus forming the
spinothalamic pathway (left). Pain information is projected to the somatosensory and anterior
cingulate cortices. The descending pathway (right) begins at the periaqueductal gray area (PAG)
of the pons (3) and terminates on serotonergic and enkephalin cell bodies in the locus coeruleus in
the brainstem (2). Seortonergic and enkephalin neurons project to the dorsal horn and inhibit the
release of Substance P from nociceptive neurons. Noradrenergic neurons from the locus coeruleus
(2) send excitatory signals to the dorsal horn where they activate inhibitory opiate interneurons.
Numerous opiate receptors are located in the PAG, the raphe nucleus, and in the dorsal horn of
the spinal cord.

participants were administered both hot and cold stimuli via a thermode. Participants were
asked to report pain thresholds, as well as intolerable pain, as temperatures applied to the skin
were adjusted. After pain measurements were recorded, participants received intravenous **naloxone** or saline. Several minutes after injections, participants received transcranial stimulation
to the dorsolateral prefrontal cortex. Subjects receiving saline prior to stimulation reported
significant analgesia, while those receiving naloxone did not. These results suggest that pain
modulation by the prefrontal cortex is mediated by endogenous opiates. It is believed that
opiate drugs, such as morphine, exert their cortical analgesia via neural inhibition within the
prefrontal cortex.

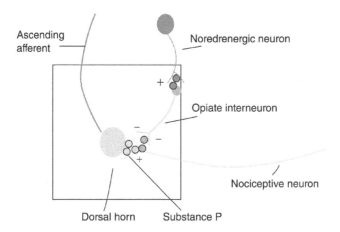

Figure 7.8 Opiate interneurons inhibit the release of pain signaling substance P in the dorsal horn of the spinal cord.

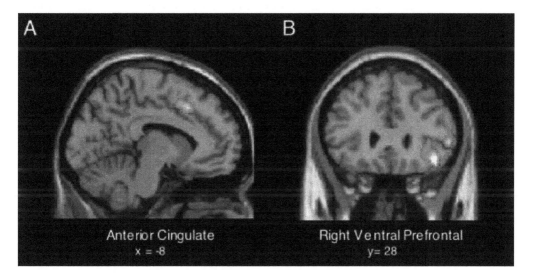

Figure 7.9 The anterior cingulate cortex (A) and the ventral prefrontal cortex (B) are active during feelings of pain. Opiate activity in the prefrontal cortex modulates pain perception.

Opiate Receptors and Endogenous Ligands

The identification and distribution of opiate receptors and their endogenous ligands began in the early 1970s with the work of Candace Pert and Solomon Snyder, who first identified opiate receptors using radioactively labeled opiate drugs. Since their discoveries, three different receptor subtypes (μ, δ, and κ) and their ligands have been identified. These receptor subtypes have distinct functions and distributions throughout the brain and spinal cord.

The μ (mu) receptor is widely distributed throughout the brain and spinal cord and is presumably the most important of the opiate receptors for pain analgesia. Morphine and related opiates have a high affinity for μ receptors while naloxone, a drug that competes for and blocks these receptors, disrupts drug-induced analgesia. μ receptors also contribute to the regulation of respiration in the ventral medulla. High doses of opiates acting on these receptors can cause **respiratory depression** by inhibiting respiratory responses triggered by carbon dioxide. A second receptor subtype, the δ (delta) receptor, is most abundant in the striatum and in the nucleus accumbens. The δ receptor is believed to play important roles in both analgesia and opiate-induced euphoria and reinforcement. The third receptor subtype, the κ (kappa) receptor is predominantly found in the amygdala, the hypothalamus, and in the pituitary gland. These receptors are also involved in analgesia, but perhaps most importantly in **dysphoria** and thermoregulation. Dysphoria is an emotional state characterized by depression, anxiety, and restlessness—a state opposite to euphoria. Dysphoria may be caused by κ antagonism of μ receptors. The κ receptor subtype will be discussed in greater detail in later sections on opiate-induced euphoria and dependence.

Endogenous ligands for the opiate receptors were discovered quickly after the receptors were described. These ligands were called **endorphins** after *endo* for endogenous and *orphan* for morphine. The endorphins are a class of opiate peptides that are produced from the breakdown of larger peptides within the cell's soma. These opiates include two **enkephalin** peptides, leu and met enkephalin, and **dynorphin**, which are stored in and released from synaptic vesicles.

All of the opiate receptor subtypes are metabotropic G-coupled receptors that have inhibitory effects on receiving neurons. Several of these inhibitory effects have been well described. First of all, opiate receptors can hypopolarize postsynaptic membranes by increasing K^+ conductance at axoaxonal synapses. As K^+ flows out of the neuron the membrane becomes hyperpolarized, making it less likely to fire. Opiate synapses in the dorsal horn inhibit the release of substance P in this way (Figures 7.7 and 7.8). Secondly, opiate activation of presynaptic heteroreceptors decreases the amount of neurotransmitter synthesized and released from these neurons. For example, in the nucleus accumbens dopamine release is regulated by inhibitory GABA heteroreceptors on dopamine-releasing neurons. Opiates bind to heteroreceptors on GABA neurons, thereby inhibiting the release of GABA. Dopamine release is increased by inhibition of inhibition (disinhibition) (see Figure 7.10). The anesthetic and reinforcing effects of opiates appear to result from these, and perhaps other, inhibitory mechanisms. The euphoric and reinforcing effects of opiates will be discussed later in this chapter.

Opiate Agonists and Antagonists

Drugs that bind to opiate receptors can exert a variety of effects depending on their molecular structure. The natural opiates heroin, morphine, and codeine all bind to opiate receptors with high affinity, and they exert the same effects as the endorphins on opiate receptors; that is, they contribute to neural inhibition. Drugs that mimic the effects of endogenous ligands are called **pure agonists**. Several of the synthetic opiates are also pure agonists, including methadone, pethadine (Demerol), and fentanyl (Duragesic, Abstral, and Subsys). Drugs that have a lower affinity for receptors than a natural ligand, or are selective in their affinity for specific receptor subtypes, are called **partial agonists**. Several partial synthetic opiate agonists are available, but they have relatively little clinical significance. Finally, several synthetic opiate drugs exert agonist effects on some receptors and antagonistic effects on others. These drugs are referred to as **mixed agonist-antagonists**. For example, it may be clinically desirable to activate kappa receptors for their analgesic effects while inhibiting mu receptors to blunt the euphoric effects of an opiate. Several mixed agonist-antagonist drugs have been synthesized, including

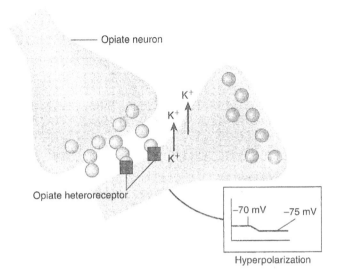

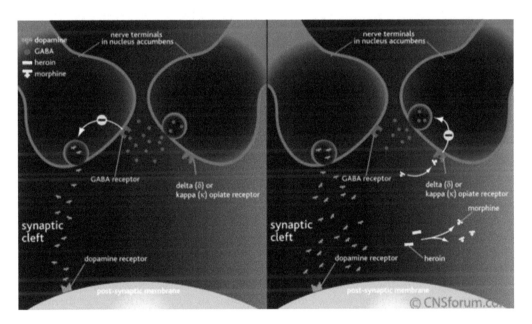

Figure 7.10 Opiate receptors cause neural inhibition in several ways: by increasing K^+ conductance the cell becomes hyperpolarized (left) and by disinhibition of catecholamine neurotransmitter release (right).

pentazocine (Talwin). Partial and mixed agonists are much less effective than pure agonists for analgesia. In fact, morphine remains to be the most effective opiate for postoperative pain, even after 50 years of research and drug development.

Drugs may also block or diminish the effects of endogenous opiates or any of the opiate agonists. A **pure antagonist** has a high affinity for receptors, but it does not exert any physiological effect on the receptor or the receiving cell. Antagonists compete with agonists as well as with natural ligands for receptor sites and may even displace an agonist that is occupying a receptor. Naloxone (Narcan) is the prototype opiate pure antagonist and it is often administered to heroin overdose victims in attempts to reverse life-threatening respiratory depression. An intravenous injection of **naltrexone** can reverse a serious heroin overdose within minutes. Naltrexone (Revia) is also a pure opiate antagonist that is typically used to treat opiate dependence. Although either naltrexone or naloxone could be used to augment treatment for opiate dependence, naloxone is preferred because it is longer acting than naltrexone. In addition to their clinical significance, these opiate antagonists have been very useful in elucidating the roles of endogenous opiates in behavior.

Mechanisms of Opiate Reinforcement

The opiate heroin is perhaps one of the most powerfully addictive drugs known. It rapidly enters the brain because of its high lipid solubility and immediately exerts its effects on synapses in the mesolimbic system as well as on synapses throughout the brain and spinal cord. The reinforcing, and addictive, effects of opiates take place within several structures of the mesolimbic system, including the **ventral tegmentum** and the nucleus accumbens. The ventral tegmentum of the midbrain is rich with dopaminergic cell bodies that project their axons to several limbic structures, including the nucleus accumbens. Axons from the nucleus accumbens project via the globus pallidus to the dorsal medial nucleus of the thalamus, which then projects to the prefrontal cortex. While most of the neurons that comprise the nucleus accumbens are GABAergic, this area is also rich with dopamine and opiate receptors.

It is well known that increases in dopamine activity in the nucleus accumbens mediate the reinforcing effects of opiates and other drugs. As illustrated in Figure 7.10, opiates bind to autoreceptors at GABAergic synapses and exert inhibitory effects on GABA release. This in turn results in decreased GABA inhibition of dopamine release in the nucleus accumbens. Just how increased dopamine activity in the mesolimbic system contributes to reinforcement is much less clear. It is speculated, however, that a major function of this pathway is to amplify stimulus salience and to motivate motor activity. From an evolutionary perspective, stimuli associated with palatable foods and sexual behaviors, for example, should themselves become highly valued for their predictive significance. Likewise, these stimuli should excite motor activities that lead to appetitive behaviors. Research from several types of experiments supports this hypothesis. For example, in animals that have been surgically prepared for recording electrical activity in mesolimbic structures, we see increased activity when they are given opportunities to eat palatable foods or engage in sexual behaviors. Furthermore, we see similar increases in electrical activity when they are in contexts where these behaviors regularly occur. Therefore, stimuli associated with feeding or engaging in sexual behaviors can themselves control dopamine activity in the mesolimbic system. As a result, these activities, and the stimuli associated with them, become highly valued.

Certain drugs, as well as stimuli associated with the onset of drug effects, can also become highly valued and therefore reinforcing. Numerous experiments report the powerfully reinforcing effects of opiates on the operant behavior of animals. For example, rats will lever press at high rates for opiate infusions into the nucleus accumbens or the ventral tegmentum (see Figure 7.11). The reinforcing effects of opiates can also be blunted by the administration of naloxone—a powerful opiate antagonist. The topic of drug **self-administration** will be discussed further in the section on opiate dependence. As we will see, research on the reinforcing properties of drugs, as well as on the properties of drug-associated stimuli, has contributed significantly to our understanding of addiction.

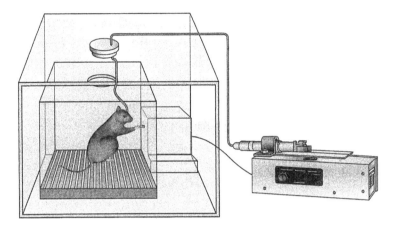

Figure 7.11 Laboratory rats fitted with a cannula, lever press for opiate reinforcement delivered by an infusion pump into the nucleus accumbens. Response rates for opiate reinforcement typically far exceed those for food or water reinforcement and can be maintained for several hours.

Opiate Tolerance

In Chapter 2, we defined drug tolerance as a shift to the right in the dose response curve. That is, after repeated drug exposure it takes larger doses to produce an effect (illustrated in Figure 7.12). It is important to remember here that although tolerance develops quite quickly to opiate drugs, the rate of tolerance development is not the same for all opiate effects. For instance, tolerance to the analgesic and reinforcing effects of opiates occur more rapidly than to the respiratory depressant effects. Because of this, overdose to opiates can be a significant concern as doses are increased over time to sustain analgesia, or to heroin patients who use increasing amounts to thwart withdrawal symptoms.

As described in some detail in Chapter 2, tolerance to opiates is complex and involves several distinct mechanisms. The primary metabolic enzyme for morphine is UGT2B7 (UDP-Glucuronosyltransferase-2B7), which converts morphine into M3G (morphine-3-glucuronide) and M6G (morphine-6-glucuronide). These metabolic byproducts account for about 70 percent of administered morphine, while the remaining 30 percent is either excreted unchanged or converted into other minor metabolites. The active metabolite of morphine, M6G, is about two to four times more potent than morphine, while M3G metabolite appears to have little pharmacological activity. These products are further metabolized and eventually excreted by the kidneys. After repeated opiate administration, the concentration of UGT2B7 in the liver increases and morphine is metabolized more quickly. This increased rate of drug metabolism is referred to as **metabolic tolerance**.

Perhaps more importantly for opiate tolerance, however, are adaptive changes to opiate-receiving neurons. While the details of these mechanisms have not been completely worked out, several adaptive changes have been described and evidence is accumulating for others. For example, chronic use of opiates is known to initially inhibit cyclic AMP (cAMP) production, which is later offset by compensatory mechanisms that return cAMP levels to normal. As you recall, cAMP is an essential second messenger for metabotropic receptors. Therefore, compensatory production of cAMP appears to be an important mechanism underlying opiate **cellular tolerance**. When opiate use is suddenly terminated, upregulated cAMP may contribute a rebound in noradrenergic cell activity in the locus coeruleus,

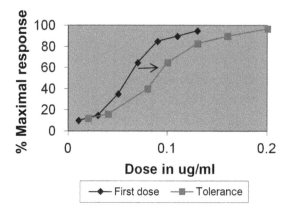

Figure 7.12 Dose response curves for Oxycodone. Tolerance can be observed as a shift to the right in the dose response curve. After repeated exposure, larger drug doses are required to produce the same magnitude of effect.

and to withdrawal symptoms (Ivanov & Aston-Jones, 2001; Punch et al., 1997; Rasmussen et al., 1990).

Metabolic tolerance and upregulation of cAMP alone, however, cannot completely account for opiate tolerance. As discussed in Chapter 2, tolerance often depends on the prior exposure to drug-associated cues. That is, tolerance may be expressed in contexts where drugs were administered, but not in another unfamiliar context. This **associative tolerance** results from the acquisition of a Pavlovian association between salient drug cues (conditioned stimuli) and drug onset cues (unconditioned stimuli). Because this kind of tolerance can be immediately expressed in the appropriate context, additional dynamic cellular adaptations must be involved. At this point, all we appear to know is that this mechanism is likely to be mediated by the NMDA receptor. Evidence from a number of studies, including those conducted by the author, indicate that associative tolerance can be both disrupted and reversed by the administration of NMDA receptor antagonists such as **dextromethorphan**.

This research has important implications for drug addiction treatment. First of all, it illustrates why recidivism may be so high for drug addiction, as drug treatment often involves controlled abstinence in a clinical setting away from drug-associated cues. Once the user returns to places or contexts where drug use occurred, conditioned responses associated with drug use (e.g., cravings and drug seeking) are elicited. Furthermore, exposure to a single dose may completely reinstate the addiction and tolerance. In our laboratory, rats demonstrated the reinstatement of tolerance and drug-seeking behaviors after several months of abstinence following a single low dose of morphine, but only if it was administered in the original drug context. Rats given morphine after abstinence in their home cages did not show reinstatement (Figure 7.13). Clearly, more research on the cellular mechanisms underlying associative tolerance is needed before we can develop effective drug treatment programs.

Pharmacological Treatment of Opiate Dependence and Addiction

The Centers for Disease Control and Prevention (CDC) estimates that approximately one million people in the United States are currently dependent on heroin or other opiates, including oxycontin, hydrocodone, and fentanyl. These opiate users are at risk for HIV, hepatitis, and liver disease, as well as a host of other disorders. As many as 70,000 of these users die from drug overdose each year. The financial costs of opiate dependence and addiction, although impossible to determine, are estimated to exceed $80 billion annually.

From the preceding discussion, it is clear that successful programs for opiate dependence must involve more than detoxification in a clinical setting. Drug-associated contextual cues can, and often do, elicit cravings and withdrawal symptoms even after months of abstinence. And, as illustrated in Figure 7.13, these drug-related behaviors can be reinstated after extinction if drug use reoccurs in familiar drug contexts. Successful programs must, therefore, employ both behavioral and pharmacological approaches to minimize the probability of recidivism, which occurs in as many as 80 percent of treated opiate users.

Most opiate treatment programs begin with a period of **methadone maintenance** where methadone is substituted for heroin, or another opiate. Methadone is the preferred substitute for heroin for several reasons. First of all, it has a very long half-life (15–22 hours) compared to other opiates. Once-daily methadone administration may be sufficient to reduce withdrawal symptoms and maintain abstinence for most patients. Methadone can be administered orally, and this route of administration does not produce the "rush" or "high" associated with IV drug use. Most patients require between 60 and 120 mg of methadone each day for at least one year, and often for a period of several years to life, for treatment at a cost of about $4,000 per patient per year. Every day, over 100,000 patients take methadone as part of a drug treatment program.

Other synthetic opiates have been developed for opiate maintenance, including **levometha-dyl** (Orlaam), which was discontinued in 2003 because of adverse cardiac side effects, and **buprenorphine** (Suboxone), approved by the FDA in 2002. Both of these synthetic opiates have long half-lives of about two and a half days, requiring dosing only three times per week. Suboxone contains buprenorphine, the synthetic opiate, and naloxone to deter illicit intravenous use. If administered intravenously, naloxone antagonizes buprenorphine effects and precipitates withdrawal symptoms. When taken orally the naloxone does not cross the blood–brain barrier and has little or no antagonistic effect.

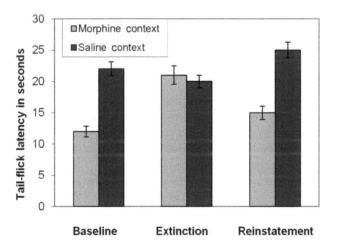

Figure 7.13 Average tail-flick latencies in response to thermal pain for animals receiving morphine in the same context where tolerance developed vs. receiving morphine in a different context. The first panel shows associative tolerance that develops to the drug administration context (shorter latencies). Panel 2 shows the extinction of tolerance following a two-week period of no drug administration. Panel 3 shows the reinstatement of associative tolerance following the single administration of 3 mg/kg morphine in context.

Source: Author's laboratory.

Methadone (or buprenorphine) by itself is not sufficient as a treatment for opiate addiction, but space in comprehensive residential treatment facilities is limited and expensive. Often methadone maintenance is initiated in an outpatient setting, while the patient is awaiting space in a residential facility. In these cases, unfortunately, many return to heroin or other drugs. The success of methadone maintenance is difficult to assess since definitions of success vary widely. Critics of methadone maintenance programs argue these programs merely substitute one addiction for another and success should be defined as complete abstinence from all drugs. Using this definition these programs fail. Advocates, on the other hand, argue that success should be measured in terms of social cost, and methadone programs do decrease the costs of crime and disease associated with illicit drug use. Regardless of definition, methadone is not a cure for opiate addiction.

Glossary

Alkaloids nitrogen-containing compounds produced by a variety of plants. Many psychoactive compounds are alkaloids.

Associative tolerance a decrease in drug effectiveness as a consequence of Pavlovian conditioning.

Buprenorphine a synthetic opiate used for the treatment of opiate dependence.

Cellular tolerance a decrease in drug effectiveness as a consequence of compensatory adaptations within receiving neurons.

Codeine a less-potent narcotic than morphine, extracted from opium or synthesized from morphine.

Controlled Substance Act passed in 1970 to regulate the manufacture, importation, possession, and distribution of certain drugs. The CTA also created drug schedules, which limit the use of certain drugs.

Dextromethorphan a drug that acts as an NMDA receptor antagonist.

Dynorphin an endorphin neurotransmitter that binds to the kappa opiate receptor.

Dysphoria an unpleasant or uncomfortable state that is the opposite of euphoria.

Endorphin a class of endogenous opiate peptides.

Enkephalin an endorphin. May be either leu or met enkephalin.

Harrison Narcotic Act passed by Congress in 1914 to regulate the manufacture and distribution of opiates and cocaine.

Heroin potent narcotic derived from morphine. Because of its abuse potential it is no longer used as an analgesic.

Levomethadyl a synthetic opiate used for the treatment of opiate dependence.

Metabolic tolerance a decrease in drug effectiveness as a consequence of an increased rate of its metabolism.

Methadone maintenance a treatment program for opiate dependence that substitutes methadone for heroin or another opiate.

Mixed agonist-antagonist a drug that exerts agonistic effects on some receptor subtypes and antagonistic effects on other receptor subtypes.

Morphine a major active compound of opium. Used as a potent analgesic.

Morphine-6-glucuronide an active metabolite of morphine and heroin.

Naloxone a pure opiate antagonist often used to treat opiate dependence.

Naltrexone a pure opiate antagonist used to treat opiate overdose.

Nociceptors pain receptors that transduce stimulation into activity in pain-signaling neurons.

Nucleus accumbens an area of the forebrain located adjacent to the head of the caudate nucleus and the putamen and below the lateral ventricles. Most of the neurons within the nucleus accumbens are GABAergic. Dopamine neurons from the ventral tegmentum terminate in the nucleus accumbens.

Opiate any natural derivative of opium as well as all endogenous compounds that bind to opiate receptors.

Opioids synthetic or partially synthetic compounds that mimic the effects of opiates.

Opium potent narcotic extracted from the poppy plant *Papaver somniferum*.

Partial agonist a drug that has a lower affinity for a receptor than an endogenous neurotransmitter but exerts similar effects on receptors.

Pure agonist a drug that mimics the effects of an endogenous neurotransmitter.

Pure antagonist a drug that has a high affinity for receptors but does not exert any physiological effect on the receptor.

Respiratory depression the inhibition of inhibiting respiratory responses triggered by carbon dioxide. Often the cause of death from drug overdose.

Self-administration an experimental procedure where an animal may control the rate of drug delivery. Typically a drug is administered through a cannula following a lever press.

Spinothalamic pathway pathway of ascending neurons from the dorsal horn of the spinal cord to the thalamus, the somatosensory cortex, and to the anterior cingulate cortex.

Substance P an excitatory neurotransmitter released in the dorsal horn of the spinal cord by pain-transmitting neurons.

Ventral tegmentum a structure containing dopamine neurons located in the midbrain. Part of the mesolimbic system.

8 Substance Abuse and the Neurobiology of Addiction

The most recent national surveys on drug abuse estimate that approximately 20 million people were diagnosed with a **substance use disorder** in 2020. This estimate is approaching 8 percent of the adult population. Over 71,000 people died from drug overdose in 2020 (SAMHSA, 2021). The annual prevalence of the use of illicit drugs is approaching 60 million people, or about 22 percent of the population, over 12 years of age. These numbers have dramatically increased over the past few years since more accurate national surveys are being used and *DSM-5* criteria have been employed. The rapid increase may also be attributed to COVID-19. While not all individuals who abuse drugs can be considered to be drug addicted, clearly many are. In this chapter, I will examine the diagnostic criteria for substance use disorders and explore the neurobiology of drug addiction. As we will see, the term **addiction** has often been used synonymously with dependence. Not all drugs that cause dependence will be defined here as addictive. While drug addiction implies a dependency, addiction is a consequence of specific neural adaptations resulting from the use of drugs that affect dopamine activity in the mesolimbic and mesocortical systems. Not all drugs that cause a dependency produce these types of neural adaptations. The drugs listed in Figure 8.1, among others, do.

Carl remembers his very first drink at age 12. His parents had a liquor cabinet in their dining room where he found a well-used bottle of gin. After consuming about eight ounces he immediately became ill and vomited in his bedroom. Hours later, Carl was punished by his parents, and they put a lock on their cabinet to prevent another occurrence. The last thing Carl wanted, however, was another drink. The illness and subsequent hangover were sufficient to deter his drinking for almost a year. While in middle school Carl befriended a young boy who was much more experienced with alcohol than he. As a son of an alcoholic father, his friend had unfettered access to alcohol. Carl remembers drinking at all times with his friend, even in the morning on the way to school. By the time Carl graduated from high school he was drinking most days. He either stole wine from a local grocery store or from the parents of his friends. Although Carl knew a few alcoholics, including the father of his friend, he didn't think of himself as one. He simply enjoyed the feeling of intoxication and was quite good at hiding it from his own parents and teachers. Carl looked forward to attending college where he anticipated the parties and binge drinking he had often heard about.

Soon after his freshman year began, Carl was involved in an automobile accident. He was charged with driving under the influence (DUI) and sentenced to a night in jail and the suspension of his driver's license for a year. In addition, Carl was required to attend weekly meetings with other alcohol users, where they discussed the symptoms and ramifications of abuse and addiction. Carl was not convinced that he had an alcohol problem, but he played along to meet the requirements of his sentence. After dismal academic performance his first year, Carl decided college wasn't for him and he accepted a salesman position at a local car dealership where he had worked the previous summer. Selling cars was easy for Carl. He enjoyed meeting people and found that working at the dealership provided numerous opportunities to meet for drinks with other salesmen. Carl believed that his performance was actually enhanced with a few drinks, since it made small conversation and sales talk much easier.

DOI: 10.4324/9781003309017-8

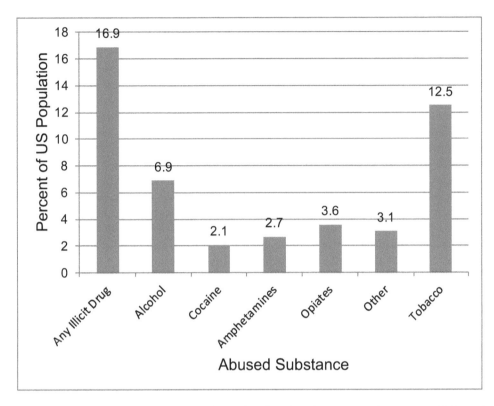

Figure 8.1 Percentage of the US population *who used an* illicit *drug during 2020*. The category All drugs does not include tobacco products. The category Amphetamine includes methamphetamine, Opiates includes prescription and non-prescription narcotics, Cocaine includes crack, and Other includes inhalants and sedatives.

Source: Compiled from SAMHSA (2021).

Within a year at the dealership Carl began drinking while at work. After several reprimands his position was shifted from a salaried one to one paid solely on sales commissions. The increased stress of earning a livable wage and being newly engaged precipitated even more drinking. By now Carl had developed tolerance to large amounts of alcohol. He also found that abstaining from drinking was increasingly difficult. When confronted about alcohol by his fiancée, Carl would get enraged in denial. He claimed he needed it to relax from the pressures of work. Once they were married Carl promised to quit and he found a new job as an insurance adjuster. Quitting drinking, however, was always just a promise.

After a mere three months Carl was fired from his new job. The reasons for his dismissal were never stated, but it was clear to his wife that drinking was the problem. Carl began each day with a glass of vodka. For lunch he would have a few drinks with a sandwich or fries. After work Carl would have a few martinis before dinner and a scotch or two immediately after. Because he never felt drunk, Carl was still convinced alcohol wasn't a problem. He knew he could quit if he wanted to—he just didn't want to quite yet.

Within a year of marriage Carl and his wife sought counseling as a last resort to save their marriage. Carl had become increasingly aggressive after drinking and was having difficulties finding work. Their social life had also deteriorated, and according to his wife, this too was because of his excessive drinking. After a few drinks Carl was prone to become belligerent and aggressive. It was during his first counseling session that Carl agreed to alcohol treatment and to attend Alcoholics Anonymous sessions. Carl abstained from alcohol for nearly three months before resuming drinking. During this time he had suffered through his first bout of alcohol withdrawals, delirium tremens, and severe alcohol cravings. This was not to be his last bout, however.

After Carl resumed drinking his wife filed for divorce and moved back with her parents. Carl moved into a small apartment since he could not afford the house payments on his intermittent salary. With another car accident and DUI, Carl was sentenced to 30 days in a residential treatment facility.

Carl's story is neither unusual nor typical of alcohol addiction. Addiction to alcohol can occur abruptly or develop gradually over many years. It may begin in adolescence, as it did with Carl, or it may begin late in life. What appears to be a common thread in substance abuse is the pattern of destruction it renders to personal and family lives. Substance abusers are often in denial about the pain they cause to others close to them. They are also in denial about the severe health and financial consequences of substance abuse to themselves. Alcohol addiction is more common in individuals with other, comorbid, psychological disorders, including depression, bipolar disorder, and anxiety disorders. Perhaps alcohol addiction is a form of self-medication for these preexisting conditions. It is also possible that alcohol abuse potentiates the development of other psychological disorders.

Substance abuse treatment is rarely successful on the first attempt and is seldom complete. Recovered alcoholics often rightly claim that addiction is just a drink away. Carl's story provides a nice introduction to substance abuse disorders; his case clearly meets the criteria for one.

The *Diagnostic and Statistical Manual of Mental Disorders* (*DSM-5*) does not make a distinction between drug dependence and addiction, and in fact the term "addiction" is no longer used. Rather, the *DSM* classifies substance use disorders by the degree of impairment caused by drug use and whether tolerance and/or withdrawal symptoms are present. According to these distinctions, an individual may be dependent on a substance without having a disorder. For example, most individuals addicted to nicotine are not considered to have a substance use disorder, even though they may meet the minimal diagnostic criteria for this disorder.

The diagnosis of substance use disorder requires that the symptoms of drug tolerance and/or withdrawal are present. This diagnosis presumes that the drug use has persisted long enough for these symptoms to develop.

The *DSM-5* identifies ten distinct substance use disorders. These include alcohol use disorder, cannabis use disorder, opioid use disorder, and stimulant use disorder among several others, including sedatives, hallucinogens, and inhalants. The criteria for many substance use disorders are similar and include the following:

A problematic pattern of substance use, leading to clinically significant impairment or distress, as manifested by three, or more, of the following occurring at any time in the same 12-month period:

1. The substance is taken in larger amounts over a longer period than was intended.
2. There is a persistent desire or unsuccessful efforts to cut down or control substance use.
3. A great deal of time is spent in activities necessary to obtain, use, and recover from the substance effects.
4. Craving, or a strong desire or urge to use the substance.
5. Recurrent substance use resulting in a failure to fulfill major role obligations at work, school, or home.
6. Continued substance use despite knowledge of having persistent or recurrent social or interpersonal problems caused or exacerbated by the effects of substance use.
7. Important social, occupational, or recreational activities are given up or reduced because of substance use.

8. Recurrent substance use in situations in which it is physically hazardous.
9. Continued substance use despite knowledge of having a persistent or recurrent physical or psychological problem that is likely to have been caused or exacerbated because of substance use.
10. Tolerance, defined as a need for markedly increased amounts of the substance to achieve intoxication.
11. Withdrawal symptoms specific to the substance.

Carl's condition clearly meets most of these criteria. He has developed tolerance to large amounts of alcohol, he suffers withdrawals with abstinence, and alcohol use has caused severe disruptions to all areas of his life. If he is like many recovering alcoholics he will be in and out of treatment for much of his remaining life. During periods of abstinence he will be tempted to drink and will experience alcohol cravings when in the presence of others using alcohol. These symptoms may diminish, but never completely disappear even after many years of abstinence.

The Neurobiology of Addiction

As stated earlier, certain drugs not only cause dependency after repeated use but they may also cause addiction. While addiction certainly implies a dependency, there are also both behavioral and neurobiological features of addiction that are not present in all cases of drug dependency. Among the most remarkable features of drug addiction is the intense desire or motivation to take a drug, even in the face of serious adverse consequences, including arrest and imprisonment, termination of employment, and even an increased risk of serious disease. Equally sinister is the enduring craving for the drug after many years of abstinence, making drug relapse a likely occurrence for most addicts. How could a substance produce such powerful control over one's behavior that one risks everything one has, including families, one's employment, one's freedom, and one's health? In order to understand how drugs could produce such powerful effects on behavior we need to explore just how addictive substances change the brain. Over the past 20 years, we have learned a great deal about the neurobiological adaptations resulting from the use of certain drugs from both human and animal experiments. It is these adaptations that will form the critical distinction between drug dependence and its more insidious form, drug addiction.

Reward Pathways

The brain's response to addictive substances may be a mere coincidence of a drug's effects on the brain's **reward pathway**. This pathway is an evolutionary adaptation that assists organisms in assigning hedonic value to stimuli. For instance, the reward pathway ensures that organisms find certain foods more appealing than others based on their caloric value. It also ensures that organisms are motivated to seek out sexual partners and reproduce. This survival-enhancing system motivates animals to seek out and to repeat whichever activities activated the reward pathway.

The essential neural structures that comprise the brain's reward pathway include the ventral tegmental area of the midbrain and the nucleus accumbens. Even simple organisms such as the earthworm *Caenorhabditis elegans* have a rudimentary version of these dopamine-containing structures. Deactivation of these neurons disrupts the worm's ability to identify food. In the laboratory, rats can be trained to lever press to obtain small amounts of a dopamine-stimulating drug (e.g., cocaine) into the nucleus accumbens. Blocking the activity of these drugs or destroying dopamine-containing cells within these structures can severely disrupt lever pressing and drug administration. Addictive drugs tap into and modify the brain's reward pathways, ensuring that the motivation to seek and use drugs persists.

The investigation of reward pathways originated in 1954 with James Olds and his student Peter Milner. In their experiments rats were implanted with electrodes into the **septum** to determine whether electrical stimulation would enhance maze learning. The septum is located centrally, deep below the basal ganglia and adjacent to the nucleus accumbens. In fact, the complete name of the nucleus accumbens in Latin is *nucleus accumbens septi*, which means "nucleus leaning against the septum." To their surprise, after stimulating a rat when it was in a particular corner of the maze it quickly returned for more. After a few applications of electrical stimulation the animals were "indubitably coming back for more" (Olds & Milner, 1954). While the exact location of their electrode is unknown, numerous other experiments have replicated their findings with electrodes located in various areas, including the septum, the **medial forebrain bundle** (the bundle of axons projecting from the VTA to the nucleus accumbens), and the nucleus accumbens. These structures illustrated in Figure 8.2 are all part of the reward pathway, and they comprise the mesolimbic system.

Since the discovery by Olds and Milner, neuroscientists have learned that electrical stimulation, like cocaine, causes an increase in the availability of dopamine in the VTA and the nucleus accumbens (see Figure 8.3). In addition, natural reinforcers such as palatable food, sucrose solution, and the availability of a sex partner all stimulate the availability of dopamine in this region (see also Figure 8.4). Therefore, it appears that certain drugs activate the same brain regions as do natural reinforcers and this activation is well correlated with positive feelings in humans (Cooper & Knutson, 2008; Knutson et al., 2001; Uhl et al., 2019). Addiction may not be solely dependent upon a drug's ability to increase dopamine activity in these mesolimbic structures, but on how quickly it does so. Drugs like cocaine, heroin, and nicotine are much more addictive when smoked or administered intravenously than when ingested orally because of how rapidly these routes of administration reach the brain.

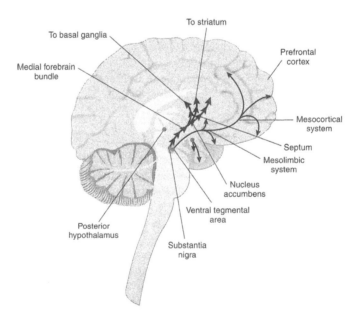

Figure 8.2 Mesolimbic and mesocortical dopamine systems. The mesolimbic system originates in the ventral tegmental area (VTA) and projects along the medial forebrain bundle to the amygdala, lateral hypothalamus, and the nucleus accumbens. The mesocortical system also originates in the VTA but projects to the prefrontal cortex. Increased activity of dopamine in these reward systems is believed to underlie reinforcement as well as drug addiction.

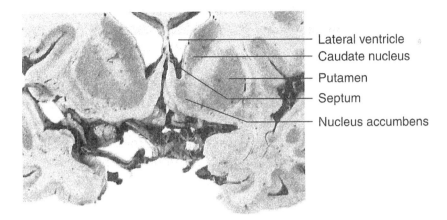

Figure 8.3 Transverse section through a human brain revealing structures of the basal ganglia and mesolimbic system. Note the close proximity of the septum and the nucleus accumbens.

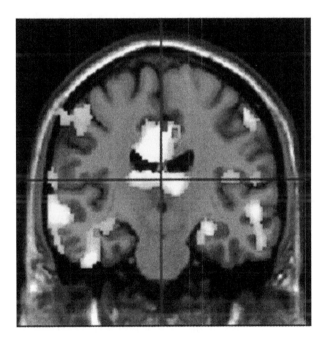

Figure 8.4 Functional MRI scan showing activity in the nucleus accumbens. Activation of the nucleus accumbens is correlated with positive subjective feelings.

Source: Knutson et al. (2001).

Drugs and Reward Pathways

Drugs that either directly (e.g., cocaine) or indirectly (e.g., heroin) increase dopamine activity in the VTA and nucleus accumbens are powerfully reinforcing and can maintain high rates of lever pressing in experimental animals. In addition, disrupting neurons in these regions, or the pathways connecting them, greatly diminishes the reinforcing effects of these drugs. The

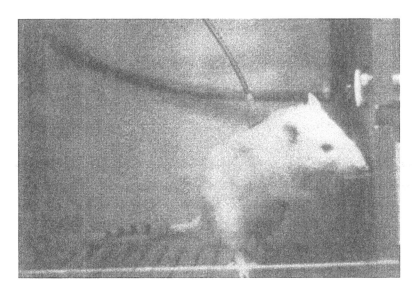

Figure 8.5 A self-administration experiment where a laboratory rat is fitted with a drug-delivery cannula. Lever presses result in small infusions of drug directly into specific regions of the brain.

strong correlation between a drug's ability to maintain **self-administration** through high rates of lever pressing and its addictive potential makes animal self-administration a useful tool to evaluate a drug's liability for addiction (Figure 8.5). However, increasing dopamine activity in these mesolimbic structures in itself is not sufficient to cause addiction. If it were, addictions to all sorts of activities and foods would easily occur. While the term addiction has been, and still is, applied to cases of severe compulsive behavior—such as eating, gambling, video gaming, and sex—to date no one has described the patterns of lasting adaptions to mesolimbic and cortical systems I describe here.

Why might the rate of drug administration determine its addictive liability? Several hypotheses have been proposed. The first hypothesis argues that the more rapidly a drug enters the brain, the more euphoric it is. Support for this comes from early studies comparing the subjective effects of cocaine when administered at different rates. At all doses investigated, cocaine and heroin produce greater euphoria when administered intravenously when compared to similar doses delivered intranasally (Comer et al., 1999; Resnick et al., 1977). Similar results were found with amphetamines (Volkow et al., 2001). These results are depicted in Figure 8.6.

While this argument seems compelling, there is only a weak relationship between a drug's subjective euphoric effects and its reinforcing effects. For example, nicotine produces little change in euphoria in smokers, but it is both reinforcing and highly addictive. In fact, intravenous nicotine produces few if any pleasurable subjective responses at all in smokers, even though it is effective in reducing nicotine cravings (Rose et al., 2000). It appears, therefore, that euphoria may be important in drug-taking behavior, but something other than euphoria must contribute to a drug's reinforcing and addictive potential.

The second and more recent hypothesis of addictive liability poses that a drug's psychomotor and incentive sensitization effects are more closely associated with its addictive potential than its ability to induce euphoria. **Psychomotor sensitization** refers to a drug's potential to increase motor activity and drug-seeking behaviors after repeated administration. These behavioral effects are easily conditioned and elicited by contexts where drugs were administered.

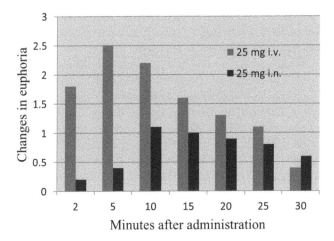

Figure 8.6 The subjective effects of 25 mg of cocaine depend on route of administration. Cocaine administered intravenously (IV) produces greater changes in euphoria than do intranasal (IN) doses.

Source: Data from Resnick et al. (1977).

Incentive sensitization, on the other hand, is an increase in the incentive value of the drug as well as drug-associated cues. For example, an animal previously exposed to nicotine, amphetamine, or cocaine demonstrates an increase in the rate of drug self-administration (increase in incentive value) and an increase in preference for drug-associated cues and contexts (as a result of conditioning) (Bradberry, 2000; Cromberg et al., 2001). Both psychomotor and incentive sensitization are observed in humans with a history of drug use.

The ability of drugs to induce psychomotor and incentive sensitization appears to depend on neurological adaptations in mesolimbic areas resulting from rapid rates of drug administration. It has been well established, for example, that the consequences of acute cocaine administration depend on its route of administration. Changes in neural activity measured by glucose utilization occur primarily to the nigrostriatal system following intraperitoneal administration as compared to increased activity in the mesolimbic and mesocortical systems following intravenous administration. The author of this report (Porrino, 1993) concluded that "cocaine activates different neuronal circuitry depending on the route by which it is administered." Furthermore, "the absence of metabolic activation in the mesolimbic system following acute intraperitoneal cocaine was not the result of the specific dose chosen or the length of time between cocaine administration and measuring glucose utilization."

Since this study a number of others have been conducted to examine the cellular adaptations resulting from rapid drug administration.

Neurological Adaptations Resulting From Rapid Drug Delivery

Because drug addiction is characterized by long-lasting behavioral changes, including drug cravings and drug seeking that can be reinstated after long periods of abstinence, the neural adaptations underlying addiction must also be enduring. The most likely candidates for these adaptations include drug-induced changes to gene expression in dopaminergic neurons within the mesolimbic and mesocortical pathways. Other neuronal adaptations, such as long-term potentiation (LTP), are too short-lived to adequately account for addiction. How then do drugs initiate gene expression in specific neurons? In attempts to answer this question, researchers have focused on a class of regulator proteins called **immediate early genes** (IEGs). Immediate early genes are proteins that are activated by stimuli that activate intracellular signaling. While many of the signaling pathways activated by IEGs may be regulatory or homeostatic, the IEGs activated by certain drugs may have profound influences on dopaminergic cell functioning. One IEG that has received considerable attention because it is activated by addictive drugs is **c-FOS**. This is a protein that is expressed in response to a variety of extracellular signals, including drugs such as cocaine, amphetamine, nicotine, and morphine. As cellular activity in response to a drug increases, **c-FOS protein** is expressed in greater amounts (Cruz et al., 2014; Harlan & Garcia, 1998; Thomas et al., 2008; Zhang et al., 2006).

In Figure 8.7, we see how receptor activation by a neurotransmitter, such as dopamine, leads to the activation of the **second messenger** cyclic AMP (cAMP), which in turn activates protein kinase (PKA). Protein kinase enters the cell nucleus where it activates a cyclic AMP response element-binding (CREB) protein. The **CREB protein** binds to a specific binding element on DNA, allowing it to turn on the gene for the synthesis of the c-FOS protein. These are transcription factors that promote the synthesis of messenger RNA (mRNA) under the direction of DNA. These proteins are essential for the cellular adaptations resulting from drug use.

Drug addiction is a result of lasting neural adaptations that alter the brain's response to dopamine. The mechanism underlying this alteration appears to be CREB-activated c-FOS. c-FOS appears to coordinate the response of dopamine $D_{1\&2}$ receptors to repeated drug exposure. $D_{1\&2}$ receptors are believed to mediate the psychomotor and incentive sensitization that follows addictive drug use.

As mentioned, the rate of drug administration is critical to these neuronal adaptations. To illustrate this, rats were exposed to doses of cocaine or saline infused through intravenous catheters. The infusion rate of intravenous cocaine was varied over 5, 25, or 100 seconds.

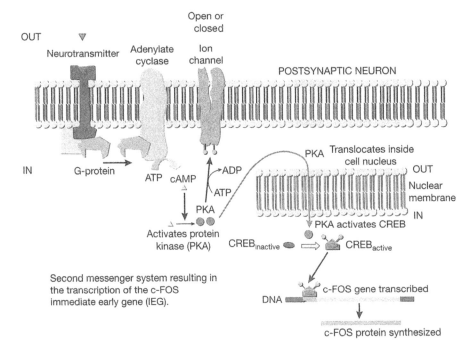

Figure 8.7 c-FOS gene transcription in response to neurotransmitter-activated second messenger system and CREB activation.

The researchers measured the density of c-FOS protein by a radioactive marker in several brain regions, including the medial prefrontal cortex and the nucleus accumbens. As shown in Figures 8.8 and 8.9, the rapid infusion (delivered within five seconds) of cocaine produced the greatest change in c-FOS expression. Rapid rates of cocaine and nicotine delivery also induced the greatest amount of locomotor activity (psychomotor sensitization) in these animals (Ferrario et al., 2008; Samaha et al., 2004; Samaha & Robinson, 2005).

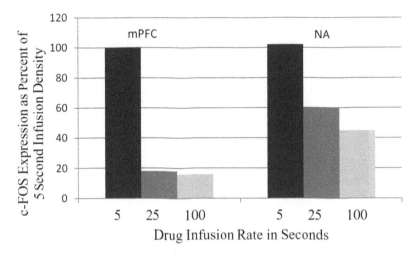

Figure 8.8 Cocaine-induced c-FOS expression in the medial prefrontal cortex (mPFC) and the nucleus accumbens (NA) following 5, 25, or 100 second drug infusion rates. Bars represent the percentage of c-FOS expression following a five-second infusion rate. c-FOS density was greatest following a five-second infusion and was approximately 18 percent of the five-second density in the mPFC and about 50 percent of the five-second density in the NA with 25 and 100 second infusion rates.

Source: Samaha and Robinson (2005).

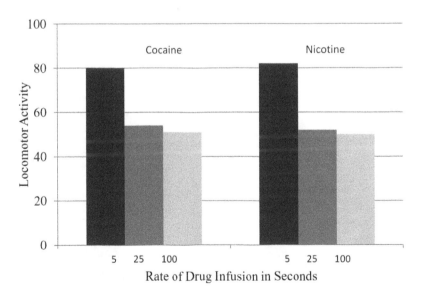

Figure 8.9 Locomotor activity of rats exposed to different rates of cocaine and nicotine administration. The rate of drug delivery influences the expression of psychomotor sensitization.

Source: Samaha and Robinson (2005).

While the consequences of rapid c-FOS expression on dopamine and other neurotransmitter function is not well understood, it has been suggested that it leads to receptor desensitization and internalization (Nestler & Aghajanian, 1997). Decreased dopamine receptor availability (downregulation) is clearly a consequence of chronic drug exposure. PET imaging studies of drug-addicted brains reveal downregulation in both mesolimbic and cortical dopamine regions and to dopamine innervation of the frontal lobe, as shown in Figures 8.10 and 8.11. c-FOS activity is also a biological marker for the conditioning of drug-associated cues, which trigger

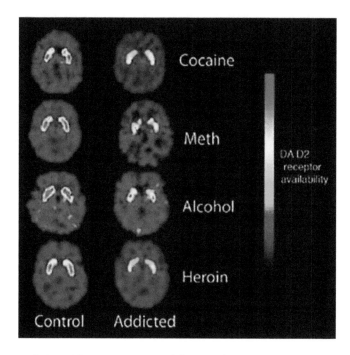

Figure 8.10 Downregulation of dopamine receptors following chronic drug exposure.

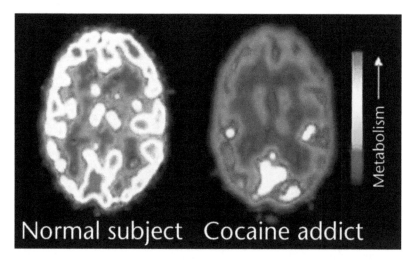

Figure 8.11 Decreased glucose utilization in the frontal lobe seen in addiction results in poor impulse control, deficient prosocial behavior, decreases in risk aversion and judgment.

both drug craving and drug-seeking behaviors (Kufahl et al., 2009). Using dopamine D_2 receptor knockout mice, Solís et al. (2021) found that incentive and psychomotor sensitization were diminished following both cocaine and amphetamine administration in these animals. Thus, behavioral sensitization appears to be dependent on adaptations to D_2 receptors following acute drug administration.

In summary, drug addiction is characterized by powerful and long-lasting behavioral changes, including drug cravings and drug seeking that can be reinstated after long periods of abstinence. Addiction occurs to a wide range of drugs that, although they have no common structural features, all contribute to increased dopamine activity in the nucleus accumbens, as well as in other structures of the mesocortical pathway. After repeated use, these addictive substances begin to alter the structure of dopamine-receiving neurons by upregulating the proteins CREB and c-FOS. A rapid rate of drug delivery and availability to the brain enhances CREB and c-FOS upregulation, but it is not essential. These proteins contribute to downregulation of $D_{1\&2}$ receptors in the nucleus accumbens. In addition, changes to mesocortical structures occur, leading to decreased frontal lobe activity (Figure 8.11), which allow for drug-associated stimuli to elicit drug-seeking behaviors, while leaving cortical inhibitory mechanisms unable to regulate them. Drug and alcohol addicts share common symptoms of those with frontal lobe dysfunction and hypofrontality. Addicts are defined by their lack of impulse control, poor judgment, decreased risk aversion, and poor social behavior. All of these are attributes of normal frontal lobe functioning.

Addiction is a complex set of neural adaptations leading to the development of tolerance, dependence, and a life-disrupting pattern of drug-related motivations and behaviors. The menacing fact that these changes are enduring and susceptible to reinstatement following abstinence makes addiction particularly difficult to treat.

The Treatment of Drug Addiction

Addiction's toll on society is estimated to exceed $300 billion each year, making it one of our most urgent social problems. Improving our understanding of the neurobiology of addiction will be critical to the development of new treatment methods. The treatment options available today are largely unsuccessful for most addicts, and those who do recover are at a continued risk of recidivism. Treatment for addiction can include drug therapy as well as behavioral therapies, including the popular 12-step program. Behavioral programs tend to target problematic patterns of behavior and the social and environmental contributions to drug use. They can also provide support as a substance abuser grapples with the pain of withdrawal. Current drug therapies, on the other hand, attempt to mimic the abused drug's effects and dampen cravings associated with withdrawal. Several of these approaches, including bupropion and nicotine replacement, are discussed in Chapter 10 on nicotine. It is important to emphasize that there are presently no cures for drug addiction. There are, however, several promising lines of research.

Immunization Against Abused Drugs

One of the most promising approaches to drug treatment research is to prevent the drug from entering the brain altogether. Two avenues of research along this line have been explored. One approach involves **passive immunization** with **catalytic antibodies** capable of rapidly degrading cocaine (Landry & Yang, 1997; Landry et al., 1993). Whether passive immunization with catalytic antibodies can effectively degrade cocaine over long periods of time has yet to be demonstrated. Passive immunization does not stimulate the production of new antibodies, and thus resistance to cocaine would be expected to diminish over time, requiring repeated immunization.

Another approach involves **active immunization** with a cocaine–protein conjugate that stimulates the formation of cocaine-specific antibodies (Ettinger et al., 1997; Johnson & Ettinger, 2000). In these experiments, cocaine molecules were actually attached to a large immunogenic protein and injected into laboratory animals. The reason for conjugating cocaine to a large protein is that organisms do not typically produce antibodies to small compounds. If they did, they (including humans) would develop antibody responses to all drugs and to foods that enter the blood supply. Attaching cocaine to a protein that is known to stimulate an immune response essentially tricks the immune system into recognizing the cocaine molecule as a foreign protein. After immunization with the cocaine-protein conjugate, antibodies are produced and attach to both the protein and to the cocaine molecule. Presumably, cocaine that is bound to a large antibody is unable to cross the blood–brain barrier, thereby resulting in lower levels of cocaine actually reaching the brain.

Figure 8.12 shows a typical western dot blot assay. Strips of assay paper are pretreated with drops of cocaine solution. Later, blood from an immunized animal is applied to the paper. If cocaine antibodies are present in the blood they will attach to the cocaine and be revealed by dark dots over the cocaine.

Research in the author's laboratory has shown that immunization with a cocaine–protein conjugate inhibits cocaine's reinforcing and analgesic properties as well as an animal's ability to discriminate cocaine from saline injections. Figure 8.13 shows the results of an experiment where laboratory rats were trained to discriminate cocaine from saline injections. After the animals learned the discrimination they were immunized against cocaine with the

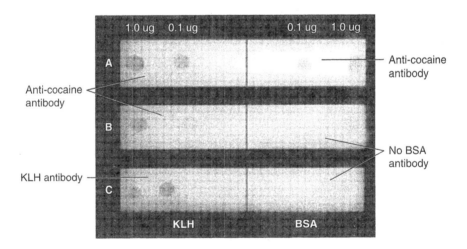

Figure 8.12 Western dot blot assays for anti-cocaine antibody. Two dilutions (1.0 ug and 0.1 ug) of cocaine-KLH were placed on the left side of strips A–C. Two dilutions of cocaine-BSA (1.0 ug and 0.1 ug) were placed on the right side of strips A and C. The right side of strip B contained two dilutions (1.0 ug and 0.1 ug) of BSA alone. Strips A and B were incubated with serum from an animal immunized with cocaine-KLH. Binding of antibodies to the strips is indicated by stain. Binding of antibody to cocaine-KLH (A and B left side), cocaine-BSA (right side of A indicated by arrows), but not to BSA alone (B right side) indicates the presence of anti-cocaine antibodies in this animal. Strip C was incubated with serum from an animal immunized with KLH alone. Binding of antibodies to cocaine-KLH (C left) indicates the presence of anti-KLH antibody. The absence of binding to the cocaine-BSA (C right) indicates the lack of anti-BSA or anti-cocaine antibody in this animal.

Source: Ettinger et al. (1997).

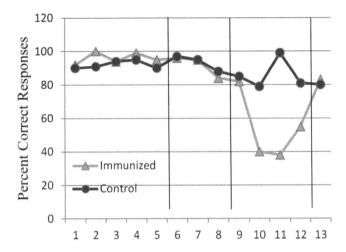

Figure 8.13 Percentage of correct responses during cocaine trials for the final five sessions prior to immunization, the three postimmunization maintenance sessions, and all five sessions after immunization.
Points to the right of the third vertical line mark the increase in cocaine dose from 5.0 mg/kg to
20.0 mg/kg for the final cocaine trial.

Source: Johnson and Ettinger (2000).

cocaine–protein conjugate. The ability of animals to accurately discriminate cocaine from
saline decreased from nearly 100 percent before immunization to approximately 50 percent
(chance levels) after immunization. High doses of cocaine could overwhelm the antibody,
however, and reinstate cocaine discrimination. Evidence from other laboratories also suggests
that immunization reduces the levels of cocaine in the brain, even following rapid routes of
delivery, such as intravenous and intranasal administration (Fox, 1997).

Other laboratories have also demonstrated effective immunization against the effects of
heroin (Bonese et al., 1974), nicotine (LeSage et al., 2006; Pentel et al., 2000), and methamphetamine (Byrnes-Blake et al., 2001) in laboratory animals. Several clinical trials evaluating
the effectiveness of cocaine immunization with humans have been conducted, but the results
are somewhat mixed. In a clinical trial with 18 cocaine-dependent subjects, anti-cocaine
vaccination apparently decreased the subjective, euphoric effects of cocaine, but most patients
relapsed to cocaine use during or immediately following treatment, in spite of their high
levels of anti-cocaine antibodies (Martell et al., 2005). Several additional clinical trials are
presently underway with cocaine and nicotine vaccines with the hopes of developing more
effective immunization methods. Presently there are no commercially available vaccines or
immunotherapies for addictive drugs, although numerous studies show promise for cocaine,
heroin, and methamphetamine abuse (Kinsey et al., 2009; Xiaoshan et al., 2020; Xu & Kosten,
2021 for a recent review).

Targeting Neural Mechanisms to Prevent Drug Relapse: Glutamate AMPA Receptors

As mentioned previously, a particularly sinister characteristic of addiction is its reinstatement
following long periods of drug abstinence. The reinstatement of cravings and drug-seeking
behavior can occur during periods of stress or upon exposure to drug-associated environmental cues. While it has long been suspected that projections from cortical neurons to the

nucleus accumbens must be involved in reinstatement, these speculations have only recently been confirmed. In a series of studies, evidence for glutaminergic neurons projecting from the prefrontal cortex to the nucleus accumbens have been established (Bossert et al., 2007; Engblom et al., 2008; Kalivas et al., 2003; LaLumiere & Kalivas, 2008; Ping et al., 2008). These glutamate neurons project to, and regulate the release of dopamine in, the nucleus accumbens (Sakae et al., 2015).

During stress, or in the presence of drug-associated cues, increased activity in the gluta-minergic pathway from the prefrontal cortex to the nucleus accumbens results in increases in glutamate release, which contributes to increased dopamine activity. A disruption of this activity caused by either dampening prefrontal glutamate neuronal activity or the blockade of glutamate AMPA receptors in the nucleus accumbens prevents the reinstatement of drug-seeking behavior in animals (LaLumiere & Kalivas, 2008). Glutamate plays an essential role in the regulation of dopamine in the prefrontal cortex elicited by drug-associated cues (Kawahara et al., 2021). Glutamate AMPA receptors control sodium channels and consequently the excit-ability of dopamine neurons (see Figure 8.14). These AMPA receptors are upregulated during drug use and are part of the set of complex neural and behavioral adaptations contributing to and maintaining drug addiction.

Given what we now know about the neural circuitry involved in drug relapse, the develop-ment of pharmacological methods to dampen this activity may be on the horizon. Blockade of glutamate AMPA receptors in the nucleus accumbens and the activation of inhibitory glutamate autoreceptors both prevent cue-induced reinstatement of drug seeking in animals. The development of drugs to target these receptors is in progress.

Targeting Neural Mechanisms to Prevent Drug Relapse: Dopamine D_3 Receptors

Research has suggested that the D_3 receptor plays a significant role in the regulation of dopa-mine release in the nucleus accumbens (Shafer & Levant, 1998). Unlike $D_{1\&2}$ receptors, D_3 receptors appear to be upregulated following chronic drug exposure. The enhanced expression of D_3 receptors appears to be critical for cue-induced cravings and drug-seeking behaviors in animals (Xi et al., 2013). Again, this neural mechanism evolved to ensure that animals would

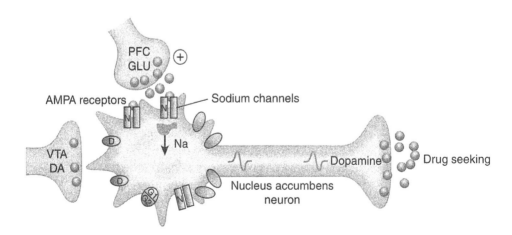

Figure 8.14 Glutaminergic involvement in the reinstatement of drug-seeking behavior following abstinence. Drug-associated cues can lead to the reinstatement of cravings and drug seeking via glutamate projections from the prefrontal cortex (PFC) to the nucleus accumbens, where they regulate the release of dopamine. Blockade of the glutamate AMPA receptor prevents reinstatement.

easily remember and seek cues associated with food and sexual partners. Addictive drugs coincidently amplify this adaptation.

Research has shown that selective D_3 antagonist may blunt DA release, via DA caused by drug-associated cues. In animal studies, D_3 antagonists disrupt amphetamine self-administration (Chen et al., 2014) and place preferences conditioned by cocaine (Hachimine et al., 2014; Song et al., 2013). A proposed treatment for stimulant addiction, therefore, is blocking these receptors with D_3 antagonists. It has been proposed that this blockade decreases cue-induced DA release, and therefore reduces drug cravings during abstinence (Guerrero-Bautista et al., 2020, 2021). At the time of writing, no human trials with D_3 antagonists had been conducted, but there is evidence of increased D_3 receptor expression in cocaine addicts (Payer et al., 2014).

Reversal of Neural Adaptations Following Abstinence

The adaptations to dopamine receptor expression described earlier may return to normal levels following extended abstinence. In animal studies, chronic exposure to cocaine resulted in depletions of both D_1 and D_2 receptor expression. After 21 days of abstinence, dopamine receptors returned to normal levels (Beveridge et al., 2009; Maggos et al., 1998). In human methamphetamine addicts, the return to normal dopamine functioning may not be as dramatic. Volkow et al. (2001) investigated dopamine receptor expression following abstinence in five methamphetamine abusers who had used meth at least five days per week for at least two years. As shown in Figure 8.15, dopamine functioning in several brain regions regained significant functioning after 14 months of abstinence. In more recent studies with human cocaine abusers, researchers found significant recovery of prefrontal cortex activity after long-term (10–14 months) abstinence (Connolly et al., 2012; Hanlon et al., 2013). It is difficult to compare human and animal studies since the duration of abuse is considerably longer in humans addicted to drugs and the methods of assessment are considerably different. While animal studies are limited to behavioral studies, human studies often use PET or fMRI

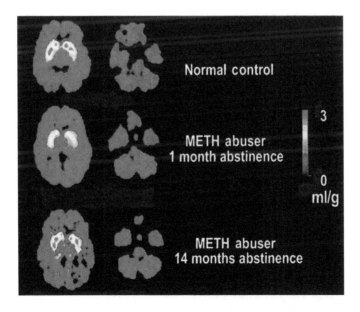

Figure 8.15 PET image studies of dopamine transporter availability following abstinence from methamphetamine. Source: Volkow et al. (2001).

brain scans. The differences in recovery rates between animals and humans described earlier may merely be a reflection of different methodologies. Clearly, these and other studies have promising implications for recovering addicts, but more research on the effects of protracted abstinence in humans needs to be done.

Are Video Games, Gambling, and Sex Addictive?

We often use the term "addiction" to describe compulsive, and occasionally destructive, behaviors like excessive video gaming, gambling, and hypersexuality. But are these behaviors really addictions? According to the definition of addiction laid out here, to label them addictions would require that we establish a pattern of neural adaptations in the mesolimbic and cortical systems similar to those resulting from repeated drug use. While there is evidence that video gaming, gambling, and sexual activity increase dopamine activity in the mesolimbic pathway, this by itself does not meet our definition of addiction. Dopamine activity in the mesolimbic pathway is involved in numerous activities, including eating, drinking, sexual behavior, behavior reinforcement, attention, and the kind of sensory-motor integration involved in video game playing (Koepp et al., 1998). Furthermore, cues associated with highly palatable foods, opportunities for reinforcement, a sexual partner, video games, and gambling can themselves increase arousal and dopamine activity. As I discussed in the previous section, the effectiveness of a substance as a reinforcer was not by itself useful in defining addiction.

In a recent study comparing the neural activity of casual video game players with excessive players, the researchers did find a difference in amplitude of electrical potentials induced by video game cues compared to those induced by neutral cues in one of nine brain areas investigated in excessive players. While the authors concluded that this represents sensitization of dopaminergic neurons in the mesolimbic pathway, they provide no compelling evidence of sensitization mediated by neural adaptations resulting from excessive game playing. In fact, the only electroencephalograph (EEG) recording that revealed differences between casual and excessive game players was recorded above the midline (Thalemann et al., 2007). Whether these recordings represent activity differences in mesolimbic structures cannot be determined by the EEG procedure (Figure 8.16).

A number of other studies have reported differences in dopaminergic activity between compulsive and non-compulsive gamblers (e.g., Bergh et al., 1997). For example, there is evidence

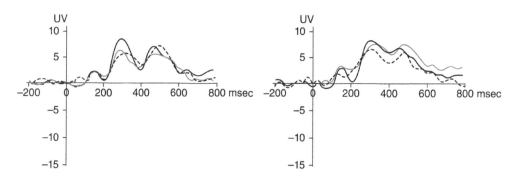

Figure 8.16 Electroencephalograph (EEG) recordings from the midline of brains in casual vs. excessive video game players. The dotted trace shows the pattern of electrical potentials evoked by video game visual cues. The dark gray trace was evoked by neutral cues and the light gray by alcohol-related cues. These EEG records were recorded from electrodes placed along the midline of the head (From Thalemann et al., 2007).

that gamblers carry an allele for the dopamine receptor gene (D_2A_1) far more frequently than non-gamblers (Comings et al., 1996; da Silva Lobo et al., 2007), which may indicate that there is a genetic disposition towards gambling. Similar results have been found with excessive video game players (Koepp et al., 1998). Again, however, an increase in dopamine activity is not evidence of a predisposition for addiction. In fact, increased densities of dopamine receptors do not appear to predispose individuals for substance abuse or addiction. A considerable amount of research is currently being conducted to uncover possible genetic contributions to addiction (see Agrawal & Lynskey, 2008, for a review). While much of this research suggests associations with genes, we still have no consensus on which genes might be involved.

In summary, compulsive gaming, gambling, and sexual behavior may share common diagnostic criteria with substance use disorders, but evidence that they share common patterns of neural adaptations that underlie drug addiction remains controversial. Labeling compulsive and sometimes life-disruptive behaviors as addictions neither advances our understanding of their causal factors nor does it elevate their status as a disease. Until we can describe patterns of neural adaptations in the mesolimbic pathway that accompany these compulsions, there is little evidence that they are addictions. Compulsive video game play, gambling, and sexual activity are each maintained by a complex set of reinforcer expectations and learned consequences that may make them much more difficult to fully describe than drug addictions.

In the following chapters I will examine the pharmacology and abuse liability of some of the most common drugs of abuse. In Chapter 9, I review the stimulants cocaine and amphetamine, the psychedelics LSD and psilocybin, and marijuana. In Chapter 10, I discuss alcohol, nicotine, and caffeine.

Glossary

Active immunization results in the stimulation of specific antibodies by the organism's immune system. Immunization against flu viruses is active immunization. Active immunization may also be used against specific drugs, such as cocaine.

Addiction a form of drug dependency that results from specific neural adaptations that affect dopamine activity in the mesolimbic and mesocortical systems.

Catalytic antibodies antibodies used in passive immunization that facilitate the degradation of a specific molecule or drug.

c-FOS a protein that is expressed in response to a variety of extracellular signals, including drugs such as cocaine, amphetamine, nicotine, and morphine.

c-FOS protein a protein transcription factor that promotes the synthesis of messenger RNA (mRNA) under the direction of DNA.

CREB protein cyclic AMP response element-binding protein. Binds to an element on DNA, thereby activating a gene for the synthesis of a specific protein.

Immediate early genes (IEGs) proteins that are activated by stimuli that activate intracellular signaling. IEGs may also be activated by certain drugs.

Incentive sensitization an increase in the incentive value of the drug as well as drug-associated cues.

Medial forebrain bundle the bundle of axons projecting from the VTA to the nucleus accumbens.

Passive immunization an immunization method using antibodies that rapidly degrade a molecule or drug by increasing enzyme activity. See also **Active immunization**.

Psychomotor sensitization refers to a drug's potential to increase motor activity and drug-seeking behaviors after repeated administration.

Reward pathway a pathway of dopaminergic neurons originating in the ventral tegmentum and projecting to the nucleus accumbens and prefrontal cortex.

Second messenger a chemical within a cell that activates a cascade of events leading to the opening or closing on an ion channel. Cyclic AMP (cAMP) is a second messenger. A neurotransmitter is considered to be the first messenger.

Self-administration an experimental procedure where animals can control the rate and amount of drug administration, usually by pressing a lever. Often used to assess the abuse liability of drugs.

Septum a structure of the mesolimbic system that is adjacent to the nucleus accumbens.

Substance use disorder a pattern of drug use that leads to significant impairment in functioning and personal relations. The *DSM-5* identifies substance use disorders by substance classification (alcohol use disorder, opiate use disorder, stimulant use disorder, etc.)

9 The Pharmacology of Scheduled Psychoactive Drugs

Psychostimulants, Psychedelics, and Marijuana

This chapter and the next examine the pharmacology of a wide range of drugs that have both clinical and recreational significance. These drugs range from the mild psychostimulant caffeine, which is found in coffee, tea, and chocolate, to some of the most addictive and destructive substances known, including crack cocaine and methamphetamine. The pharmacology of the opiates was described in an earlier chapter.

Katherine had a relatively normal childhood. She grew up in a family of four. Her father was a successful real-estate broker in Seattle and her mother, who was an elementary school teacher before she had children, remained at home during the early years before she and her twin brother started school. Late in elementary school Katherine discovered she could easily influence those around her using her popularity and good looks. She matured more quickly than other girls her age and took advantage of the attention she drew. By middle school Katherine was attracted to older boys and enjoyed the thrills of occasional cigarettes and alcohol that they could provide. She was able to evade most of the trouble her risky lifestyle taunted until she became pregnant during her junior year of high school. Her gothic style of dress kept this a secret from her friends and parents through the first four months of pregnancy. The secret ended when Katherine developed a serious infection from gonorrhea and needed medical attention. Because of the advanced stage of infection Katherine was encouraged to have an abortion. After this, Katherine's life began to change in significant ways. Her relationship with her parents deteriorated quickly, and she was no longer attending school. Katherine found the company of an older boy who could afford a nice downtown apartment by selling marijuana, methamphetamine, and crack cocaine whenever it was available. It wasn't long before Katherine was using meth regularly and assisting her friend in its distribution.

By the time she was 18, Katherine was addicted and no longer a desirable partner to her companion and business partner. Once their relationship ended Katherine found it more and more difficult to obtain the meth she craved. She returned home for a few weeks and convinced her father she needed a loan to begin cosmetology school and to secure an apartment near its campus. With $8,000 Katherine moved back downtown and quickly reestablished a source for meth. Her stint at school lasted less than a month, and it was clear that $8,000 wouldn't last much longer. At this point Katherine's life was consumed by methamphetamine. Most of her days began late, after shrugging off a drug hangover and trying to locate methamphetamine or crack cocaine. Even though Katherine knew the streets well, her drug cravings often pushed her for miles in the rain to finally locate a seller. On days drugs were unavailable Katherine returned to her apartment to fight off the severe headaches and nausea of withdrawals, and hopefully sleep. In order to keep her apartment, and the drug supply that now cost almost $100 per day, Katherine turned to petty theft and prostitution. At first she found it easy to attract high-paying clients through an agency in Seattle. However, as the meth began to take its toll, her appearance deteriorated quickly and her agency and once-easy clients were no longer interested.

Predictably, Katherine, along with several other young girls, was arrested late one night in a prostitution sting. Not knowing who else to call, she woke her mother who was able to secure her release. Shocked by her appearance and stuporous condition, her mother rushed her to a hospital. Katherine had lost over 30 lbs from her previously healthy weight, her forearms had scars from numerous injections and scratching,

DOI: 10.4324/9781003309017-9

and she had hepatitis from contaminated needles and unprotected sex. In the course of just over 18 months Katherine had transformed from an attractive and popular high school student to a young woman hovering over death with a methamphetamine addiction. Katherine was admitted to a private recovery clinic in Seattle where she spent the next 30 days living at the facility with few opportunities to leave. The exceptions were brief excursions with her parents for dinner or a quick shopping spree. After her in-house stay Katherine was allowed to move back to her parent's home and to attend college part time. She is now in her second semester with plans to study psychology.

During our interview Katherine admitted that, although she hasn't used drugs since her release, she has felt the intense urge. While recently driving the streets she had once walked in search of meth, the frightening and exhilarating anticipation of seeing a seller all rushed back to her. The next few hours were filled with the confusion of racing thoughts and the severe temptation to use just one more time. In all likelihood Katherine's addiction will win out within a year, as it unfortunately does with most drug addicts. The recidivism rate for meth addiction is over 80 percent within the first year of abstinence. Most recovered addicts will have sought help several times before finally quitting meth for good.

Katherine's case is neither surprising nor is it typical, as there is no characteristic course or set of experiences that leads one to drug addiction. Katherine flirted with risky behavior from early in middle school, but other drug addicts may begin using at a much older age, even after they have started a career and family. We begin this chapter, however, by reviewing the pharmacology of a wide range of drugs with potential for abuse in addition to their significant clinical importance.

The use of drugs by youth in our country had been rising at an alarming and steady rate prior to 2000. At that time, approximately 41percent of high school seniors had used an illicit drug during the previous year. Since the early 2000s, however, illicit drug use by teenagers has slightly declined (see Figures 9.1 and 9.2). The most recent statistics, from the National Survey on Drug Use and Health (Elflein, 2022), estimate the annual prevalence of illicit drug

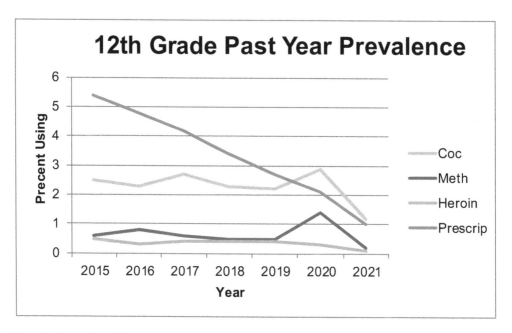

Figure 9.1 Annual prevalence of drug use by 12th graders from the highest prevalence rates recorded in 2000 through 2021. Since 2010, there has been a very slight decline in overall illicit drug use.

Source: SAMHSA (2022).

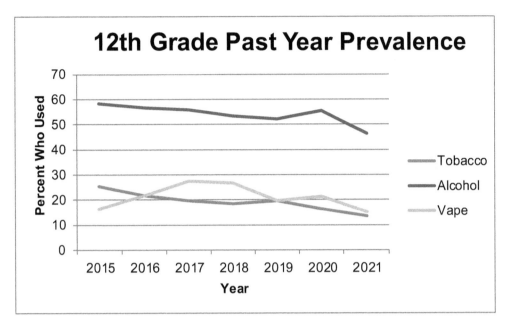

Figure 9.2 Annual prevalence of alcohol, tobacco, and vaping use by 12th graders. Both alcohol and tobacco use have declined about 1 percent each year for the past 10 years, while vaping has increased.

Source: SAMHSA (2022).

use by 12th graders to be approximatly 32 percent. A similar but steeper descending trend over these years has also been observed with alcohol and tobacco use. The only upward trends have been increases in vaping and **marijuana** use, which corresponds with a decrease in marijuana perception of risk, as well as marijuana's legal status in many states (see Figure 9.3).

The use of psychoactive drugs is not a recent phenomenon, as many of the drugs discussed in this chapter have uses dating back hundreds or even thousands of years. Caffeine, nicotine, cocaine, opium, **psychedelic** mushrooms, marijuana, and alcohol all have uses that can be traced back to ancient times. Other, more modern drugs are either derivatives of these ancient substances or they have been discovered or synthesized more recently. For example, amphetamines were more recently extracted from the Ephedra plant; **LSD** from the ergot fungus, which grows on grain; and morphine extracted from opium. For convenience, these psychoactive drugs will be separated into two categories: scheduled drugs and unscheduled drugs and substances.

The term **drug schedule** refers to a drug's classification based on its potential for abuse, as described by the **Controlled Substance Act** of 1970. The Controlled Substance Act identified five schedules, or classifications, of drugs ranging from Schedule I to Schedule V. Schedule I drugs, for instance, were those with little or no clinical significance but with a great potential for abuse. Included in Schedule I are LSD, marijuana, and heroin. Schedules II through V classified drugs with decreasing abuse potential and with some clinical importance. The drug schedules created by the Controlled Substance Act are summarized in Table 9.1 with a few examples within each classification. The use of scheduled drugs is highly regulated by the **Drug Enforcement Administration** (DEA), and they are only available by prescription from a licensed practitioner or through a special license issued by the DEA to scientists and laboratories for the purpose of conducting research.

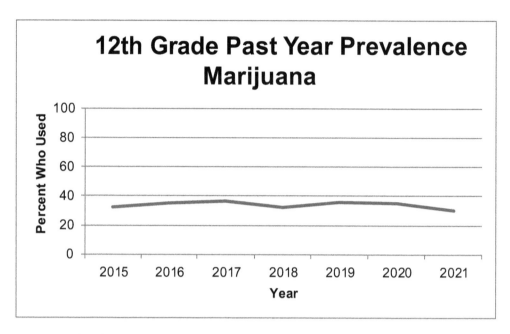

Figure 9.3 A relatively stable pattern of marijuana use since 2015 among 12th grade students.
Source: National Institute on Drug Abuse (2021).

Table 9.1 The classification of controlled substances by the Controlled Substance Act of 1970.

Schedule	Description	Examples of drugs and substances
I	Drugs have a high potential for abuse, have no accepted medical use, and there is a lack of safety information regarding their use.	Heroin, LSD, mescaline, psilocybin, marijuana
II	Drugs have a high potential for abuse, have accepted medical uses, but their use may lead to severe dependence.	Morphine, codeine, cocaine, amphetamine, methamphetamine, nabilone (synthetic THC)
III	Drugs have a potential for abuse, have accepted medical uses, and their use may lead to low or moderate dependence.	Anabolic steroids, pentobarbital, Marinol (synthetic THC)
IV	Drugs have a low potential for abuse, have accepted medical uses, and they have a lower risk of dependence than Schedule III drugs.	Benzodiazepines, Phenobarbital, and Ambien and similar sleep aids
V	Drugs have a low potential for abuse, have accepted medical uses, and have a lower risk of dependence than Schedule IV drugs.	Codeine and opiate preparations for cough or diarrhea

Note: A complete list of scheduled drugs is available from the Drug Enforcement Administration (www.usdoj.gov/dea).

Scheduled Psychoactive Drugs

The scheduled drugs discussed in this section include cocaine, amphetamines, marijuana, and psychedelic drugs. All of these drugs fall into either Schedule I or II for controlled substances. It is important to point out that the assignment of a drug schedule may be more influenced by politics than by pharmacology. Marijuana and LSD are two such examples. Neither of these drugs has been shown to have a high abuse potential and marijuana, arguably, has medical benefits. The barbiturates and benzodiazepines that fall into Schedules III and IV were described in Chapter 5 on anxiety disorders, and the opiates in Schedules I and II were described in Chapter 7.

Psychostimulants: Cocaine

Cocaine is extracted from the coca plant (*Erythroxylum coca*), which readily grows in the mountainous regions of South America (Figure 9.4). Although most of the illicit cocaine comes from Columbia and Peru, significant amounts are also grown in Bolivia and Ecuador.

Coca leaves have been used by the indigenous people of South America for thousands of years. These leaves, when chewed, produce a sense of well-being and confidence, as well as relief from fatigue. The practice of chewing coca leaves appears to have been widespread in South America, and evidence for its use has even been found in ancient Peruvian tombs. While chewing coca is still popular in some South American regions, most cocaine is exported as cocaine sulfate or cocaine hydrochloride.

Cocaine compounds are extracted from the coca leaf by crushing the leaves in a solvent such as kerosene, benzene, or alcohol to extract the cocaine. Traditionally the leaves were crushed by stomping on them in large vats, but mechanical crushing has essentially replaced stomping, as it is a much quicker and more efficient way to macerate the leaves for cocaine extraction. The liquid mixture that is produced is processed with heat and sulfuric acid to isolate the cocaine alkaloids and remove the waxy residue from the leaf extract. This process results in a cocaine sulfate paste that can contain as much as 60 percent cocaine. Cocaine paste can be further processed with diluted hydrochloric acid to produce a water-soluble crystalline compound called cocaine hydrochloride (see Figure 9.5).

Not only have large cocaine processing facilities in South America provided customers around the world with cocaine, they have begun to devastate the ecology of streams and rivers where these solvents are dumped after cocaine extraction. Numerous formerly pure streams in Columbia and Peru are now polluted with extraction solvents such as kerosene, gasoline, and benzene, as well as sulfuric and hydrochloric acids.

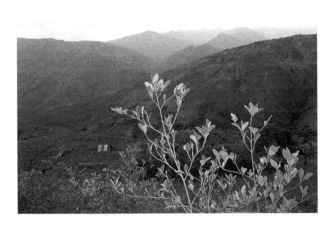
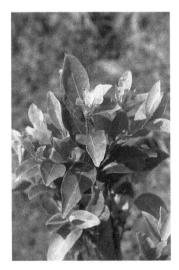

Figure 9.4 Coca shrubs grow readily in mountainous regions throughout South America. The coca leaves from these shrubs can be harvested several times each year.

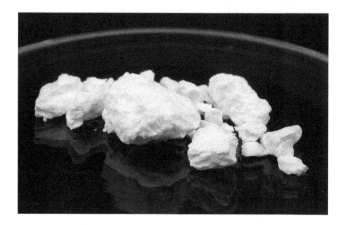

Figure 9.5 Processed cocaine hydrochloride. This water-soluble compound can be snorted, injected, or converted into crack cocaine for smoking.

As shown in Figure 9.1, the use of cocaine among high school seniors has been essentially stable for the past 10–15 years. However, in 2021 it was estimated that over 14 percent of Americans over age 12 had used cocaine at least once and that there are about 2 million regular users of cocaine. In the United States, a gram of cocaine hydrochloride (about 60–70 percent pure) costs just over $175, but the price can vary widely depending on location. This is enough cocaine to provide about 5–10 doses of snorted, or 10–15 doses of intravenous, cocaine to users who have not developed significant tolerance.

While the amount of cocaine produced in South America is difficult to determine, the Office of National Drug Control Policy estimates that 2,000 metric tons were produced in 2020, and most of this was bound for the United States. In that year, over 73 metric tons (73,000 kilos) were seized by law enforcement agencies in the United States. These numbers have remained relatively stable over the past decade.

History of Cocaine Use

The stimulant effects of coca were recognized and well described long before cocaine was identified as its active ingredient. The cocaine alkaloid was first isolated in 1855 by the German chemist Friedrich Gaedcke, who named it erythroxyline. It was another German scientist, Albert Niemann, who actually named it cocaine after carefully describing its extraction and purification process. Soon after its isolation, cocaine became widely used as a local **anesthetic**, particularly for surgeries of the eyes and nose. Cocaine was also added to tonics and beverages because of its stimulating effects. In 1863, the wine tonic Vin Mariani was marketed in the United States, and soon after cocaine was added to the original Coca-Cola recipe, thus its name. By the early 1900s, cocaine could be purchased in local drugstores and was included in a variety of tonics and remedies.

Sigmund Freud's interest in cocaine began in the early 1880s after reading scientific reports about its effects. Freud claims to have used cocaine frequently during this period: "I take very small doses of it regularly against depression and against indigestion, and with the most brilliant success." His experiences as well as recommendations for its uses were soon published in a series of scientific papers and letters called the *Cocaine Papers*. The first of this sequence,

"Über Coca" (About Cocaine), was published in 1884. A selection from this work describes some of his experiences:

> The psychic effect of cocaïnum muriaticum in doses of 0.05–0.10g consists of exhilaration and lasting euphoria, which does not differ in any way from the normal euphoria of a healthy person. The feeling of excitement which accompanies stimulus by alcohol is completely lacking; the characteristic urge for immediate activity which alcohol produces is also absent. One senses an increase of self-control and feels more vigorous and more capable of work; on the other hand, if one works, one misses that heightening of the mental powers which alcohol, tea, or coffee induce. One is simply normal, and soon finds it difficult to believe that one is under the influence of any drug at all.

Freud enthusiastically promoted the use of cocaine to his friends and his fiancée, in spite of concerns by those close to him that he may have become addicted to it. Freud continually denied that cocaine had any harmful effects, and whether he was actually addicted during this time remains unknown:

> It seems to me noteworthy—and I discovered this in myself and in other observers who were capable of judging such things—that a first dose or even repeated doses of coca produce no compulsive desire to use the stimulant further; on the contrary, one feels a certain unmotivated aversion to the substance.

It wasn't until the passage of the **Harrison Narcotic Tax Act** in 1914 that cocaine was prohibited in all its forms and mistakenly described as a dangerous narcotic. After its prohibition, cocaine was only available to licensed practitioners for medicinal and research uses. Its use as a **local anesthetic** continues to the present, although other local anesthetics, like lidocaine (Xylocaine) and procaine (Novocaine), are much more commonly used.

Pharmacology of Cocaine

Cocaine hydrochloride (cocaine-HCl) is a water-soluble compound that, once administered, readily separates into cocaine-H^+ and Cl^- ions in the blood. The protonated (positively charged) cocaine ion (cocaine-H^+) quickly passes through cell membranes and enters the brain. How rapidly cocaine enters the brain depends on its route of administration. Snorted and orally ingested cocaine enter the brain more slowly and incompletely than either intravenous administration or the inhalation of vaporized cocaine. For example, peak levels of cocaine are reached within five minutes of an IV injection compared to nearly an hour after intranasal administration.

Crack Cocaine

In the 1980s, cocaine users began converting cocaine hydrochloride (an acid) into a base by dissolving it in a mild ammonia (NH_3) solution. This results in the compound **methylbenzoylecgonine**, which could be vaporized for inhalation. During the production process a cracking sound is made, thus the name **crack**. Crack cocaine can also be manufactured by heating cocaine hydrochloride in water and sodium bicarbonate (baking soda). The cocaine rocks (called freebase cocaine) produced by these methods are then heated until they vaporize. Inhaling the vapors of freebase cocaine is an efficient and rapid method of cocaine delivery. Peak plasma levels are reached within five minutes by inhalation (Figure 9.6).

Cocaine is widely distributed throughout bodily tissues and is metabolized quickly by both blood and liver enzymatic hydrolysis. The metabolic half-life of cocaine varies between one and one and a half hours. The principal metabolites of cocaine are **benzoylecgonine** and **ecgonine**, both of which can be detected in the blood and other tissues for several weeks. Benzoylecgonine can also be detected in the hair of regular users for the life of a particular hair cell or until it is cut and only sections grown since the last drug use are exposed. If cocaine is used with alcohol the active compound **cocaethylene** is formed, which is believed to be an even more potent euphoric than cocaine itself. Cocaethylene has a half-life of approximately two and a half hours, nearly doubling the duration of the toxic and psychoactive effects of cocaine. Cocaethylene is particularly toxic to cardiac functioning. It causes severe hypertension, ventricular arrhythmia, and decreased blood flow—any of which can have unpredictably fatal consequences to otherwise healthy individuals (Wilson & French, 2002).

Mechanisms of Cocaine Action

Cocaine readily passes through cell membranes in the brain and acts by binding to the **dopamine transporter** (DAT) on the presynaptic membrane. Because of its high affinity for the transporter protein, cocaine blocks the normal reuptake of dopamine from the synaptic gap, resulting in prolonged dopamine activity on postsynaptic receptors. Cocaine has similar effects on transporters for both norepinephrine and serotonin. However, cocaine's effects on the dopamine transporter are believed to be the most important for its psycho-stimulating and reinforcing effects. In human studies, the subjective, euphoric effects of cocaine appear to be directly related to its degree of DAT binding (shown in Figure 9.6). At least 47 percent of dopamine transporters need to be blocked before subjects perceive the euphoric effects of cocaine, and doses that typically induce euphoria in cocaine users occupy between 60 and 80 percent of DATs (Volkow et al., 1997).

It is important to note, however, that DAT blockade by itself is not sufficient to account for cocaine's euphoric effects. The drug methylphenidate (Ritalin), which was described in the chapter on attention disorders, also blocks DATs to an extent similar to that of cocaine. The critical difference between methylphenidate and cocaine is how rapidly DAT blockade occurs after administration. Cocaine quickly enters the brain and blocks DATs, while orally administered methylphenidate only does so slowly (Volkow et al., 2003). A rapid increase in dopamine activity in the **mesolimbic system** is believed to be critical for the euphoric and reinforcing potential of cocaine and other addictive substances.

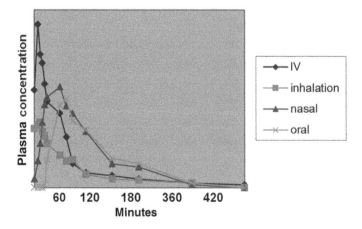

Figure 9.6 Plasma cocaine levels. Cocaine concentrations in plasma depend upon the route of administration. The highest concentrations follow IV administration or inhalation in about five minutes.

As stated, cocaine also blocks norepinephrine and serotonin transporters, and these systems may also contribute to cocaine's reinforcing and euphoric effects. To examine this, mice with genetic deletions of the DAT gene (knockout mice) have been tested for cocaine's reinforcing effects. If cocaine reinforcement is mediated solely by dopamine transporter blockade, DAT knockout mice would not be expected to demonstrate cocaine reinforcing effects. A popular method to investigate drug reinforcement is to repeatedly administer cocaine to animals in the same side of a dual-chambered apparatus (see Figure 9.8). Later, animals are given a choice to explore both chambers, and the time animals spend on each side is a measure of their conditioned place preference. This procedure is referred to as **place preference conditioning** (PPC). Typically, animals prefer spending time in the chamber associated with cocaine administration.

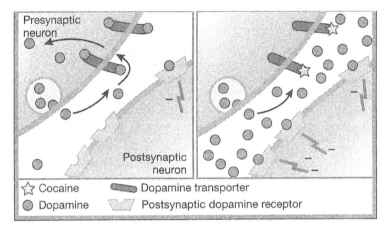

Figure 9.7 Model of how cocaine affects dopamine system. Cocaine acts by blocking the reuptake transporters for dopamine, serotonin, and norepinephrine on the presynaptic terminal.

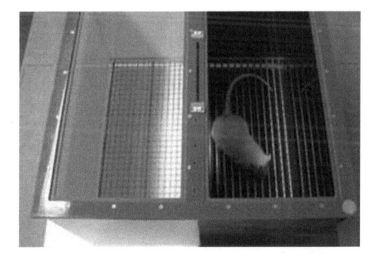

Figure 9.8 Place preference conditioning (PPC) apparatus used to investigate the reinforcing effects of drugs. Animals tend to prefer spending time in the chamber associated with cocaine administration. Place preference conditioning is a demonstration of Pavlovian conditioning where context cues serve as conditioned stimuli (CSs) and drug onset serves as an unconditioned stimulus (US). Conditioned responses (CRs) are increases in motivation and arousal expressed as preferences for the drug-associated context.

Dopamine transporter knockout mice retain cocaine's reinforcing effects in spite of the fact that they don't express the dopamine transporter. It is believed that in these mice cocaine effects on serotonin neurons within the **ventral tegmental area** (VTA) contribute to enhance dopamine activity in the mesolimbic system, particularly in the **nucleus accumbens** (Hnasko et al., 2007; Mateo et al., 2004; Sora et al., 2001; Thanos et al., 2008).

In summary, cocaine's euphoric and reinforcing effects are primarily mediated by enhanced dopamine concentrations in synapses in the nucleus accumbens and in the basal ganglia. In DAT **knockout animals** these effects appear to be mediated upstream of the nucleus accumbens, in the ventral tegmental area (VTA) of the midbrain where these dopamine neurons originate. Serotonin in the VTA appears to regulate dopamine activity and may contribute to increased dopamine release in the nucleus accumbens (see Figure 9.9).

Cocaine as a Local Anesthetic and Na⁺ Channel Blockade

Cocaine has a long history of use as an anesthetic for surgery of the eyes, mouth, and nose (see Figure 9.10). Its ability to not only dull pain but to constrict local blood flow makes it ideal for these uses. Cocaine disrupts the propagation of action potentials by blocking voltage-gated Na^+ channels. As action potentials propagate along an axon, voltage-gated sodium channels open as the membrane depolarizes, allowing Na^+ influx and a continuation of the action potential. When cocaine enters these channels it effectively blocks Na^+ influx and prevents further depolarization (Figure 9.11). Because protonated cocaine (cocaine-H^+) more easily enters a sodium channel when it is open, the anesthetic effects of cocaine are greatest when local pain-transmitting neurons are rapidly firing. Cocaine is most often used as a local anesthetic whenever its actions are to be restricted to its site of administration. In surgery of the eye, for example, cocaine may either be applied directly to the eye or injected to tissues surrounding the eye. Cocaine does have **analgesic** properties when administered systemically (an IV injection, for example), but these effects are not considered local anesthetic effects, even though the anesthetic effects is still mediated by Na^+ channel blockade.

Cocaine use is occasionally associated with cardiac toxicity, including myocardial infarction, arrhythmias, and occasional sudden death. It is believed that Na^+ channel blockade in neurons controlling cardiac functioning may be a contributing factor in these abnormalities. Cocaine's respiratory depressant effects are also believed to be mediated by Na^+ channel blockade in neurons within the chemosensitive sites of the medulla. Normally, these neurons respond to decreases in blood pH by triggering ventilatory responses. Cocaine, as well as the opiates, barbiturates, and alcohol can all inhibit respiratory responses, although by different means, and can lead to respiratory failure and sudden death.

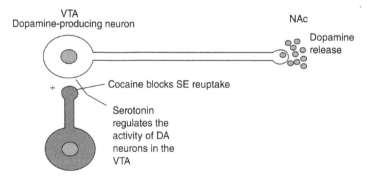

Figure 9.9 Serotonin–dopamine interactions in the ventral tegmental area (VTA). Serotonin, and perhaps norepinephrine, regulates the activity of dopamine neurons in the VTA and can contribute to increased dopamine release in the nucleus accumbens (NAc).

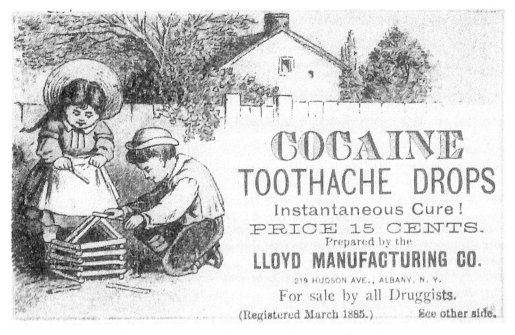

1885 Advertisement for cocaine toothache drops

Figure 9.10 Cocaine was widely used as a local anesthetic before 1914, when it was prohibited in tonics and remedies.

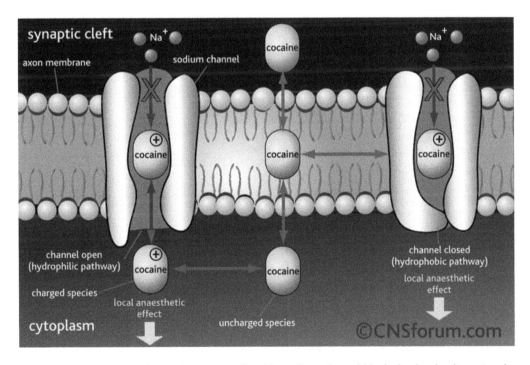

Figure 9.11 Cocaine's anesthetic effects are mediated by sodium channel blockade, thereby disrupting the propagation of action potentials. Protonated cocaine (cocaine-H$^+$) readily enters Na$^+$ channels when pain-transmitting neurons are firing.

Psychostimulants: Amphetamine and Methamphetamine

The amphetamines are a collection of closely related compounds that resemble the neurotransmitter dopamine in chemical structure (see Figure 9.12). The first of these compounds to be used was ephedrine, which is extracted from the *ephedra sinica* plant, also known as ma huang from ancient Chinese medicine. Ma huang has been used as an herbal remedy for at least 5,000 years to treat a variety of ailments, including asthma and allergic reactions as well as congestion resulting from the common cold.

More recently, **ephedra** has been marketed as a diet aid for weight loss, to increase wakefulness, and as a performance enhancer. Its effectiveness as a weight loss and performance-enhancing supplement remain controversial, but it has nevertheless been banned by many sport organizations as well as by the International Olympic Committee. Because of several highly publicized fatalities related to ephedra in the late 1990s, it was finally banned altogether by the FDA in 2004.

Amphetamine was first synthesized by the Romanian chemist Lazăr Edeleanu in 1887. It wasn't until the mid-1930s, however, that amphetamine was finally marketed as an inhalant antihistamine under the trade name Benzedrine. Soon after, the structurally related amphetamine **dextroamphetamine** (Dexedrine, shown in Figure 9.13) was introduced to treat narcolepsy, attention disorders, nasal congestion, and obesity. By the late 1940s, amphetamines were used to treat nearly 40 different disorders, including depression, fatigue, obesity, narcolepsy, drug addiction, and even the hiccups. It was also widely used by the US military to thwart fatigue and sleepiness in combat during both world wars. By the 1960s, amphetamine production surged as it was mass marketed as a weight loss aid. During this time of easy availability it was used by many college students to facilitate long study sessions in lieu of caffeine.

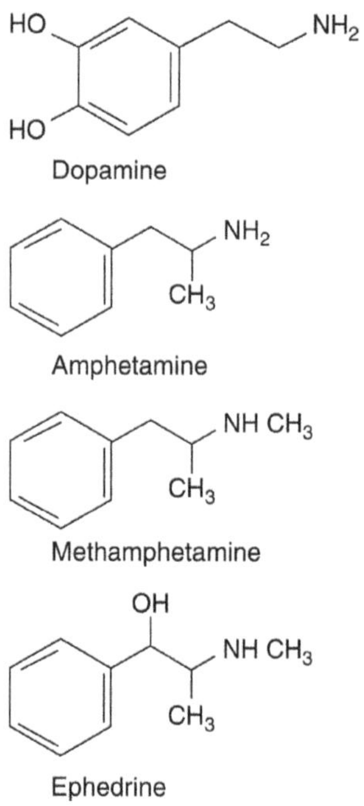

Figure 9.12 Molecular structures of dopamine, amphetamine, methamphetamine, and ephedrine. All of these compounds share a similar core structure.

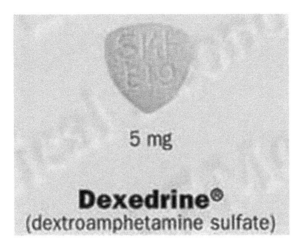

Figure 9.13 Dexedrine, dextroamphetamine sulfate, is available in either tablet or capsule form.

Endurance athletes, particularly competitive cyclists, found amphetamines useful to enhance training and competition. Sadly their use in sports led to a number of unfortunate deaths related to cardiac toxicity. In the early 1970s, amphetamine production reached its all-time high of over 10 billion tablets. Because of the widespread abuse of amphetamines, Benzedrine was replaced with propylhexedrine as the active ingredient in the Benzedrex inhaler, and Dexedrine became more restricted as it was classified as a Schedule II drug with high abuse potential and limited medical use. Dexedrine and other amphetamines are still prescribed to treat narcolepsy and some attention disorders.

As amphetamine became less available, and users demanded an even more powerful drug, illicit amphetamine sales and the manufacture of methamphetamine surged. **Methamphetamine** was first synthesized from ephedrine in 1893, but its popularity in the United States emerged in the 1980s as users quickly discovered its powerful euphoric effects. The name methamphetamine comes from its chemical name methyl-amphetamine (**desoxyephedrine**). Methamphetamine is easily produced by the chemical reduction of ephedrine (loss of the hydroxyl group, shown in Figure 9.12). Clandestine laboratories perform this reduction by various methods requiring chemicals that are easily obtained (as depicted in the popular HBO series *Breaking Bad*). Methamphetamine differs structurally from amphetamine by the additional methyl group (CH_3), which increases its lipid solubility, allowing it to cross the blood–brain barrier within seconds of an injection. As the illustration in Figure 9.14 shows, pure methamphetamine is in a crystal form, thus the name **crystal meth**.

Pharmacology of the Amphetamines

Amphetamines can be administered by various methods, including the oral ingestion of pill forms, nasal inhalation (snorting), smoking, or by IV injection. Peak plasma levels are reached in about two to three hours after oral administration and within five minutes after an IV injection or smoking. Once administered, amphetamine is rapidly distributed to body tissues, including the brain. Because of its greater lipid solubility, methamphetamine crosses the blood–brain barrier more quickly, allowing larger concentrations of the drug to enter the

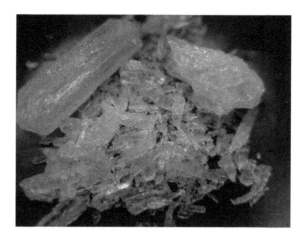

Figure 9.14 Methamphetamine (desoxyepherdine) is derived from several precursor compounds, including ephedrine and pseudoephedrine. This crystalline form is typically called crystal meth.

brain. For this reason, methamphetamine produces a greater "high" and users prefer it over other forms of amphetamine.

The metabolic half-life of the amphetamines varies between approximately 10 and 15 hours. Amphetamine is metabolized into p-OH-amphetamine and norephedrine, both of which are inactive. Methamphetamine is first metabolized into amphetamine before it is more completely metabolized and excreted by the kidneys.

Mechanisms of Amphetamine Action

Amphetamines, including methamphetamine, have perhaps some of the most complex and wide-ranging synaptic effects of any psychoactive drug (see Figure 9.15). They increase synaptic concentrations of both norepinephrine and dopamine by several different mechanisms. First of all, amphetamines block the **reuptake transporters** for norepinephrine, as well as increase the amount of norepinephrine (NE) released into the synapse during neuronal firing. Both of these effects contribute to enhanced norepinephrine activity in both the brain and the peripheral nervous system.

Amphetamines contribute to increased dopamine activity by several different mechanisms. First, they bind to the vesicular transporter and cause dopamine to be released from its storage vesicles into the cytoplasm of the terminal button. This "free" dopamine is then transported into the synaptic cleft by amphetamine-induced reversal of the dopamine transporter (DAT). Amphetamines also increase the amount of dopamine released from synaptic vesicles during neuronal signaling. These combined mechanisms enhance extra cellular concentrations of dopamine significantly.

The mechanisms by which the amphetamines contribute to behavioral stimulation, euphoria, and to cortical arousal appear to be complex as well. Dopamine agonism contributes to both euphoria and to increased cortical arousal via the **mesolimbic–mesocortical pathways** originating in the ventral tegmental area (VTA). Dopamine projects from the VTA to the nucleus accumbens as well as several other limbic structures, including the amygdala and hypothalamus. It is believed that the euphoria caused by amphetamine is mediated in these regions of the brain. Dopamine neurons from the VTA also project to the frontal cortex (the mesocortical pathway).

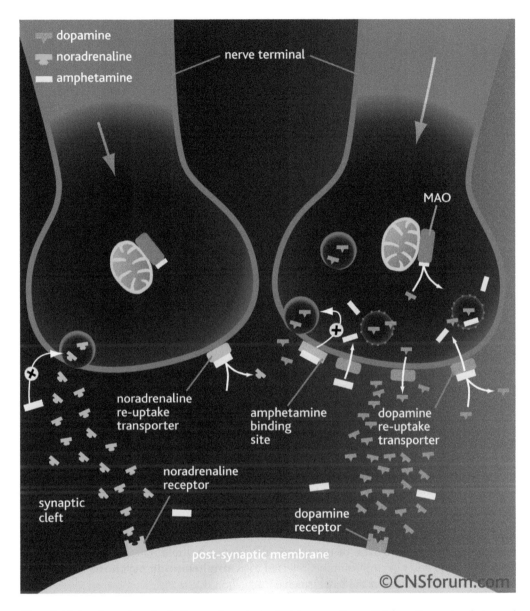

Figure 9.15 Amphetamines (including methamphetamine) increase the availability of norepinephrine and dopamine in several different ways, including: (1) by binding to the presynaptic membrane of dopaminergic and noradrenergic neurons it increases the release of both norepinephrine and dopamine from synaptic vesicles; (2) by causing the transporters for dopamine to act in reverse, transporting vesicular dopamine back into the terminal, and to transport this "free" dopamine into the synaptic cleft; and (3) by blocking the reuptake transporter for norepinephrine.

Amphetamines also increase dopamine activity and release in the **nigrostriatal system**, which originates in the substantia nigra and projects to regions of the basal ganglia. The motor-stimulating effects of amphetamines are mediated by increased dopamine activity in these regions. At high doses amphetamines can induce **stereotyped behavior** and hallucinations, resembling behaviors observed in some schizophrenic patients. In fact, researchers have

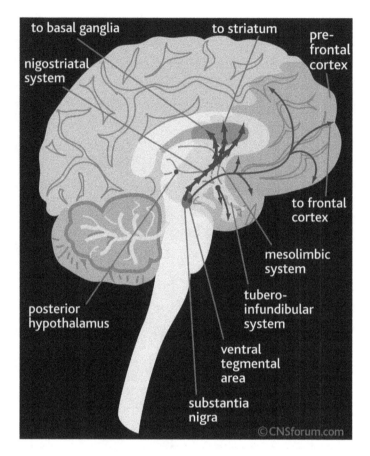

Figure 9.16 Dopamine pathways originate in the substantia nigra and ventral tegmental area of the midbrain. The nigrostriatal system innervates the basal ganglia while the mesolimbic-cortical system projects to the nucleus accumbens and to the frontal cortex.

used this observation to induce psychotic states in animals with amphetamine as a method to investigate the effectiveness of novel antipsychotic medication. The psychotic symptoms caused by toxic doses of amphetamine, referred to as **amphetamine psychosis**, are believed to involve structures within the basal ganglia.

In summary, amphetamines cause a wide array of effects mediated by enhanced dopaminergic and noradrenergic activity in all three of the major dopamine and norepinephrine pathways in the brain. These effects include enhanced or stimulated cognitive abilities, increases in motor activity, and states of euphoria and well-being.

As illustrated in Figures 9.16 and 9.17, amphetamines cause increased norepinephrine and dopamine activity, which also contribute to cortical arousal via the **reticular activating system** originating in the brainstem. Increased activity in the reticular activating system increases cortical arousal, vigilance, and attention. These neurotransmitters also contribute to amphetamines' anorectic (decreased appetite) effects. Amphetamines increase the expression of the appetite-suppressing peptide **CART** (**cocaine and amphetamine-regulated transcript**) in the **arcuate nucleus** of the hypothalamus. CART is believed to play a significant role in the hypothalamic regulation of feeding and satiety. Certainly CART is at least partially involved in the appetite-suppressing effects of both cocaine and amphetamine.

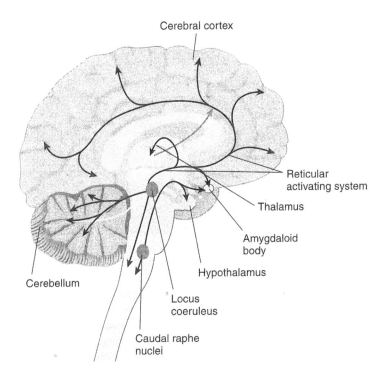

Figure 9.17 Cell bodies of norepinephrine neurons are predominantly located in the locus coeruleus and project along the reticular activating system to the hypothalamus, the thalamus, and to the frontalcortex.

Other Amphetamine-Related Compounds

A number of other compounds that are structurally related to the amphetamines also have powerful euphoric effects. Perhaps the best known of these is **ecstasy**, or methylenedioxymethamphetamine (**MDMA**), shown in Figures 9.18 and 9.19. Another, but less familiar, compound is 3,4 methylenedioxyamphetamine (**MDA**).

MDMA, also referred to as ecstasy or Molly, first gained popularity in the 1970s as a drug used to assist psychotherapy. Therapists who promoted its use claimed it facilitated communication and allowed patients to more directly experience their inner self. MDMA quickly spread to recreational use before it was banned by the FDA in 1985. MDMA is now listed as a Schedule I drug with no accepted medical use and a high potential for abuse. The use of MDMA peaked in the early 2000s as its popularity as a "club drug" soared. By 2014, an estimated 15 percent of 18–25-year-olds had used ecstasy. Since 2003, there has been a slight decline in MDMA use, but about 7 percent of the adult population used ecstasy in 2015 (NIDA, 2016).

Users of MDMA report that it produces euphoria, increased self-perception, enhanced sensations, and that it promotes intimacy with others. Ecstasy also produces some very troubling side effects, including increased heart rate and blood pressure, intense sweating, and teeth grinding so forceful broken teeth were not uncommon. To prevent tooth damage users often chew on baby pacifiers. Perhaps the most troubling effect of MDMA, however, is its powerfully neurotoxic effects.

In animal studies, short-term MDMA administration is known to cause significant damage to cortical serotonergic neurons (Hatzidimitriou et al., 1999; Mechan et al., 2006). These

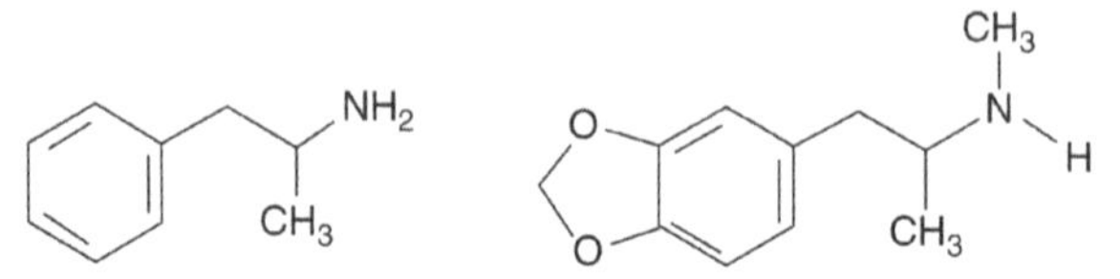

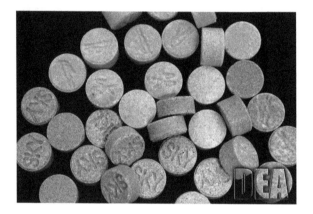

Amphetamine   Methylenedioxymethamphetamine (MDMA)

Figure 9.18 Methylenedioxymethamphetamine (MDMA), also referred to as ecstasy, is structurally similar to amphetamine.

Figure 9.19 Tablets of methylenedioxymethamphetamine (MDMA), used as a club drug, have been banned since 1985.

degenerative effects appear to persist for many years after acute MDMA use (see Figure 9.20). By all indications the use of MDMA by humans is also associated with neurotoxicity, including decreased serotonin synthesis in the frontal cortex (Booij et al., 2014). Two recent reviews of research studies that have examined the effects of MDMA use on cognitive functions both concluded that even low to moderate drug use was associated with decrements in a number of cognitive domains, including attention, concentration, and memory (Kalechstein et al., 2007; Mustafa et al., 2020; Zakzanis et al., 2007).

MDMA is a potent serotonin and dopamine agonist. It directly increases serotonin activity by both enhancing serotonin release during neuronal signaling and preventing its reuptake. MDMA appears to enhance dopamine activity in the nucleus accumbens by blocking DAT and perhaps indirectly by activating serotonergic neurons, which regulate dopamine activity in the ventral tegmental area (Amato et al., 2007; Federici et al., 2007). MDMA is predominantly a serotonin agonist, but dopamine activity plays a significant role in its euphoric and behavior-stimulating effects. Dopamine is also believed to mediate MDMA's reinforcing effects in animal **self-administration** studies (Ball & Slane, 2014; Daniela et al., 2006).

Psychedelic Drugs: LSD and Psilocybin

Of all of the psychotropic drugs, LSD (lysergic acid diethylamide) causes perhaps the most astonishing psychological effects. Most notable are LSD's powerful hallucinogenic effects. Hallucinations, which are profound distortions of a person's perceptual experiences, can occur in any sense modality. The most striking hallucinations caused by LSD are visual. These hallucinations

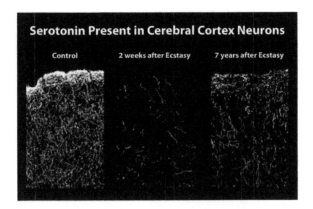

Figure 9.20 Serotonin present in cerebral cortex neurons. Cortical serotonergic axons in a squirrel monkey after saline (control) or 5 mg/kg MDMA twice daily for four days. Animals were sacrificed and examined after two weeks or after seven years. Some cortical regeneration can be seen after seven years.

Source: Hatzidimitriou et al. (1999).

typically involve color and movement elaboration. For example, while observing clouds a person under the influence of LSD may see complex distortions in their color and movement. Sounds or music may be heard with greater intensity and complexity. For instance, because of sound exaggeration, a person may describe hearing a piece of music for the first time when in fact they have heard it on many occasions. Some LSD users describe their hallucinations as **synesthesia**, where sensations in one modality are experienced or mixed with another. For instance, visual hallucinations may occur to the sound of music. Users of LSD typically describe their perceptual experiences as pleasurable and amusing, but these hallucinations can be disturbing to some.

Lysergic acid diethylamide (LSD) was first synthesized in 1938 by Dr. Albert Hofmann (1906–2008), who was working as a chemist for the Swiss pharmaceutical company Sandoz laboratories (Figure 9.21). Hofmann was investigating the pharmacological properties of a variety of alkaloids extracted from plants and the ergot fungus, which grows on grain. Because of other research projects, Hofmann placed the LSD on a shelf only to return to it five years later.

In 1943, Hofmann began investigating the properties of his previously synthesized LSD, known as LSD-25 because it was the 25th lysergic acid compound synthesized in his laboratory. Hofmann reported in his journal that after working with LSD-25 he became "remarkably restless, combined with a slight dizziness." He returned home, where he further reported "fantastic pictures, extraordinary shapes with intense, kaleidoscopic play of colors."

Hofmann believed that he must have absorbed a small amount of LSD through his skin. Several days later he ingested 250 ug of LSD to experiment with it further. Soon after ingesting this dose Hofmann began to get dizzy again. He found it difficult to speak but managed to get his assistant to escort him home on his bicycle:

> On the way home, my condition began to assume threatening forms. Everything in my field of vision wavered and was distorted as if seen in a curved mirror. I also had the sensation of being unable to move from the spot.

Once home Hofmann found his surroundings both unfamiliar and frightening. He believed that there was no other known substance that evoked such profound psychic effects:

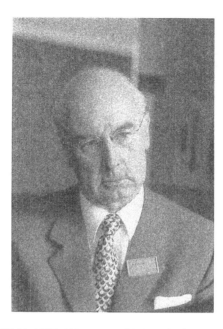

Figure 9.21 Albert Hofmann (1906–2008). Discoverer of LSD and advocate of its responsible use.

> Everything in the room spun around, and the familiar objects and pieces of furniture assumed grotesque, threatening forms. *They were in continuous motion, animated, as if driven by an inner restlessness.*

Albert Hoffman continued taking LSD (usually on his birthday) for the remainder of his life. He remained an advocate of its responsible use and founded a nonprofit foundation dedicated to furthering the investigation of psychedelic substances.

Pharmacokinetics of LSD

LSD is rapidly absorbed after oral administration and peak plasma levels are reached within about two hours. LSD readily crosses the blood–brain barrier and is quickly distributed to tissues throughout the body. The half-life of LSD ranges between two and three hours, but its effects may last as long as 12 hours. LSD is the most potent of all the psychoactive drugs. Effective doses begin at approximately 25 ug (25 millionths of a gram), which is about 1,000 times more potent than amphetamine or cocaine, which have effective doses of approximately 25 mg (thousandths of a gram). A popular form of LSD administration in the 1960s and 1970s is illustrated in Figure 9.22. Ironically, even though LSD is extremely potent, there appears to be no confirmed lethal dose. In 1977, a case of possible overdose was reported where it was estimated upon autopsy that the user had ingested 320 mg (320,000 ug) of LSD. However, no cause of death was reported (Griggs et al., 1977). Other estimates for lethal overdose in humans range between 50,000 and 100,000 ug or between 2,000 and 4,000 doses.

LSD Toxicity and Side Effects

LSD is characterized by its remarkable hallucinogenic effects, but several noticeable side effects are also common. These include increased body temperature, heart rate, and blood pressure,

Figure 9.22 A popular way to deliver and administer LSD is on small stamps that contain 50–100 ug of LSD. These stamps are placed on the tongue, where the drug is rapidly absorbed.

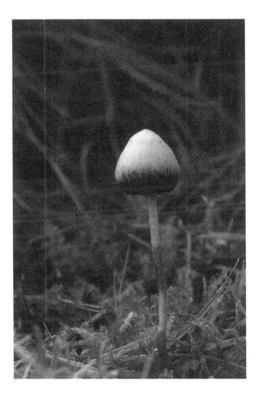

Figure 9.23 Psilocybin mushroom (Psilocybe semilanceata). A common species of psilocybin mushroom found in the Pacific Northwest and in the northeastern United States.

pupil dilation, dizziness, and occasional nausea. The psychological side effects can include confusion, acute panic, and noticeable distortions in both space and time. Occasionally LSD users report that their experience was disturbing or frightening and that their experience was a "bad trip." In addition, a few users report that they experience flashbacks of these disturbing experiences. While there is no known pharmacological mechanism that could cause flashback experiences, these unpleasant perceptual experiences more likely correspond to memories of these experiences rather than to some residual drug effect. Nevertheless, because a number of LSD users have reported flashbacks that have persisted long after drug use, a separate category was created in the *DSM* for **Hallucinogen Persisting Perception Disorder**.

The *DSM-5* criteria for Hallucinogen Persisting Perception Disorder (HPPD) require that the person has not recently used a hallucinogenic drug and shows no present signs of any drug intoxication. The following diagnostic criteria must be met:

A. The re-experiencing, following cessation of use of a hallucinogen, of one or more of the perceptual symptoms that were experienced while intoxicated with the hallucinogen (e.g., geometric hallucinations, false perceptions of movement in the peripheral visual fields, flashes of color, intensified colors, trails of images of moving objects, positive afterimages, halos around objects).
B. The symptoms cause clinically significant distress or impairment in social, occupational, or other important areas of functioning.
C. The symptoms are not due to a general medical condition (e.g., anatomical lesions and infections of the brain, visual epilepsies) and are not better accounted for by another mental disorder.

In a recent review of the literature on HPPD (flashbacks) it was concluded that while the disorder is likely to be genuine and can persist for months after LSD use, it is an uncommon occurrence with no known pathology. In addition, there is no consensus on how, or whether, HPPD should be treated (Halpern et al., 2002).

Pharmacology of LSD

Lysergic acid diethylamide and psilocybin are partial serotonin (5-HT) agonists that bind with high affinity to a number of 5-HT receptor subtypes. If you recall from Chapter 2, **partial agonists** are drugs that have an affinity for a receptor site but may exert less of an effect on the receptor than the endogenous ligand—in this case serotonin. The affinity of LSD and psilocybin for 5-HT receptors is believed to be a consequence of their similar molecular structure. All three of these substances share a common indole structure, which is illustrated in Figure 9.24.

Research with laboratory animals suggests that the hallucinogenic effects of LSD are mediated by the 5-HT_{2A} receptor subtype specifically. For example, drugs that block 5-HT_{2A} receptors also disrupt the ability of laboratory animals to discriminate between LSD and saline administrations (Appel et al., 2004). Blocking other serotonin receptors does not disrupt the discriminative properties of LSD. Animals lacking the serotonin transporter gene (SERT knockout animals) also fail to discriminate LSD from saline, providing further support for the role of 5-HT_{2A} receptors in LSD's hallucinogenic effects (Krall et al., 2008; Ly et al., 2018).

Understanding the action of LSD on serotonin receptors only partially explains its profound perceptual effects. What is clearly needed is a better understanding of how serotoninergic systems in the brainstem and the cortex modulate sensory information and perception. Several lines of research are beginning to elucidate how hallucinations may be caused. One approach is to evaluate how serotonin systems regulate sensory information projected from the brainstem to the thalamus and then to cortical sensory areas. Possibly, LSD disrupts the normal filtering of extraneous sensory information, resulting in overstimulation of cortical sensory areas. LSD does increase the activity of sensory neurons to stimulation (Aghajanian et al., 1999; Preller et al., 2019). Additionally, LSD may alter the activity of several cortical areas, including the

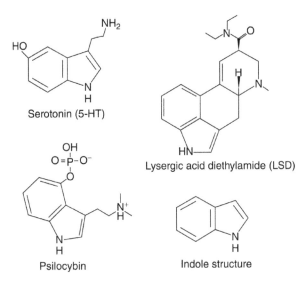

Figure 9.24 Lysergic acid diethylamide (LSD) and psilocybin share a common indole molecular structure with serotonin.

medial prefrontal cortex and the anterior cingulate by agonizing 5-HT$_{2A}$ receptors there. To demonstrate this, researchers have investigated the increased activity of cortical neurons in response to LSD administration (Gresch et al., 2002). More recent research has shown that LSD effects are mediated by specific pathways within the somatosensory cortex that express the 5-HT$_{2A}$ receptor. Activating these signaling pathways may be sufficient to induce hallucinations independently of sensory input via the thalamocortical pathways (González-Maeso et al., 2007; López-Giménez & González-Maeso, 2018).

LSD also interferes with dopamine neural transmission. In animal studies, drugs that block 5-HT$_{2A}$ receptors block the ability of rats to discriminate the immediate effects (within an hour) of LSD administration. However, the more delayed effects of LSD were only disrupted by haloperidol—a potent antagonist of DA$_2$ receptors (Borroto et al., 2014; Marona-Lewicka et al., 2005). These results suggest that LSD acts in two phases—an immediate phase mediated by serotonin agonism and a delayed effect mediated by dopamine agonism. The effects of LSD on dopamine appear to be mediated by the activation of serotonin in the cortex (De Gregorio et al., 2016). The role of dopamine in the hallucinogenic effects of LSD are unknown at this time.

Pharmacology of Psilocybin

Psilocybin is a psychedelic compound found in a variety of mushrooms in the *Psilocybe* genus (see Figure 9.23). One common North American species is *Psilocybe semilanceata*, which can be found in cattle or sheep pastures in the Pacific Northwest, as well as in several northeastern states. Recreational doses of psilocybin range from 1 to 5 grams of dried mushrooms. They can be eaten raw or boiled in water for tea. Once ingested, psilocybin is quickly metabolized into the psychoactive metabolite psilocin. The psychoactive effects of psilocin are typically observed within 20–30 minutes after ingestion. These effects include visual hallucinations, synesthesia, intensified hearing, loss of coordination, increased heart rate, and increased blood pressure. Psilocybin also appears to cause long-lasting changes in mood and a sense of well-being. These positive effects are currently being investigated for psilocybin's therapeutic effects (discussed in

Chapter 3). The psychedelic effects of psilocybin usually last between four and six hours but may last up to eight hours in rare instances. The therapeutic effects of psilocybin may last up to six months, suggesting that psilocin may produce long-lasting structural adaptations to limbic and cortical neurons. While psilocybin's hallucinogenic effects are believed to be mediated by agonism of serotonin 5-HT$_{2A}$ receptors (as with LSD), the mechanism of its therapeutic effects remains unknown (Ling et al., 2022). The physiological effects of psilocin are believed to be caused by central activation of the sympathetic system. Psilocybin and psilocin have very low toxicity (as does LSD)—the LD50 dose is believed to be 2,000–3,000 times a typical dose in humans (Passie et al., 2002).

In summary, LSD and psilocybin's hallucinogenic effects are believed to be mediated by partial agonism of 5-HT$_{2A}$ receptors. The 5-HT$_{2A}$ receptors in the brainstem, the thalamus, and in several cortical areas—including the medial prefrontal cortex, the anterior cingulate, and in the somatosensory cortex—appear to mediate its hallucinogenic effects. How alterations in 5-HT$_{2A}$ activity in these brain regions cause hallucinations remains unknown, but several possibilities have been proposed. First, 5-HT$_{2A}$ agonism in the brainstem appears to disrupt normal filtering of sensory information to the thalamus and cortex, resulting in sensory overload. And secondly, increased cortical activity by 5-HT$_{2A}$ receptor agonism independently of sensory stimulation may cause hallucinations. Research on both the neurophysiological and the behavioral effects of hallucinogens is typically done with laboratory animals. Whether the patterns of neuronal signaling induced by these substances in animals resemble the hallucinations reported by humans may never be known.

Marijuana (Cannabinoids)

Marijuana is the common name for the hemp plant ***Cannabis sativa*** (shown in Figure 9.25). Archeological evidence for the use of cannabis by the Chinese dates back to around 10,000 BC. From China, cannabis apparently spread to India and other regions of the Middle East where its resin, known as hashish, was and still is widely used. From Egypt, cannabis use continued to spread throughout Europe and finally to the United States. During the colonial period the hemp plant was considered a valuable agricultural commodity and was used primarily for the production of rope. Whether the colonists were aware of the intoxicating effects of cannabis is still controversial. Certainly by the mid-1800s cannabis was being used for its pharmacological effects in the United States. In the mid-1800s a number of popular European writers were describing their experiences with cannabis, including the French authors Victor Hugo and Pierre Gautier, who established the then famous Club des Hashischins in Paris. In the early

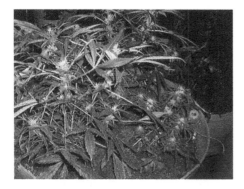
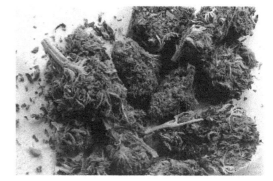

Figure 9.25 Marijuana plant (top) and dried mature flower (bottom).

1900s, cannabis was being touted for its medicinal properties in Western medicine and an assortment of cannabis products were available. In the 1930s, at least 28 different cannabis products were available to American physicians, including a variety of pills, syrups, and even drug mixtures. Further investigations into the pharmacological properties and uses of cannabis were cut short, however, by the **Marihuana Tax Act** of 1937, which essentially banned cannabis altogether by an elaborate code of costly tax provisions. Legal historians have argued that had it not been for numerous unfounded claims that cannabis caused insanity, murder, and death, the Act may not have passed. Cannabis was further regulated by the Controlled Substance Act of 1970, which listed cannabis as a Schedule I drug. Since 1970, a number of states have attempted to decriminalize marijuana use, but all legal efforts to reschedule it for medicinal purposes have failed. A few states, however, do allow patients with specific medical conditions to grow or purchase small amounts of marijuana for medicinal use. In addition, a number of states have recently passed legislation allowing for the possession, sale, and recreational use of marijuana.

Pharmacokinetics of Marijuana (Δ^9- Tetrahydrocannabinol)

With the isolation of the active compound in marijuana by two Israeli chemists in 1964, and its synthesis a year later, the pharmacological properties of cannabis were quickly pursued (Gaoni & Mechoulam, 1964; Mechoulam & Gaoni, 1965). Prior to the isolation of Δ^9—**tetrahydrocannabinol** (Figure 9.26) by Gaoni and Mechoulam, it had been assumed that the psychoactive properties of cannabis were due to a combination of cannabinols, which had been first extracted from marijuana in 1846 by the Smith brothers in Edinburgh, Scotland. The Smiths were pioneers of modern pharmacology who produced a variety of plant extracts for medicinal purposes. Using traditional methods of their time, they tested their cannabis extract on themselves and reported that "two thirds of a grain of this resin acts upon ourselves as a powerful narcotic, and one grain produces complete intoxication" (From Iversen, 2000; 1 grain is approximately 65 mg).

Smoking marijuana is perhaps the most effective method of administration. Upon heating, the Δ^9- tetrahydrocannabinol (THC) in marijuana is vaporized and readily passes through the surface of the lungs into the blood. Within seconds of inhalation THC passes through the blood–brain barrier and enters the brain. Peak plasma levels are typically reached within a few minutes of smoking. While plasma concentrations vary depending on the amount administered, typical doses in experienced users result in concentrations between 100 and

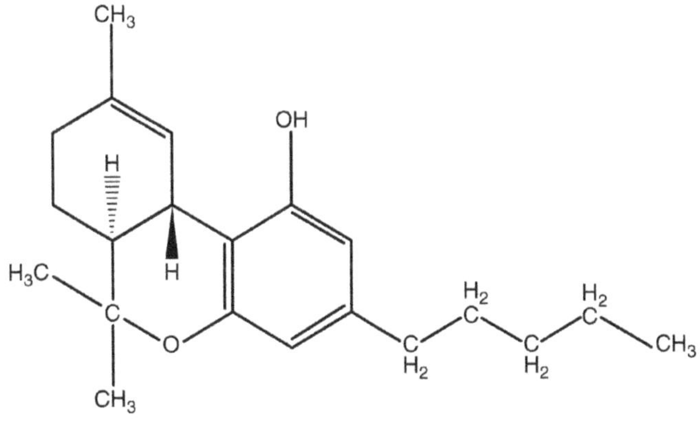

Figure 9.26 Molecular structure of Δ^9- tetrahydrocannabinol (THC).

200 ng/mL of plasma. The THC concentration of marijuana is highly variable, depending upon the variety of cannabis and how it is grown. Concentrations of THC in the dried flowering top of the plant average about 8.5 percent but can range from about 3 percent to as high as 25 percent for some varieties that have been developed through selective breeding. If a typical marijuana cigarette contains about 0.5 g of plant material with a THC content of about 8.5 percent, it would contain approximately 42.5 mg of THC. The amount of this dose that is actually inhaled may only be as high as 10–20 percent, with the remaining going up as side stream smoke or exhaled before complete absorption. Thus, the bioavailability of THC in a cigarette may be only about 5 mg.

After administration, THC is rapidly metabolized into the active metabolite 11-hydroxy-THC in the liver and then into the inactive metabolite 11-nor-9-carboxy-THC before excretion. Relatively small amounts of THC are excreted unchanged. The subjective effects of THC peak at about the same time as plasma levels and persist for about one to two hours, or when plasma levels decline below about 5.0 ng/mL. The elimination half-life of THC ranges between 24 and 72 hours.

Orally ingested marijuana is absorbed much more slowly and incompletely and can depend heavily on what else is available in the stomach and digestive system, since THC can be absorbed by dietary fats. In addition, orally ingested THC must first pass through the liver, where much of it is metabolized by liver enzymes. Peak plasma levels are reached between one and four hours after consumption. Because THC and its metabolites remain in the body for such long periods, sensitive drug tests can detect a single use for up to two weeks after exposure. Frequent users of marijuana may have detectable levels of metabolites for three to four weeks after abstinence, as the THC that had accumulated in tissues is gradually metabolized.

Pharmacodynamics of Marijuana (Δ^9- Tetrahydrocannabinol)

Before THC was isolated it was assumed that cannabis acted on nerve cells in some nonspecific way that interrupted normal cell functioning. For example, an active substance might enter and distort the cell's membrane and thereby alter cell firing. We'll see later on that alcohol can exert these kinds of nonspecific effects. After the discovery of THC, however, it became clear that it must interact directly with neuronal signaling systems. One clue to this hypothesis was that doses of THC that produce noticeable effects are extremely small. If an average marijuana cigarette delivers about 5 mg of THC, only a very small fraction of this amount actually enters the brain. To exert its effects, therefore, it is presumed that THC must be acting directly on cell receptors rather than by some unknown nonspecific effect, such as altering the conformation of cell membranes.

In 1988, researchers using a radioactive labeling technique identified **cannabinoid receptors** in the brains of laboratory rats. In their experiments, radioactive tritium was attached to the synthetic cannabinoid compound CP-55,940 (Devane et al., 1988). By labeling cannabinoid receptors with a radioactive marker, scientists were now able to locate the distribution of these receptors throughout the brain. Numerous cannabinoid receptors (CB$_1$ receptors) are now known to be located in the basal ganglia, cerebellum, hippocampus, amygdala, thalamus, and the cortex (see Figure 9.27). The distribution of these receptors will at least partially account for many of marijuana's behavioral effects. A second type of cannabinoid receptor has since been found outside the brain in lymphatic tissues of the immune system. These receptors are classified as CB$_2$ receptors to distinguish them from the CB$_1$ receptors located in the brain.

Cannabinoid CB$_1$ receptors are located on the presynaptic terminals of several different types of neurons (see Figure 9.28). All of these receptors are metabotropic G-protein coupled receptors that regulate the formation of cAMP. In fact, it is believed that CB$_1$ receptors are the most widely expressed G-protein coupled receptors in the brain. Activation of the G-protein

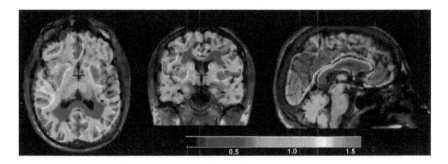

Figure 9.27 PET images of a brain following the injection of a radioactive CB₁ receptor ligand. High densities of cannabinoid receptors are expressed in the cerebral cortex, cerebellum, caudate nucleus, putamen, globus pallidus, substantia nigra, and in the hippocampus.

Source: Burns et al. (2007).

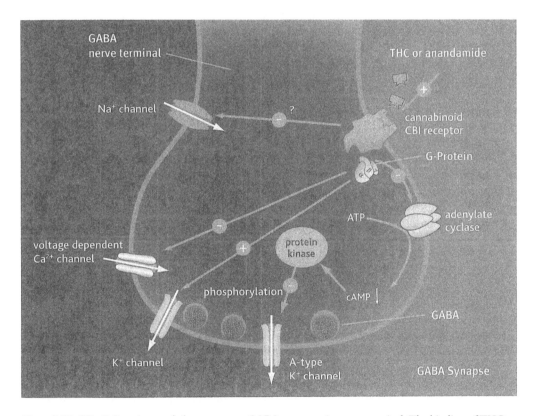

Figure 9.28 CB₁ G-Protein coupled receptors on GABA presynaptic nerve terminal. The binding of THC or anandamide to the CB₁ receptor inhibits GABA release by preventing Ca⁺⁺ influx.

by THC inhibits cAMP formation, inhibits voltage-dependent Ca^{++} channels, and facilitates K^+ efflux, all of which contribute to neural inhibition. In the hippocampus THC binds to CB_1 receptors on glutamate neurons exerting inhibitory control over glutamate activity. The activation of these CB_1 receptors inhibits glutamate activity in hippocampal pyramidal cells. Conversely, THC binds to CB_1 receptors on GABA neurons in the frontal cortex, which regulate glutamate activity there. This decrease in GABA activity results in increased (disinhibited) glutamate and dopamine activity. Similarly, in the ventral tegmental area THC binds to CB_1 receptors on GABA neurons, which exert inhibitory control over dopamine activity (Szabo et al., 2002). This form of neuronal suppression appears to be a common type of short-term neuronal plasticity, where depolarization of a neuron causes a decrease in GABA-mediated neural inhibition.

Following the discovery of cannabinoid receptors in 1988, the search for endogenous ligands intensified. In 1992, William Devane (the discoverer of the cannabinoid receptor) and his colleagues in Israel also isolated an endogenous cannabinoid, arachidonoyl ethanolamine. They named this substance **anandamide** after the Sanskrit word *ananda*, which means bliss. Anandamide is enzymatically synthesized on demand by neurons from the precursor fatty acid arachidonic acid. It is now recognized that anandamide plays an important role in regulating neural activity that mediates memory formation, appetite, pain signaling, motor activity, and reward. Other endogenous ligands for the cannabinoid receptor have yet to be found. The euphoric effects of marijuana are believed to be mediated in part by disinhibition of dopamine activity in the mesolimbic system (Bloomfield et al., 2016; Fadda et al., 2006; Lecca et al., 2006; Solinas et al., 2008). Whether cannabis use is sufficient to cause the kinds of adaptations to dopaminergic neurons that underlie addiction remains unclear. In fact, recent studies have shown that typical recreational doses of THC (the amount administered by a standard cannabis cigarette) do not significantly increase dopamine activity in the striatum (Stokes et al., 2009), whereas chronic treatment with repeated high doses of THC does appear to increase activity in the mesolimbic and cortical dopamine systems (Bloomfield et al., 2016; Kolb et al., 2006; Ginovart et al., 2012).

Medicinal Uses for Cannabinoid Compounds

In the past decade, a number of states have passed legislation to allow marijuana for medicinal and recreational uses. Presently 37 states permit physicians to prescribe marijuana for medical use and 19 of these states also allow recreational use.

Drug manufacturers have created several synthetic THC drugs that are available by prescription. Dronabinol (Marinol) is a synthetic THC that is extracted from marijuana. Originally listed as a Schedule II drug, Marinol was recently rescheduled as a Schedule III drug. It has been approved by the FDA to treat nausea and vomiting associated with cancer chemo and radiation therapy as well as appetite loss in patients with AIDS. Advocates for the medicinal use of marijuana claim, however, that Marinol is not as effective as marijuana, perhaps because synthetic drugs lack the nearly 60 other cannabinoids that are present in marijuana. In addition, users of Marinol often complain about its delayed onset and its excessive intoxicating effects that are much more difficult to regulate than smoked marijuana.

Nabilone (Cesamet) is an entirely synthetic THC that was originally approved by the FDA in 1985, but marketing actually began in 2006. It was approved to treat nausea and vomiting related to cancer therapy as well as to treat anorexia and weight loss associated with AIDS. Nabilone is presently a Schedule II drug.

A number of other medical conditions may also respond well to marijuana treatment. These include the vision-threatening increase in ocular pressure associated with glaucoma, as an analgesic for chronic and phantom limb pain, to treat withdrawal symptoms associated with opiate and alcohol addictions, and for treating muscle spasms in patients with multiple sclerosis, Huntington's disease, and Parkinson's disease. Marijuana may also be useful in treating bronchial constriction in asthmatics and in treating certain kinds of cancer by inhibiting cell proliferation and metastasis (Dariš et al., 2019; Kogan, 2005; Preet et al., 2008). Clearly more research on thepotential therapeutic benefits of marijuana is needed.

Pharmacological Effects of Marijuana, Dronabinol, and Nabilone (THC)

Memory and Cognition

Marijuana and synthetic THC compounds exert significant effects on both the central and peripheral nervous systems. The central effects of THC include mild euphoria, anxiolysis, and distortions in the perception of time. In some users, THC can cause confusion and a heightened sense of anxiety, but these effects tend to dissipate after repeated administration or use. In addition, THC impairs both cognitive and motor functioning—effects that do not typically persist beyond the period of intoxication. The deleterious effects of marijuana on memory and cognitive functioning have long been known, and recent research has revealed that these effects are mediated, at least in part, by cannabinoid CB_1 receptors in the hippocampus and frontal lobes. Cannabinoids act by suppressing glutamate activity and **long-term potentiation (LTP)** in hippocampal neurons and by disinhibiting glutamate neurons in the frontal cortex (Colizzi et al., 2016; Hoffman et al., 2007; Kang-Park et al., 2007a; Ranganathan et al., 2006).

Motor Control and Coordination

Cannabinoids are also known to disrupt motor control and performance (refer to Figures 9.29 and 9.30). These effects appear to be mediated by two distinct mechanisms. First, there is an abundance of cannabinoid receptors on glutamate neurons within the basal ganglia. High doses of THC inhibit the release of glutamate in afferent neurons in the basal ganglia, causing disrupted movement and even cataplexy. Animals administered high doses of THC exhibit immobility as well as symptoms characteristic of Parkinson's disease (Gerdeman et al., 2001). In addition, cannabinoids disrupt normal cerebellar control of movement independently of

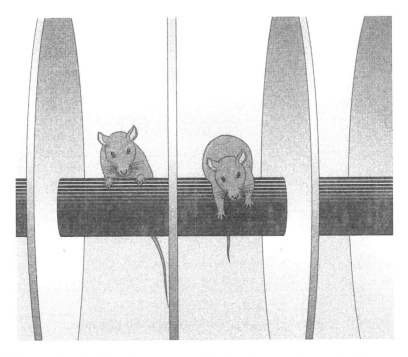

Figure 9.29 Rota-rod treadmill test for motor coordination. Rats or mice are placed on a rotating rod. Time spent on the rod is a measure of motor coordination.

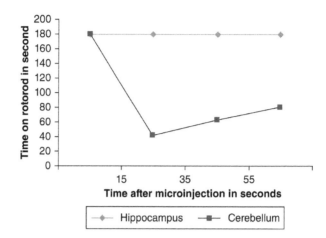

Figure 9.30 Time mice spent on a rota-rod as a measure of motor coordination after a microinjection of the CB_1 agonist CP55,940 into either the hippocampus (control) or the cerebellum. Cerebellar injections of the CB_1 agonist sharply disrupted performance.

Source: Data from DeSanty and Dar (2001).

central dopamine motor pathways (DeSanty & Dar, 2001; Patel & Hillard, 2001). Taken together, cannabinoids have the potential to disrupt movement and coordination by activating CB_1 receptors in both the cerebellum and in the nigrostriatal dopamine system. Paradoxically, activation of these cannabinoid receptors seems to have therapeutic effects for individuals with degenerative motor diseases, including multiple sclerosis, Parkinson's, and Huntington's disease (Koehler et al., 2014; Patel et al., 2019; Rekand, 2014). Cannabinoids may also offer protection from further neurodegeneration associated with these diseases by inhibiting the cytotoxic effects of excessive Ca^{++} influx into neurons in the motor pathways (Battista et al., 2006; Sagredo et al., 2007; Wang et al., 2022).

Antiemetic Effects: Nausea and Vomiting

Chemo and radiation therapy–induced nausea remains to be a significant problem for most patients undergoing treatment for cancer. While several **antiemetic** (antinausea) drugs, including benzodiazepines, are often useful, a significant number of patients prefer marijuana over the alternatives. Cannabinoids may not only be more effective than benzodiazepines for nausea, the side effects of cannabinoids are also more tolerable to many patients. Nausea and vomiting are triggered as toxic drugs and cellular debris stimulate receptors in the **area postrema** of the brainstem. Cannabinoids appear to act directly on CB_1 receptors in the area postrema, inhibiting the vomiting reflex (Sharkey et al., 2007; Van Sickle et al., 2001).

Cannabinoids also have significant peripheral effects, including effects on the cardiovascular and immune systems. Additionally, cannabinoids exert a significant effect on the intraocular pressure associated with glaucoma.

Cardiovascular Effects

The cannabinoids have notable effects on both heart rate and blood pressure. While initial use may cause both an increase in blood pressure and heart rate in some users, repeated use typically produces a significant decrease in blood pressure as a result of vasodilation. This vasodilating effect is mediated peripherally through CB_1 receptors located on the heart and blood vessels. As blood pressure drops, heart rate increases moderately to compensate for a drop in blood flow. This increase in heart rate may be problematic for some with severe cardiovascular disease, but there is little evidence that moderate cannabis use is associated with adverse cardiovascular events. There is conflicting evidence about the risk of ischemia, a restriction in blood supply to the heart, which can lead to a heart attack, associated with cannabis use. Several studies report an increased risk (e.g., Viswanathan et al., 2019), while others found that cannabinoids may protect the heart against ischemia, (Banaszkiewicz et al., 2022; Kollins et al., 2015; Lépicier et al., 2006, 2007). Most studies linking marijuana use to increased cardiovascular disease are retrospective and correlational, thus limiting conclusions about risk. Because of its listing as a Schedule 1 drug, cannabis research will continue to be limited.

Immune System Effects

As noted earlier, cannabinoids interact with both CB_1 and CB_2 receptor types. While CB1 receptors are expressed on both central and peripheral neurons, CB_2 receptors appear to be localized almost exclusively on cells of the immune system. The role of these cannabinoid receptors in immunoregulation remains obscure. Recent research has revealed, however, that cannabinoids, and CB_2 agonists specifically, inhibit immune responses and inflammation (Henshaw et al., 2021; Lombard et al., 2007; McKallip et al., 2002). The development of specific CB_2 agonists, therefore, may prove useful in treating a variety of inflammatory and autoimmune disorders. As of yet, the immunosuppressive properties of cannabis have not been demonstrated to be a significant concern for patients or users. There is no evidence that cannabis use is associated with an increased risk of infectious disease or the progression of cancer.

Tolerance and Dependence

In laboratory animals, repeated administration of high doses of THC can produce tolerance to the cardiovascular and behavioral responses to THC. For example, in a recent study with mice, researchers administered THC twice a day for seven days on an escalating dose schedule beginning with 10 mg/kg and increasing to 60 mg/kg. Animals on the increasing dose schedule developed tolerance to THC's locomotor and analgesic effects, while mice treated with 10 mg/kg twice each day did not. The mechanism underlying tolerance in these animals was a decrease in cannabinoid receptor activation in several brain regions, including the hippocampus, cingulate cortex, periaqueductal gray area, the caudate nucleus, nucleus accumbens, and in the cerebellum (McKinney et al., 2008). Other researchers have shown that cannabinoid receptor internalization may mediate this decrease in CB_1 receptor activation during tolerance (Wu et al., 2008).

Changes in the rate of THC metabolism may also contribute to cannabis tolerance, but this alone would not be sufficient to account for tolerance to such high THC doses.

It is important to consider that while tolerance to THC has been demonstrated in humans and in animals that have been given extremely high doses of THC, tolerance may not occur to the doses most users and patients receive. A typical dose of Marinol, for example, would be approximately 5–20 mg/day for a patient being treated for nausea or glaucoma, and as stated earlier, a typical marijuana cigarette may contain about 5mg of THC. The doses required to demonstrate tolerance in mice would be equivalent to approximately 300–500 mg of THC for a person.

Chronic use has been reported to produce dependence in some cannabis users, and abstinence can cause symptoms of withdrawal. These symptoms may include cravings, depressed mood, aggressiveness, and irritability—all symptoms associated with other drug dependencies, including nicotine and caffeine. Because not all users experience withdrawals upon abstinence, whether cannabis causes dependence or addiction remains quite controversial. Proponents of marijuana use argue that it does not cause dependence, nor does it contribute to addiction, while those opposing marijuana use argue that it does. Research with animals may at least partially resolve this controversy. One way researchers investigate a drug's abuse potential is to determine whether animals will administer the drug or substance to themselves. Typically such self-administration experiments involve training animals to press levers to receive small injections of a drug.

Self-Administration of THC

Drugs that have a high abuse potential, such as cocaine, heroin, amphetamine, and nicotine, easily maintain lever pressing by animals when these drugs are injected as reinforcers. In a self-administration experiment, animals are trained to lever press for drug administration intravenously or directly into the brain via a cannula, upon each completion of the schedule requirement. For example, on a fixed ratio 10 (FR10) schedule a small amount of drug would be administered after each tenth lever press response. After each drug administration there is typically a brief delay before lever presses are counted for a successive trial. Over the course of an experimental session an animal may earn 20–30 microinjections of a particular drug. In one such study, researchers trained squirrel monkeys to self-administer 4 ug/kg of THC per injection on a fixed ratio 10 schedule. Over the course of a one-hour experimental session, animals received between 40 and 50 injections of THC. After five one-hour sessions the reinforcer was switched from THC to the saline vehicle solution for another five sessions and then again to THC for the final five sessions (Justinova et al., 2003). The results of this experiment are presented in Figure 9.31. Clearly, THC maintained high levels of self-administration in this experiment, suggesting that THC does have abuse potential.

To illustrate how complicated interpreting the research on the abuse potential of cannabis can be, let us consider an alternative method to evaluate a drug's abuse potential. It is widely accepted that addictive drugs produce sensitization to dopamine neural circuits in the mesolimbic reward system. These adaptations can be observed as behavioral sensitization and increased locomotor activity. In a recent experiment, the behavioral sensitizing effects of THC after repeated administration in mice were compared to those following methamphetamine administrations. As seen in Figure 9.32, methamphetamine produced behavioral sensitization, while THC did not (Varvel et al., 2007). Whether the lack of behavioral sensitization is a consequence of THC's known motor-depressing effects in the basal ganglia is not known.

In summary, cannabinoids can, under certain conditions, produce tolerance and dependence in both animals and humans. Tolerance appears to be mediated by receptor internalization and a subsequent decrease in receptor activity. The controversy about the abuse and addictive potential of cannabis and the synthetic THC compounds remains unresolved at the time of this writing. Part of the controversy may be because addiction is defined differently in different contexts. We defined addiction in Chapter 8 as both structural and functional adaptations to mesolimbic and mesocortical systems, resulting from rapid increases in dopamine activity. There is no evidence that THC causes these adaptations. It has been

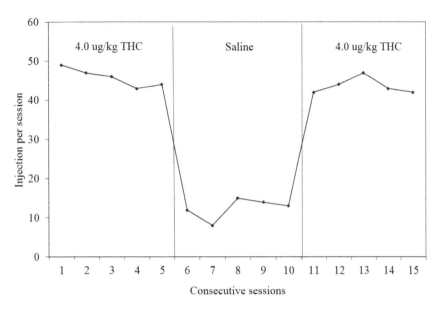

Figure 9.31 Number of THC or saline vehicle injections per training session on an FR 10 schedule for squirrel monkeys self-administering THC. THC maintained high rates of self-administration when compared to the saline vehicle solution.

Source: Data from Justinova et al. (2003).

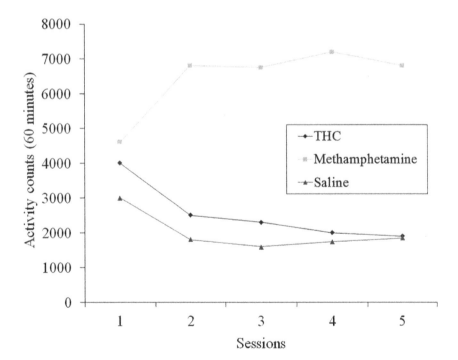

Figure 9.32 Behavioral sensitization as measured by activity in mice observed following methamphetamine treatment but not after THC or saline treatment.

Source: Data from Varvel et al. (2007).

estimated that about 3 percent of regular cannabis users develop a cannabis use disorder as defined by *DSM-IV* or *DSM-5* criteria (Chen et al., 2005; Compton et al., 2019; SAMHSA, 2021), a number that is far lower than the frequency of dependency to other drugs of abuse. If cannabis use can lead to dependence, this risk is certainly much lower than it is for other abused drugs.

Glossary

Δ9- tetrahydrocannabinol (THC) the psychoactive compound in marijuana.

Amphetamine psychosis a psychotic state induced by the stimulants amphetamine and cocaine. Symptoms include paranoid delusions and hallucinations.

Analgesic a class of drug that blocks ascending pain signals in the spinal cord and brainstem.

Anandamide an endogenous ligand for the cannabinoid receptor.

Anesthetic a class of drugs used for anesthesia. Anesthetics produce a lack of awareness of body sensations and are used to sedate patients for surgery.

Antiemetic a class of drug used to treat nausea.

Arcuate nucleus a structure within the hypothalamus implicated in feeding regulation.

Area postrema an area of the brainstem that controls the vomiting reflex. The area postrema has a relatively weak blood–brain barrier so it can detect toxins in the blood.

Benzoylecgonine a principal metabolite of cocaine.

Cannabinoid receptors a class of receptors specific for endogenous cannabinoids such as anandamide. There are two distinct forms of the cannabinoid receptor, CB_1 and CB_2.

Cannabis sativa a variety of hemp plant commonly known as marijuana.

CART see **Cocaine and amphetamine-regulated transcript**.

Cocaethylene a compound that results from mixing the administrations of cocaine and alcohol.

Cocaine a powerful stimulant drug extracted from the coca plant (*Erythroxylum coca*).

Cocaine and amphetamine-regulated transcript (CART) a peptide neurotransmitter found in the arcuate nucleus of the hypothalamus. Believed to be involved in feeding.

Controlled Substance Act enacted in 1970 to control the manufacture, distribution, and use of certain drugs with abuse potential.

Crack a cocaine product that is produced by dissolving cocaine hydrochloride in ammonia or a solution of sodium bicarbonate.

Crystal meth a crystalline form of methamphetamine.

Desoxyephedrine see **Methamphetamine**.

Dextroamphetamine (Dexadrine) an amphetamine compound used to treat narcolepsy, attention disorders, and obesity.

Dopamine transporter (DAT) a protein that selectively transports dopamine from the synaptic gap back into the terminal button.

Drug Enforcement Administration an agency within the Department of Justice that oversees and enforces the **Controlled Substance Act**.

Drug schedule a drugs classification based on its potential for abuse as described by the Controlled Substance Act of 1970. Drugs with the highest abuse potential and lowest medicinal value are Schedule I drugs. There are five drug schedules (I–V).

Ecgonine a principal metabolite of cocaine.

Ecstasy see **MDMA**.

Ephedra a mild stimulant that is extracted from the *ephedra sinica* plant.

Hallucinogen persisting perception disorder a *DSM-IV-TR* disorder characterized by the reexperience of hallucinogenic effects caused by psychedelic drugs long after drug intoxication.

Harrison Narcotic Tax Act enacted in 1914 to control the manufacture, distribution, and use of certain drugs with abuse potential. Superseded by the Controlled Substance Act of 1970.

Knockout animals an experimental animal that has been genetically altered to not express certain genes.

Local anesthetic a drug that blocks the conduction of nerve signals in a localized area for surgery.

Long-term potentiation (LTP) a long-term change in the excitability of a neuron induced by high-frequency stimulation of its receptor. LTP is most often investigated in NMDA receptors.

LSD (lysergic acid diethylamide) a potent psychedelic drug that produces visual hallucinations. Discovered by Dr. Albert Hoffman.

Marihuana Tax Act enacted in 1937 to regulate the distribution and use of marijuana by taxation.

Marijuana the common name for the hemp plant *Cannabis sativa*.

MDA (3,4 methylenedioxyamphetamine) a compound structurally related to amphetamine and similar to MDMA. Produces a state of euphoria.

MDMA (methylenedioxymethamphetamine) a compound structurally related to amphetamine with euphoric effects. Also known as ecstasy.

Methamphetamine (desoxyephedrine) an amphetamine compound that can be produced by the reduction of ephedrine.

Methylbenzoylecgonine a compound produced by dissolving cocaine hydrochloride in ammonia. Also known as crack cocaine.

Mesolimbic-mesocortical pathways neural pathway originating in the ventral tegmental area of the midbrain and projecting to the nucleus accumbens and to the prefrontal cortex.

Mesolimbic system a pathway of dopaminergic neurons originating in the ventral tegmentum projecting to the nucleus accumbens.

Nigrostriatal system a system of brain structures and neurons originating in the substantia nigra projecting to the striatum of the basal ganglia.

Nucleus accumbens a structure of the mesolimbic system that receives dopaminergic input from the ventral tegmental area.

Partial agonist a drug that has an affinity for a receptor site but may exert less of an effect on the receptor than the endogenous ligand.

Place preference conditioning an experimental procedure where animals are tested for their preference for an area in an experimental apparatus where drugs had been administered over other areas within the apparatus. A form of Pavlovian conditioning where a place becomes associated with drug effects.

Psilocybin a psychedelic compound found in a variety of mushrooms in the *Psilocybe* genus.

Psychedelic a class of drug that causes disturbances in perception.

Reticular activating system a system of neurons originating in the brainstem projecting to the thalamus. Involved in behavioral arousal and is crucial for maintaining the state of consciousness.

Reuptake transporters proteins embedded on the presynaptic terminal of neurons that transport neurotransmitter substances into the terminal button.

Stereotyped behavior rigid repetitive movements observed in experimental animals after the administration of psychomotor stimulants such as cocaine or amphetamine.

Synesthesia a perceptual phenomenon where sensations in one modality are experienced or mixed with another.

Ventral tegmental area an area of the midbrain that is the origin of dopaminergic cell bodies that comprise the mesolimbic system.

10 The Pharmacology of Nonscheduled Psychoactive Drugs

Alcohol, Nicotine, and Caffeine

Alcohol

Alcohol is the most widely abused drug in the United States and throughout the world. By the time American students graduate from high school, over 88 percent will have used alcohol, and nearly 30 percent of these students will have used it heavily. Because alcohol is so readily available and used by such a large proportion of the population, it is no wonder that it leads to the most prevalent of all substance abuse disorders. According to the National Institute on Alcohol Abuse and Alcoholism (2022), approximately 7 percent (over 15 million) of the population over 18 years of age has an alcohol abuse problem, and alcohol continues to contribute to nearly 31 percent of all automobile fatalities and 20 percent of all emergency department visits.

While we may never know when alcohol was first produced and consumed, it was most likely the result of fruit or grain fermentation by a fortuitous incident. The earliest evidence of the intentional fermentation of an alcoholic beverage comes from the discovery of large Stone Age jugs for the making of beer about 12,000 years ago. Wine production in China may be dated back more than 9,000 years, and wine making is depicted in Egyptian pictographs dating back as far as 6,000 years. Clearly, the production of alcoholic beverages from the fermentation of grains and fruits has a long history.

The distillation of alcohol from grains appeared much later, during the second millennium BC, in the region now known as Iraq, while large-scale distillation of alcohol for *spirits* probably didn't occur until the first century AD in Greece. The modern distillation of spirits began in the early 1400s in Ireland, where whiskey making was first described by monks. Soon after, a variety of drinks, including gin, vodka, and rum, were produced by distillation in different regions around the world. Prior to modern distillation, the alcohol content of alcoholic beverages remained between 3 and 15 percent. With the wide implementation of distillation processes, the alcohol concentration in beverages increased dramatically, and so too did its abuse potential.

Distillation is essentially a separation process rather than a chemical process. In alcohol distillation, alcohol is separated from other fermentation products by heating. Because alcohol has a lower boiling point it evaporates early in the heating process. This alcohol vapor is then cooled as purified alcohol. Although distillation can result in pure **ethyl alcohol (ethanol)**, most hard liquors and spirits are about 40–50 percent alcohol. Typically, the alcohol content of hard liquors is represented as **proof** alcohol. The term "proof" may have originated in the eighteenth century, when British sailors were paid with provisions of rum. To prove that the rum was not diluted with water it was mixed with gunpowder and ignited. If the mixture burned this was proof that the alcohol content was at least 50 percent (actually closer to 57 percent). Thus, rum that was at least 57 percent alcohol was 100 percent proven to be undiluted. Today, alcohol proof is exactly two times the alcohol percent by volume. For example, a spirit that is 40 percent alcohol is considered 80 proof.

DOI: 10.4324/9781003309017-10

Pharmacology of Alcohol

Absorption

Alcohol (ethanol, illustrated in Figure 10.1) is both water and fat soluble and it readily diffuses across all cell membranes. Once ingested, ethanol rapidly passes through the blood–brain barrier, allowing neural tissues to reach blood alcohol levels quickly. Peak blood levels are typically reached between 30 and 60 minutes, depending on both alcohol concentration and whether other substances are present in the stomach and digestive tract. Higher alcohol concentrations (stronger drinks) diffuse more rapidly than lower concentrations, and the availability of foods in the stomach and intestines delays distribution, since most alcohol (about 80 percent) is absorbed through the walls of the small intestine while the rest is absorbed by the stomach or excreted through sweat, respiration, and urine immediately after absorption. Because alcohol is so readily absorbed by all tissues, a pregnant woman exposes her fetus to the same blood levels as herself, since alcohol easily passes through the placenta.

Blood alcohol concentration (BAC) is typically expressed as grams of alcohol in 100 milliliters of blood. For example, 80 milligrams of alcohol in 100 milliliters of blood is equivalent to 0.08 grams per 100 ml. Sometimes this is expressed as a percentage of alcohol by weight in blood (see Figure 10.2). The somewhat arbitrary legal limit for intoxication in most states is 0.08 or 0.08 percent. Rather than measure the alcohol content of blood directly, most sobriety tests rely on the strong correlation between blood alcohol and the alcohol expired

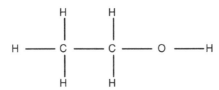

Figure 10.1 Molecular structure of ethanol (CH_3CH_2OH or C_2H_5OH).

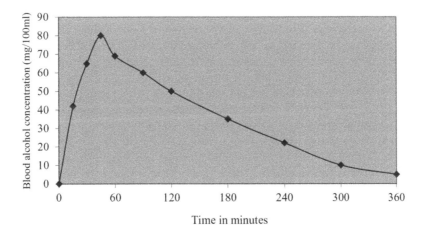

Figure 10.2 Blood alcohol concentrations (BAC) are typically measured in milligrams of alcohol per 100 milliliters of blood. After consuming 100 ml of a 90 percent alcohol (180 proof) solution peak blood levels are reached within 45 minutes in this example. A blood alcohol concentration of 80 mg/100 ml would be the same as 0.08 percent (0.08 grams per 100 ml), which is the legal limit for intoxication in most states.

Table 10.1 Common behavioral and cognitive effects of different levels of alcohol intoxication.

BAC %	Common behavioral and cognitive effects
0.01–0.05	Increased heart and respiration rates Moderate detrimental effects on cognitive and motor tasks Mild sense of euphoria and anxiolysis Reinforcement
0.06–0.10	Moderate sedation Decreases in attention, increased reaction time, impaired motor coordination Significant cognitive impairment Depression and irritability
0.10–0.15	Significant increases in reaction time and impairment in cognition and judgment Agitation and irritability (aggressiveness) Significant impairment of balance and movement Impaired vision Slurred speech Nausea and vomiting
0.16–0.29	Severe sensory impairment, including reduced awareness of external stimulation Severe motor impairment, e.g., frequently staggering or falling
0.30–0.39	Non-responsive stupor and loss of consciousness Significant anesthesia Respiratory depression and possible death
0.40 and up	Unconsciousness Respiratory depression Death for most individuals at these levels

through respiration. A breathalyzer can immediately estimate blood alcohol concentrations by analyzing a sample of your breath, which contains alcohol passed from the blood stream into the lungs. A common misconception is that this alcohol can be concealed by breath mints that mask the odor of alcohol.

The level of intoxication an individual experiences at a particular BAC varies significantly. While some may be considerably impaired at a BAC of 0.04 percent, another may function quite normally. Table 10.1 describes some of the effects typically observed at different blood alcohol concentrations in percentages.

Metabolism of Alcohol

The metabolism of alcohol begins immediately after consumption. Approximately 90–95 percent of ingested alcohol is metabolized by the enzyme **alcohol dehydrogenase**, while the remaining 5–10 percent is excreted through perspiration and respiration or metabolized by another liver enzyme **P450**. P450, or cytochrome P450, is an essential enzyme found in most biological systems that is essential to oxidative reactions involved in metabolism. Some alcohol is metabolized by this oxidative reaction. Only a small fraction of alcohol is excreted in the urine unmetabolized. Small amounts of alcohol dehydrogenase in the stomach begin to metabolize alcohol immediately. If the stomach is full, alcohol absorption is delayed and more of it is metabolized in the stomach. Once alcohol enters the small intestine it is quickly absorbed into the blood supply, which carries it to the liver where the remaining portion (80–85 percent) is metabolized by liver alcohol dehydrogenase. Alcohol that is metabolized by stomach and liver enzymes before it has had a chance to enter tissues is called **first-pass metabolism**. Approximately 25–30 percent of ingested alcohol is metabolized before or during its first pass through the liver. Once tissue and blood levels have equilibrated, metabolism continues at a slower rate. On average about 17 mg of alcohol per 100 ml of blood is metabolized each hour. This is essentially equivalent to the amount of alcohol in a shot of 40 percent alcohol (whiskey), a 4 oz glass of 12 percent wine, or a 12 oz bottle of beer. The amount of alcohol metabolized each hour depends on the availability of alcohol dehydrogenase and its coenzyme **nicotinamide adenine dinucleotide** (NAD). Nicotinamide adenine dinucleotide is considered a rate-limiting enzyme because its availability determines the rate of alcohol metabolism. As a coenzyme in alcohol metabolism, NAD^+ (positively charged) facilitates a reduction reaction (the transfer of an electron) that results in the release of energy. In alcohol metabolism NAD^+

is reduced to NADH during the production of adenosine triphosphate (ATP), which is a source of cellular energy.

Because men and women have different levels of alcohol dehydrogenase, they metabolize alcohol at quite different rates. Women have less stomach alcohol dehydrogenase than men do and may metabolize 50 percent less alcohol in their stomach than men. In addition, women typically have a greater fat to muscle ratio than men, meaning that they have less blood for a proportional body weight, as fat has a lower blood supply than muscle. Both of these factors contribute to greater blood concentrations in women than in men for equivalent doses of alcohol.

During its first phase of metabolism, alcohol is converted into acetaldehyde, which is highly toxic. Acetaldehyde is quickly metabolized by the enzyme **aldehyde dehydrogenase** into acetic acid (refer to Figure 10.3). Genetic variations in both the expression and form of aldehyde dehydrogenase have profound effects on alcohol metabolism. For example, a small proportion of the Asia population codes for an inactive form of aldehyde dehydrogenase, meaning that acetaldehyde is not further converted into acetic acid in these individuals. Even small amounts of alcohol result in toxic levels of acetaldehyde, which causes nausea, vomiting, sweating, dizziness, and severe headaches—more severe forms of the symptoms many have experienced as a hangover. The drug **dilsulfiram** (Antabuse) inhibits aldehyde dehydrogenase and causes these same symptoms in alcoholics who use it to discourage drinking. Acetic acid is oxidized into CO_2 and water.

Mechanisms of Alcohol Action: Pharmacodynamics

Although alcohol is a simple molecule its pharmacodynamics are far from simple. As mentioned, alcohol is both water and fat soluble and because of this it exerts effects on a wide range of cellular functions and systems. To describe the pharmacodynamics of alcohol we will consider both its nonspecific and specific effects on neuronal functioning.

Alcohol's nonspecific effects include its effects on all cellular membranes. By its ability to dissolve into the lipid cell membrane, alcohol disrupts several cell processes. In the past, it was believed that alcohol's main mechanism of action was membrane **fluidization**. Alcohol was presumed to act as a neuronal depressant and as an anesthetic by dissolving in cell membranes and making them more fluid. This fluidization disturbs several membrane processes, including the movement of ions through channels, the conductance of membrane potentials, and the release and storage of neurotransmitter substances (Figure 10.4, 1–3). Membrane fluidization seems to account for many of alcohol's generalized depressant and analgesic effects at higher doses.

Fluidization does not, however, account for many other effects of alcohol. These effects, typically at lower doses, include cognitive and motor disruptions, euphoria, anxiolysis, and reinforcement. To account for these effects we will examine how alcohol specifically alters the synaptic activity of several neurotransmitter systems.

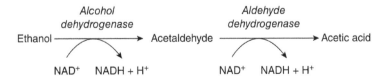

Figure 10.3 The metabolism of alcohol into acetaldehyde and further into acetic acid depends on the availability of the enzymes alcohol dehydrogenase and aldehyde dehydrogenase and the coenzyme nicotinamide adenine dinucleotide (NAD^+).

Alcohol Effects on Neurotransmitter Systems

GABA

Perhaps the most important of alcohol's specific actions is its agonistic effect on GABA receptors, specifically the GABA$_A$ receptor. It has long been known that many of alcohol's behavioral effects are mediated by enhanced GABA activity. Early evidence for this comes from studies showing that alcohol effects are dependent upon both increased GABA binding to its receptors as well as the influx of Cl$^-$ that the GABA$_A$ receptor controls. What is not well understood is whether alcohol binds to a specific receptor site, as do the barbiturates and benzodiazepines, or whether it acts in some other facilitative way. Because GABA synapses control the activity of many neuronal systems, including glutamate, dopamine, and the opioids, a description of alcohol effects on GABA receptors is essential for a complete understanding of alcohol's behavioral effects.

Recent evidence does suggest that alcohol may bind to specific GABA$_A$ receptors, including the delta Δ receptor (see Figure 10.5). Some of the strongest evidence for alcohol's specificity for delta receptors comes from studies using the drug **Ro15–4513**, which is a powerful competitive antagonist for alcohol effects. When Ro15–4513 is administered to intoxicated animals the behavioral effects of alcohol intoxication are immediately reversed. Because Ro15–4513 is known to competitively bind to the delta Δ receptor, it is presumed that alcohol also has an affinity for this receptor subtype (Borghese et al., 2014; Olsen et al., 2007; Santhakumar et al., 2007).

Chronic exposure to alcohol during pregnancy has long been known to cause damage to developing brains and to cause **fetal alcohol syndrome (FAS)**. One contribution to these deleterious effects of prenatal alcohol exposure is an upregulation of fetal GABA$_A$ receptor expression in the cerebral cortex and the hippocampus. Chronic alcohol exposure typically leads to the downregulation of specific GABA$_A$ receptor subtypes and an upregulation of others (see the following section on tolerance). Alterations in GABA$_A$ receptor expression have

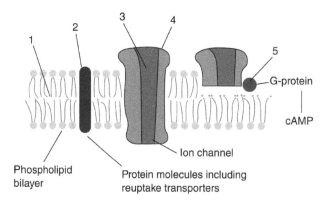

Figure 10.4 Specific and nonspecific effects of alcohol on neuronal membranes. (1) Fluidization alters lipid composition and distorts cell membrane. This affects the conductance of membrane potentials. (2) Interacts with proteins imbedded in cell membrane. Altering the function of membrane proteins disrupts internal cell processes, including the synthesis and storage of neurotransmitters and disrupting neurotransmitter reuptake. (3) Interacts with ion channel. Fluidization interferes with the movement of ions across cell membranes. (4) Binds to receptor sites on receptor complex. Alcohol acts as an acetylcholine antagonist, as a glutamate antagonist, and as an agonist at GABA receptors. (5) Stimulates the G-protein that regulates the activity of the second messenger cyclic adenosine momophosphate (cAMP).

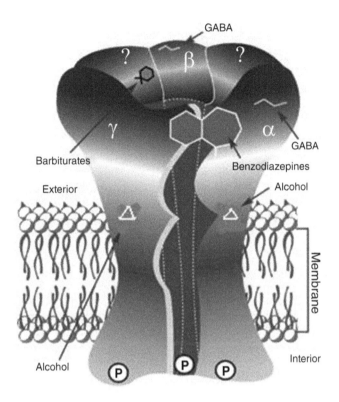

Figure 10.5 GABA$_A$ receptor complex controls an ion channel for Cl$^-$. Several distinct receptor subtypes on the GABA$_A$ complex have been identified. These include receptor subtypes for barbiturates, benzodiazepines, steroids, and perhaps alcohol. The drug Ro15–4513 and alcohol appear to bind to the delta Δ receptor.

been shown to contribute to cognitive and behavioral deficits in experimental animals (Iqbal et al., 2004). Additionally, alcohol consumption during pregnancy can lead to disruptions in normal GABAergic cell migration in fetal brains because of increased GABA availability in the cerebral cortex (Cuzon et al., 2008). A characteristic symptom of FAS is abnormal cortical morphology and development. Alcohol is also a potent antagonist of glutamate, which also contributes to is neurodegenerative effects during early neural development (Baggio et al., 2017, 2022; Olney et al., 2001).

Glutamate

At high concentrations alcohol is a powerful antagonist of the **N-methyl-D-aspartate (NMDA)** subtype of glutamate receptors. These receptors are widely distributed throughout the brain and spinal cord and play important roles in learning and memory, as well as the general excitability of cortical neurons. The activation of NMDA receptors results in the opening of ion channels for Na$^+$ and Ca^{++} influx and K$^+$ efflux, all of which produce excitatory postsynaptic potentials in receiving neurons. NMDA receptors are all **ligand-gated** receptors, meaning that ion flow only occurs when neurotransmitter is bound to receptors.

The antagonism of NMDA receptors by alcohol contributes to its impairment of learning and memory as well as to its amnesiac effects during intoxication at moderate doses and memory *blackouts* at higher doses. Chronic exposure to alcohol use contributes to NMDA receptor upregulation and appears to account for intensified CNS activity and seizures often observed in alcoholics during abstinence and alcohol withdrawal.

Dopamine

Alcohol has a powerful effect on dopamine activity in the mesolimbic system. Injections of alcohol directly into the ventral tegmental area (VTA) increase dopamine release in the nucleus accumbens (NA) (Doyon et al., 2004; Rodd et al., 2004; Sciascia et al., 2014). Additionally, alcohol ingestion at intoxicating doses also increases dopamine release in these regions. It is widely accepted that alcohol's euphoric and reinforcing effects are mediated by increased mesolimbic dopamine activity. Drugs that block dopamine binding also disrupt the self-administration of alcohol in laboratory animals (Cowen et al., 2005; Gonzales et al., 2004). The mechanisms by which alcohol increases dopamine release remain unknown.

Dopamine neurons in the VTA are regulated by a large population of GABAergic neurons within this region. Increasing GABA activity by alcohol would therefore inhibit dopamine activity in the VTA and the subsequent release of dopamine in the NA. Indeed, $GABA_A$ receptor blockade in the VTA results in increased mesolimbic dopamine activity. Recent evidence by Theile et al. (2008) suggests that alcohol causes a biphasic effect on dopamine activity. First, alcohol causes an initial increase in dopamine excitability in the mesolimbic system followed by GABA-mediated inhibition. Therefore, the effects of alcohol on mesolimbic dopamine release may be limited by neural inhibition in the VTA. It is also quite possible that there are two distinct populations of VTA dopamine neurons with different sensitivities to GABA inhibition, as there appear to be for opioid neurons in these same brain regions (Ford et al., 2006).

Although it is clear that alcohol does alter dopamine activity, at least initially, and it does support limited self-administration by animals, its abuse and addictive potential is certainly less than that of the psychostimulants like cocaine and the amphetamines. A significant proportion of the population uses alcohol frequently, and only a small fraction of these become addicted.

Opioids

Acute alcohol administration is also known to increase opioid activity in several brain regions, including the VTA. As described in Chapter 8, opioids contribute to increased dopamine activity in the VTA by inhibition of GABAergic inhibitory control over dopamine release (inhibition of inhibition). At least part of alcohol's effects on dopamine neurons is mediated by opioid suppression of GABAergic inhibition (Job et al., 2007; Kang-Park et al., 2007b; Xiao et al., 2007). Drugs such as the opiate antagonist naloxone significantly blunt alcohol-induced dopamine release while opiate agonists enhance it. This indirect mechanism of enhanced mesolimbic dopamine activity appears to contribute significantly to alcohol's reinforcing properties.

In summary, alcohol affects the activity of most major neurotransmitter systems either directly, as it does with GABA and glutamate, and/or indirectly, as it does with dopamine and the opiates. Because of alcohol's widespread nonspecific effects on these systems, just exactly how alcohol exerts its behavioral effects remains somewhat unclear. To complicate this already confusing picture, long-term exposure to alcohol contributes to a host of cellular adaptations, including receptor downregulation. These adaptations appear to play roles in alcohol tolerance as well as dysphoria and seizures associated with abstinence.

Alcohol Tolerance and Dependence

The development of tolerance to alcohol depends on both one's pattern of drinking (sporadic binge drinking or frequent drinking), and the amount of alcohol consumed during a drinking bout (one or two drinks or numerous drinks leading to heavy intoxication). Individuals who consume a few drinks sporadically develop little or no tolerance to alcohol, while heavy, frequent drinkers develop it quite rapidly. Another factor that influences alcohol tolerance is the use of other drugs in the sedative or antianxiety classes. For example, the use of barbiturates or benzodiazepines can contribute to alcohol tolerance by a process referred to as **cross tolerance**. Cross tolerance occurs when drugs share similar mechanisms of action. In this case $GABA_A$ agonism is the common mechanism. Individuals who have developed tolerance to benzodiazepines, for example, will demonstrate tolerance to alcohol even when they have no history of alcohol use. Tolerance to alcohol, and to other drugs, develops with contributions from several different mechanisms.

Metabolic Tolerance

Metabolic tolerance occurs as the liver produces compensatory increases in alcohol dehydrogenase and P450. Because over 90 percent of all alcohol is metabolized by these enzymes, even small increases in their availability can increase alcohol metabolism significantly. It is estimated that metabolic tolerance contributes to about 25 percent of all tolerance to alcohol. The remaining mechanisms for tolerance include cellular tolerance and behavioral tolerance.

Cellular Tolerance

Cellular tolerance includes several distinct adaptations to neuronal functioning, including receptor and cAMP downregulation. Chronic exposure to alcohol contributes to excessive GABAergic activity followed by receptor internalization (downregulation). Tolerance appears to result as specific $GABA_A$ receptor subtypes are no longer expressed on cell surfaces. $GABA_A$ receptors fall into several subunit classes, including alpha, beta, gamma, and delta subtypes. Each of these subtypes has several additional forms that are traditionally numbered (e.g., 1–4). Chronic alcohol intake appears to contribute to significant internalization of the alpha 1 $GABA_A$ receptors (Kumar et al., 2003, 2004; Liang et al., 2007). Alpha 1 $GABA_A$ receptors are widely expressed in the cortex and the mesolimbic system, which may account for tolerance to alcohol's cognitive and motor effects as well as to its reinforcing effect. Not all $GABA_A$ receptors are downregulated by chronic alcohol exposure. In fact, alpha 2 and 4 subtypes appear to increase with chronic exposure. These differences in $GABA_A$ receptor expression may account for different symptoms observed during alcohol abstinence after chronic exposure (Olsen & Liang, 2017).

Behavioral Tolerance

Animals and humans demonstrate significant motor impairment during alcohol intoxication. If, however, animals are allowed to practice difficult motor tasks under the influence of alcohol they develop tolerance to these disruptive effects. Tolerance to these motor effects of alcohol is called **behavioral tolerance**, and it can be distinguished from cellular, metabolic, and **associative tolerance** in animal experiments. For instance, in one experiment a group of rats was trained to run on a treadmill to avoid small electric foot shocks under the influence of alcohol, while other rats were given the same amount of alcohol but after the training sessions. During testing, all animals performed the avoidance task under the influence of alcohol, but only the group of animals that were trained under the influence of alcohol demonstrated good avoidance. Experiments like this one show that behavioral tolerance to alcohol can be learned (Wenger et al., 1981). This learning appears to involve adjustments to motor coordination (operant conditioning) in the presence of alcohol onset cues.

Another term for behavioral tolerance is **state dependent learning**, since animals tend to perform better when tested under the same physiological or drug state as they were in during training (see Figure 10.6). In this case, performance is dependent upon the animal's alcohol state during training.

Associative Tolerance

It is important to point out here that behavioral tolerance (a learned behavioral adaptation to alcohol's motor effects) is not the same as the associative tolerance discussed in previous chapters. Associative tolerance refers to Pavlovian conditioned responses elicited by drug onset cues—often the drug administration context. It is presumed that these elicited responses include the rapid internalization of receptors, making fewer available for drug or neurotransmitter binding. Associative tolerance to alcohol effects has been demonstrated by Siegel (1987). The details of synaptic adaptations that underlie associative tolerance have not been completely worked out, but they do seem to involve glutamate NMDA receptors.

Dependence

Dependence on alcohol is expressed by a pattern of symptoms typically observed during abstinence after chronic alcohol use. The duration and severity of these symptoms depends on several factors, including the duration of heavy alcohol use, the amount of alcohol used, and genetic factors that control for the neuronal adaptations that occur during alcohol exposure. The symptoms of **dependence** include nausea and vomiting, headache, sweating, tremors, and seizures during alcohol abstinence. In severe cases of long-term alcohol (or benzodiazepine or barbiturate) abuse, **delirium tremens** (DTs) can occur. Symptoms of DTs include

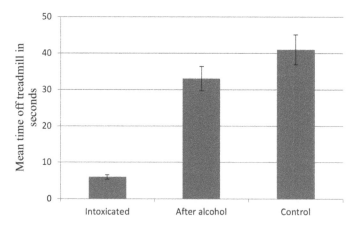

Figure 10.6 Avoidance performance as measured by time off the treadmill under the influence of alcohol. Intoxicated animals received alcohol before daily training sessions, the alcohol after group received the same amount of alcohol after daily training sessions, and the control group received saline. All animals were tested under the influence of alcohol.

Source: Data from Wenger et al. (1981).

confusion, agitation, fever, tachycardia, and hypertension. If left untreated, DTs may be fatal in as many as 35 percent of cases. Delirium tremens are typically managed by sedation with benzodiazepines, which can be gradually tapered off over the course of treatment. It is believed that the symptoms of dependence are the result of neural adaptations to GABA$_A$ receptor expression that occur during chronic alcohol use. In the absence of alcohol, these adaptations (primarily GABA$_A$ receptor downregulation) cause perturbations in the regulation of a variety of physiological systems.

Pharmacological Treatment of Alcohol Dependence

The prevalence of severe alcohol dependence and alcohol use disorder in the United States is between 6 and 7 percent of the population, but as high as 10 percent among young adults between the ages of 18 and 29. Alcohol toxicity is also the main cause of death in over 88,000 people each year. The pharmacological treatment of alcohol dependence begins during the early stages of withdrawal by managing these symptoms with benzodiazepines. Because of the similarity in mechanism of action, benzodiazepines can diminish the severity of these symptoms as neuronal systems begin to revert back to pre-alcohol states. In addition to benzodiazepine treatment, a number of other drugs have been used to diminish cravings that also occur during alcohol withdrawal. The opiate antagonist naltrexone seems to be the most effective. Table 10.2 summarizes several of the most common drugs used to treat alcohol dependence and addiction. Although several appear to withstand rigorous treatment outcome studies, many have limited value in treating alcohol abuse.

A promising new line of research is investigating the role of the cannabinoid (CB1) receptor in substance abuse. A number of animal studies suggest that the CB1 receptor plays a significant role in alcohol preference. For example, CB1 knockout mice that lack the CB1 receptor show increased sensitivity to alcohol and a diminished alcohol-reinforcing effect. Additionally, deleting the CB1 receptor gene eliminates voluntary alcohol intake by laboratory animals. The CB1 receptor antagonist, **Rimonabant (SR141716)** also reduces voluntary alcohol intake in both humans and experimental animals (Basavarajappa, 2007; Soyka et al., 2008; De Ternay

Table 10.2 Pharmacological treatment options for alcohol dependence and addiction.

Drug	Mechanism of action	Effectiveness (recent reviews)
Diazepam (Valium)	GABA$_A$ receptor agonist, benzodiazepine	Effective in reducing the severity of withdrawal symptoms (Lejoyeux et al., 1998).
Naltrexone	Opiate antagonist	Effective in reducing the severity of cravings. Does not reduce recidivism rates (Richardson et al., 2008).
Acamprosate	GABA$_A$ agonist, NMDA antagonist	Limited effectiveness in reducing cravings and recidivism rates (Richardson et al., 2008).
Fluoxetine (SSRIs)	Selective serotonin reuptake inhibitor	Limited effectiveness when alcohol abuse is comorbid with depression or anxiety (Cornelius et al., 2008).
Disulfiram (Antabuse)	Inhibits conversion of acetaldehyde into acetic acid. Causes nausea and vomiting when used with alcohol	Effective in compliant patients, but compliance is low unless supervised (Suh et al., 2006).
Bupropion (Wellbutrin)	Dopamine agonist, antidepressant	Limited effectiveness (Torrens et al., 2005).
Rimonabant (SR141716)	Cannabinoid (CB1) antagonist	Effective in a limited number of studies (Le Foll et al., 2005; Soyka et al., 2008).

et al., 2019). The use of experimental CB1 antagonists in further research will be needed to substantiate these findings and to demonstrate its clinical effectiveness in treating substance abuse.

Nicotine

Nicotine is a pharmacologically active alkaloid produced by the tobacco plant Nicotiana tabacum, shown in Figure 10.7. The tobacco plant appears to have been indigenous to the Americas but has spread around the world. Evidence for its first cultivation and use by the natives of South America date back at least 5,000 years. Tobacco use played an important role in the culture and medicinal practices of indigenous Americans. Europeans were first introduced to tobacco after the return of Columbus, who received dried tobacco leaves as gifts from the inhabitants of the West Indies. By the early 1500s, tobacco was being planted and cultivated in Europe, where it had a great appeal. Shortly after its arrival in Europe, American settlers were introduced to tobacco by North American Indians, who smoked it in small pipes. By the 1700s, tobacco use had spread around the world.

In 2005, the Centers for Disease Control (CDC) estimated that the prevalence of smoking in the United States was 21 percent in adults over the age of 18. This was approximately 42 million smokers. In 2021 this number had decreased significantly to about 12.5 percent. Smoking still contributes directly to roughly 480,000 deaths each year in the United States, and to an annual health care cost of over $167 billion dollars. Each year about 60 percent of current smokers attempt to quit, but fewer than 5 percent of these will be successful. On the bright side, nearly half of all American smokers will eventually quit, and the prevalence of smoking in the United States continues to decline from its all-time high of just over 50 percent of adults 50 years ago to fewer than 13 percent now.

A more recent, and increasing, trend worldwide is the use of electronic cigarettes, known as e-cigarettes (Figure 10.8). In 2010, less than 1 percent of adults in the United States had used e-cigarettes. That number increased to about 15 percent in 2019 and is estimated to continue to rise. E-cigarettes are battery-powered devices that heat liquid nicotine to vaporize

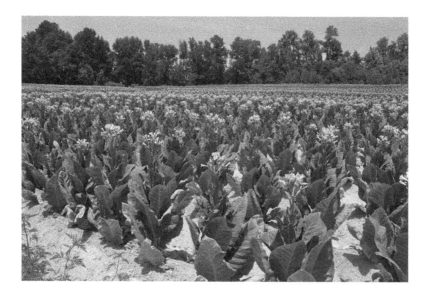

Figure 10.7 A field of tobacco plants (Nicotiana tabacum) growing in North America.

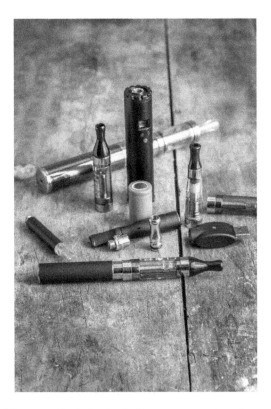

Figure 10.8 E-cigarettes deliver vaporized nicotine in lower concentrations than traditional cigarettes.

it. E-cigarettes are designed to deliver nicotine in doses similar to smoking, but the ranges of nicotine delivery are highly variable, depending on the brand. A study of nicotine absorption from e-cigarettes found that most devices delivered one third to one fourth the amount of nicotine delivered by traditional cigarettes (Farsalinos et al., 2014). While e-cigarettes eliminate many of the toxic compounds found in traditional cigarettes, the adverse health effects of their use are presently unknown.

Cigarette sales worldwide continue to increase, and smoking is now considered to be the second major cause of death and the leading preventable cause in the world. Thirty percent of the world's smokers live in China where it is promoted by the government, which produces, controls, and profits from cigarette sales. Over 350 million Chinese citizens smoke tobacco, which is more than the entire US population. The World Health Organization (WHO) considers smoking tobacco to be a global epidemic.

Pharmacology of Nicotine

Absorption

The typical cigarette contains between 0.5 and 2.0 milligrams of nicotine. Only a small percentage of this actually reaches the bloodstream, as the rest goes up in side stream smoke, is captured by filters, or is destroyed by burning. Nicotine is highly lipid soluble and readily

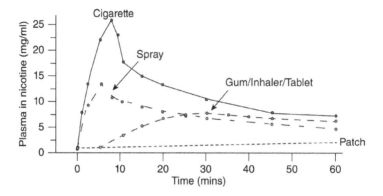

Figure 10.9 Time course of blood plasma levels of nicotine after several different routes of administration. Cigarette smoking yields the highest plasma levels.

enters the circulatory system through the linings of the mouth and lungs, as well as all skin and mucosal surfaces. Once in the blood, nicotine easily crosses the blood–brain barrier. The inhalation of smoked tobacco produces the highest plasma levels of nicotine, which begins to enter the brain within 5–10 seconds of inhalation (see Figure 10.9). Other routes of administration, including IV injections, produce substantially lower peak levels, but within 30–45 minutes the blood levels of nicotine are essentially the same for all methods of administration. The metabolic half-life of nicotine is approximately 90–120 minutes in adults. In a fetus or newborn exposed to maternal nicotine, however, the half-life can be three to four times longer. Chronic smokers regulate their blood levels by adjusting the interval between cigarette smoking. During long periods of abstinence, as during sleeping, blood levels drop and symptoms of withdrawal may begin to emerge. Regular smokers experience the most severe cravings upon waking during the night or early in the morning.

Most nicotine is metabolized by the P450 liver enzyme **CYP2A6** and aldehyde oxidase during first-pass metabolism. About 80 percent of nicotine is metabolized into **cotinine**, which is excreted along with several other minor metabolites in the urine (refer to Figure 10.10).

A genetic variation in the gene that codes for the expression of CYP2A6 has been identified in about 20 percent of the population. This deficit decreases the rate of nicotine metabolism, since most nicotine is metabolized by CYP2A6. Interestingly, these individuals tend to smoke less and they have a lowered risk of tobacco dependence and tobacco-associated disease (Pianezza et al., 1998; Siu & Tyndale, 2008). Presumably this decreased risk of dependency is a consequence of more stable, but lower blood levels of nicotine, similar to wearing a nicotine patch. This conclusion is supported by animal studies showing that the rate of nicotine self-administration is positively associated with increased rates of nicotine metabolism (Siu et al., 2006).

Mechanisms of Nicotine Action: Pharmacodynamics

Nicotine has a high binding affinity for a subtype of the ionotropic acetylcholine receptor. This receptor subtype was in fact named the **nicotinic acetylcholine receptor** (nAChR) because of nicotine's binding affinity. The nicotinic acetylcholine receptor is constructed from a number of subunits referred to as alpha 2 through 10 and beta 2 through 4 (shown in Figure 10.11). These subunits are arranged around a central ion channel that controls the

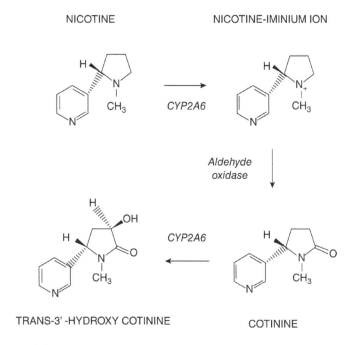

Figure 10.10 The metabolism of nicotine into its principal metabolite cotinine by the P450 enzyme CYP2A6.

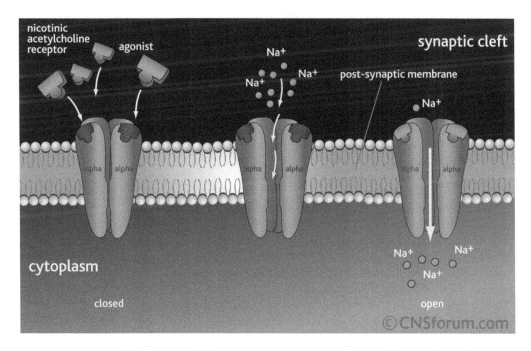

Figure 10.11 Nicotine binds to acetylcholine nicotinic receptors (nAChRs), which control ion channels for Na^+, K^+, or Ca^{++} influx.

influx of positively charged ions. While some nAChR configurations control K^+ and Ca^{++} channels, the majority control an ionotropic Na^+ channel. Once nicotine or acetylcholine bind to the receptor complex, the ion channel opens rapidly. The ion channel returns to its closed configuration after nicotine diffuses away. Typically nicotine remains bound to the nAChR for only 1–2 milliseconds. High doses of nicotine, however, can have prolonged receptor-activating effects, as high levels of the drug remain in proximity to the receptor. These nAChRs can be found both pre- and postsynaptically. Presynaptic nAChRs cause an increase in the release of neurotransmitter from the receiving neuron. When nicotine binds to a receptor controlling the influx of Ca^{++} it activates a Ca^{++}-dependent second messenger system. These metabotropic synapses are much slower and their actions longer sustained than ionotropic receptors. These receptors have been found presynaptically, where they function to increase the synthesis and release of neurotransmitters.

Nicotinic acetylcholine receptors are widely distributed throughout the central and peripheral nervous systems. In the peripheral nervous system, nicotinic receptor sites are located in neuromuscular junctions of voluntary muscles. Nicotine stimulates these receptors and can cause muscle tremors. Nicotine also increases heart rate and blood pressure, decreases body temperature, stimulates the release of epinephrine from the adrenal glands, increases muscle contraction and activity of the bowel, and causes a constriction of blood vessels in the skin. This latter effect may be what causes premature wrinkling of the skin in smokers and why facial wrinkles associated with aging can be diminished with acetylcholine antagonists (e.g., **Botox**). In the central nervous system, nAChRs are found in the cerebral cortex, the thalamus, the hippocampus, the ventral tegmental area, and regions of the basal ganglia. Nicotinic receptors are also located in the brainstem raphe nuclei and in the locus coeruleus.

Because of the wide distribution of nicotinic receptors we would be correct in presuming nicotine has significant effects on a variety of behavioral and physiological functions. For example, nicotine increases arousal and cognitive functioning in both humans and in laboratory animals. These effects are observed as increased cortical arousal measured by electroencephalograph (EEG), decreases in motor reaction time, and improved recall memory. Because of these effects, nicotine and other cholinergic drugs, such as donepezil and galantamine have been used to treat the cognitive deficits associated with Alzheimer's disease and other forms of dementia (Hernandez et al., 2005; Levin et al., 1998; Marucci et al., 2021; Murray et al., 2002). Nicotine may also be used to improve symptoms in individuals with attention-deficit/hyperactivity disorders (ADHD). In a study of young, non-smoking ADHD adults, nicotine administered by a skin patch was shown to decrease excessive behaviors and to improve several cognitive and reaction time measures (Potter et al., 2008). Other cholinergic drugs are also being investigated to treat ADHD without the use of stimulants (Fleisher & McGough, 2014).

Nicotine Tolerance and Sensitization

Tolerance to nicotine is both complex and incomplete. Tolerance to several of nicotine's physiological and behavioral effects is observed following repeated nicotine administration in both humans and animals. In fact, tolerance may need to occur to its aversive effects before nicotine's reinforcing effects may be experienced. For instance, early exposures to nicotine produce dizziness and nausea, which quickly disappear following repeated administration. Smokers would likely cease smoking if tolerance to these effects didn't occur quickly. These effects may also occur in laboratory animals. Nicotine self-administration is often difficult to obtain in experimental animals and very dependent upon the procedures for administration. The most effective method to establish self-administration in animals is to initially force-administer nicotine. After a period of forced consumption, animals will respond for injections of nicotine on intermittent schedules of infusion. The initial period of forced administration may be sufficient to induce tolerance to nicotine's aversive effects.

Nicotine's effects are complicated by the fact that both tolerance and **behavioral sensitization** occur following repeated exposure. Numerous studies have demonstrated that repeated nicotine exposure contributes to tolerance to its behavior-activating effects. While initial treatment causes decreases in locomotor activity, chronic treatment produces behavioral sensitization. Tolerance to nicotine is typically lost after several days of abstinence (e.g., Stolerman et al., 1973). In an experiment conducted by Collins et al. (1990), rats were given subcutaneous infusions of either saline or nicotine for seven days. After chronic nicotine or saline administration, all animals were given nicotine and exposed to an open field to measure locomotor activity. Control animals given prior exposure to saline demonstrated behavioral suppression, while nicotine-treated animals developed behavioral sensitization. As tolerance develops to nicotine's behavior-suppressing effects, animals show increased locomotor activity. These results are depicted in Figure 10.12.

Tolerance and sensitization to nicotine occurs in two stages. The first stage is referred to as acute tolerance, which occurs rapidly during the course of administration or immediately following it. **Acute nicotine tolerance** appears to result from rapid nAChR desensitization, resulting in a closing of the cation channel. This desensitization essentially attenuates further nicotine effects on its receptor. After repeated administration the second stage of sensitization develops, which is represented by upregulation of specific subtypes of nAChRs (see Figure 10.13). This effect of nicotine appears paradoxical since repeated administration of most receptor agonists leads to receptor downregulation, while repeated nicotine administration appears to lead to upregulation. A widely expressed subtype of nAChR that undergoes upregulation is the alpha 4 beta 2 ($\alpha 4\beta 2$) receptor type. The $\alpha 4\beta 2$ receptor exists in two activational

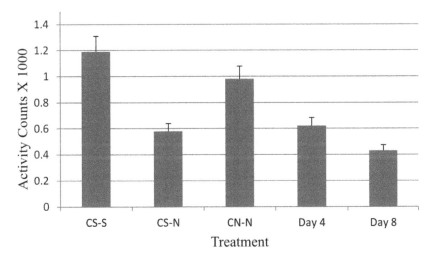

Figure 10.12 Tolerance to nicotine's behavior-depressant effects. Animals received either chronic saline treatment followed by saline during open field testing (CS-S), chronic saline treatment followed by nicotine before testing (CS-N), or chronic nicotine treatment followed by nicotine before testing (CN-N). The effects of nicotine on activity in the open field was also examined four days (Day 4) and eight days (Day 8) after nicotine abstinence. Tolerance to nicotine is observed as an increase in activity (behavioral sensitization) in the nicotine-treated animals (CN-N) but not in the saline pre-treated animals (CS-N). Tolerance was lost after four days of abstinence.

Source: Collins et al. (1990).

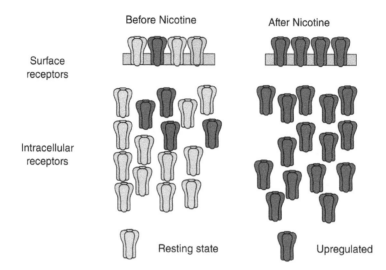

Figure 10.13 Exposure of the α4β2 nicotinic receptors to nicotine changes their state from a resting, low-
     affinity state (white) to an upregulated high-affinity state (gray). Because nicotine readily crosses
     cellular membranes, both surface and intracellular receptors undergo structural changes.

Source: Vallejo et al. (2005).

states. In its resting state, nicotine only binds with low affinity to the α4β2 receptor, but in
an upregulated state nicotine binds with a much higher affinity (see Figure 10.13). Nicotine
exposure appears to induce structural changes to α4β2 receptors on the cell's surface as well as
the intracellular receptors that may become expressed on the surface. Once in the upregulated
state, these receptors have an increased affinity for nicotine (Sallette et al., 2004; Vallejo
et al., 2005; Walsh et al., 2008). Other nicotinic receptor subtypes may also undergo similar
structural changes.

It is believed that nicotine's behavioral sensitization effects (Figure 10.14) may be mediated
by upregulation of nAChRs in the ventral tegmental area and its projections to the nucleus
accumbens, the prefrontal cortex (the mesolimbic-cortical system), and the striatum, and by
nicotine's agonistic effect on dopamine release in these regions (Buisson & Bertrand, 2001;
Li et al., 2008; Tapper et al., 2004; Vann et al., 2006). Imaging studies, like the one shown in
Figure 10.15, show upregulation and sensitization after repeated nicotine use. Upregulation of
the α4β2 receptors in the mesolimbic system may underlie dependence and addiction.

Nicotine Dependence

From the preceding discussion, it is clear that even brief exposure to nicotine induced structural changes to the nicotinic α4β2 receptor. These changes to their high-affinity state underlie
behavioral sensitization and nicotine dependence. In some individuals, with presumably different genetic propensities for these structural changes, upregulation and sensitization may
occur after smoking one or two cigarettes (DiFranza, 2008; Scragg et al., 2008). Upregulation
of nicotinic receptors has been shown to occur within minutes of nicotine exposure (Walsh
et al., 2008).

Upregulation of nicotinic receptors induces increased dopamine release from neurons in
the mesolimbic-cortical system. Prolonged nicotine exposure causes downregulation of these

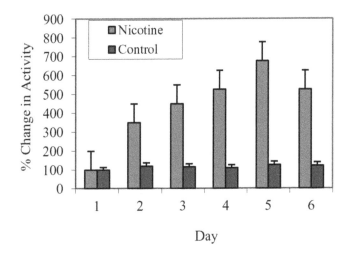

Figure 10.14 Behavioral sensitization as expressed as increased activity to single and repeated nicotine injections in rats.

Source: Data from Li et al. (2008).

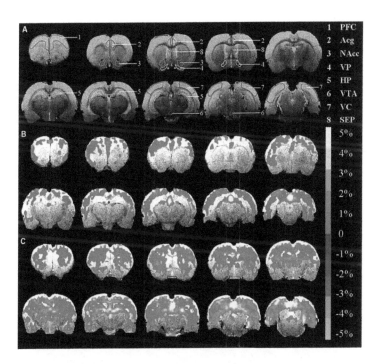

Figure 10.15 (A) MRI images showing eight brain regions. (1) PFC = prefrontal cortex; (2) Acg = anterior cingulate gyrus; (3) NAcc = nucleus accumbens; (4) VP = ventral pallidum; (5) HP = hippocampus; (6) VTA = ventral tegmental area; (7) VC = visual cortex; (8) SEP = septum. (B) Activation in many brain structures in response to a single dose of nicotine. (C) Increased activation in response to the fifth dose of nicotine shows upregulation and sensitization. Color version available in plate section.

Source: Li et al. (2008).

dopamine receptors and is believed to underlie nicotine dependence and the cravings associated with withdrawal. Like other drugs of abuse, including cocaine, the amphetamines, the opiates, and alcohol, nicotine stimulates dopamine release, which contributes to its dependence and addictive potential. During abstinence, and cravings, neural activity in a number of brain regions, including the orbital frontal cortex, the prefrontal cortex, the cingulate cortex, and the nucleus accumbens, is increased. Increased activity of these mesolimbic-cortical structures mediates cravings to smoke and maintain nicotine addiction (Fehr et al., 2008; McGranahan et al., 2011; Wang et al., 2007).

Pharmacological Treatment for Nicotine Dependence

The health consequences of using tobacco products are both well known and numerous (despite Figure 10.16). They include lung, esophageal, pancreatic, kidney, and oral cancer; pulmonary disease; heart disease; increased risk of stroke; and numerous complications to pregnancies, just to name the most common. Although the numerous mechanisms by which tobacco products cause these diseases are not the topic of this text, some of the treatment options are.

As stated at the beginning of this section, of the 42 million tobacco users in the United States, about 60 percent will attempt to quit each year. Of these, only about 5 percent will be successful for a full year or more. The good news is that about half of everyone who has ever used tobacco will eventually be successful in quitting, but typically after many unsuccessful attempts.

To assist those who need help there are several pharmacological alternatives. These include **nicotine replacement therapy (NRT)**, bupropion (Zyban), varenicline (Chantix), and potentially nicotine immunization.

Nicotine Replacement

Nicotine replacement therapies include over the counter (OTC) nicotine transdermal patches (Nicoderm, Habitrol, and Nicotrol), nicotine gum (Nicorette and Polacrilex), and nicotine lozenges (Commit). Because these products contain doses of nicotine, the cravings associated

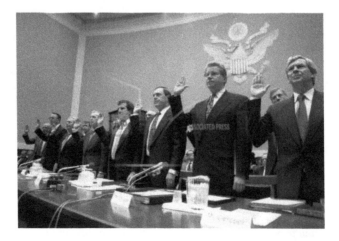

Figure 10.16 Even though there has been little debate among scientists about the addictive potential of nicotine since the early 1950s, executives from major tobacco companies testified before Congress in 1994 that nicotine was not addictive.

with tobacco abstinence are blunted. The idea behind NRT is to transfer the delivery of nicotine from tobacco products to a method of administration that can be gradually tapered off and eliminated. In addition, many of the health hazards associated with tobacco use can be avoided. Smokers often find, however, that NRT is not always effective. The slower absorption of nicotine from these products is not a substitute for the rapid absorption of nicotine inhalation. Furthermore, smokers find that it is more difficult to regulate nicotine doses with these products than with smoking.

There are also several prescription nicotine supplements, including nicotine sprays (Nicotrol, NicoNovum) and nicotine inhalers (Nicotrol). These methods were designed to deliver nicotine more quickly and in a manner similar to smoking than transdermal nicotine patches. Nicotine replacement therapies are all more effective than placebos when compared in randomized clinical trials. In some studies, NRT nearly doubled the success rate of quitting (Burns & Levinson, 2008; Eisenberg et al., 2008; Hartmann-Boyce et al., 2018).

Bupropion (Zyban)

Bupropion was briefly discussed with the antidepressants. As you may recall, bupropion had an unusual mechanism of action for an antidepressant. Rather than block the reuptake of serotonin and/or norepinephrine, bupropion preferentially blocks the reuptake of dopamine. Increasing dopamine activity by reuptake blockade appears to decrease the severity of cravings associated with nicotine abstinence. A long-acting form of bupropion (Zyban) has been approved for smoking cessation.

Varenicline (Chantix)

The newest drug to be approved for smoking cessation is varenicline (Chantix), which is a partial agonist for the nicotine α4β2 receptor, and it appears to weakly agonize other nicotinic receptors as well. Varenicline has a half-life of about 24 hours. In clinical trials varenicline has been demonstrated to be as effective as NRT and bupropion in reducing the severity of cravings and in maintaining abstinence from smoking (Eisenberg et al., 2008; Niaura et al., 2008). However, the FDA recently issued an alert suggesting that varenicline may be associated with an increased risk of psychiatric symptoms. The Federal Aviation Administration also announced that varenicline was not approved for pilots and air traffic controllers for these same reasons. Whether varenicline remains approved for treating symptoms of smoking cessation remains to be seen.

Nicotine Immunization

Although still not approved by the FDA, animal studies and clinical trials indicate that nicotine immunization may be a promising therapy for nicotine dependence. At the present, two approaches to nicotine vaccination are being investigated. One approach is to immunize with a catabolic antibody that increases the rate of nicotine metabolism. This method of immunization is referred to as passive immunization, since it does not recruit the production of antibodies by the body, but rather it works by increasing nicotine's enzymatic metabolism significantly. Another approach is to use active immunization against the nicotine molecule itself. In active nicotine immunization, the nicotine molecule is conjugated with an immunogenic protein and administered by injection. This conjugate stimulates the production of antibodies against the protein as well as against nicotine. Nicotine-specific antibodies attack nicotine in the blood and prevent its passage through tissue membranes into the brain. Both active and passive immunization have been shown to be effective in eliminating self-administration of nicotine in animals (LeSage et al., 2006; Pentel et al., 2014) and to decrease nicotine-induced dopamine release in the nucleus accumbens (de Villiers et al., 2002).

A major difference between immunotherapy for nicotine dependence and drug treatment for nicotine withdrawal is that immunization only prevents the drug from entering the brain; it does not thwart withdrawal. In fact, immunization alone would precipitate withdrawal symptoms. Whether nicotine vaccination can be used to effectively treat smoking dependence remains to be seen. A potential problem with all immunotherapies against drugs (cocaine, amphetamine, or nicotine) is that users can overwhelm the antibody with increased doses of the drug (Johnson & Ettinger, 2000).

Caffeine

Caffeine, an alkaloid found in a variety of plants, including coffee shrubs (Figure 10.17), tea plants (Figure 10.18), and cocoa plants, is the most widely used psychoactive drug in the world.

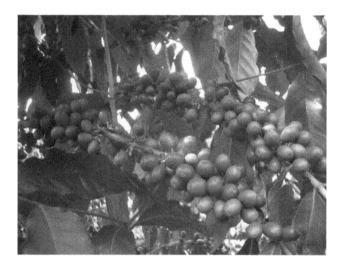

Figure 10.17 Coffee (Coffea) is a genus of small trees or shrubs native to Africa and southern Asia. Of the more than 90 species of Coffea, Coffea arabica is considered to be the most suitable for making fine coffee. The fruits or beans of the Coffea plant are dried and roasted for brewing.

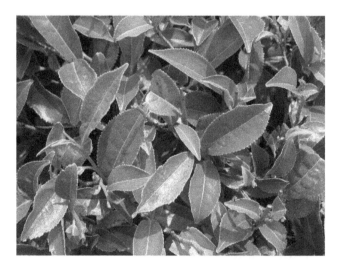

Figure 10.18 Tea plants are evergreens of the *Camellia* family native to China, Tibet, and northern India. The two main varieties of the tea plant are *Camellia sinensis*, which is grown in the mountainous regions of central China and Japan, and *Camellia assamica*, which grows in tropical climates of northeast India and the Szechuan and Yunnan provinces of China.

Table 10.3 Approximate caffeine amount in several common caffeinated beverages. The amount of caffeine in coffees, teas, and espresso drinks varies widely and depends on variety and preparation methods.

Beverage	Caffeine in milligrams
Red Bull (8.2 oz)	80
Jolt (12 oz)	71.2
Coca-Cola (12 oz)	34
Brewed coffee (8 oz)	100–200
Espresso (2 oz)	100–150
Tea (8 oz)	40–60
Hot chocolate (8 oz)	10–15

Table 10.4 Caffeine amount in several common over-the-counter remedies.

Product (1 tablet)	Caffeine in milligrams
Vivrin	200
NoDoz	200
Excedrine	65
Anacin	32

While caffeine is primarily consumed in naturally caffeinated beverages, such as coffee and tea, it is added to a number of other beverages; over-the-counter analgesics, including Excedrin and Anacin; and alertness-promoting drugs like NoDoz and Vivarin (refer to Tables 10.3 and 10.4). A small amount of caffeine is also available in products containing chocolate.

Pharmacology of Caffeine

Absorption and Metabolism

Caffeine (Figure 10.19) is readily absorbed by the stomach and small intestine within 30–60 minutes following ingestion. After absorption it is distributed to all bodily tissues, including the brain. Because of its water solubility, caffeine is freely distributed throughout all body fluids. Peak plasma concentrations are reached within two hours. Caffeine is metabolized by the hepatic enzyme P450 into two active metabolites and one inactive metabolite. Caffeine is eliminated from the body after metabolism and its metabolites are excreted through the urine. Only about 2 percent of caffeine is excreted unchanged.

The half-life of caffeine is approximately three to four hours. Its half-life is increased to about ten hours in women taking oral contraceptives or who are pregnant. Caffeine readily crosses the placental barrier and reaches comparable levels in a fetus, where its half-life may be much longer. In newborns and infants the half-life of caffeine is as long as 80 hours. This can lead to significant blood levels in infants of mothers who drink caffeinated beverages while breastfeeding.

Pharmacological Effects of Caffeine

Consumers of caffeinated beverages are familiar with many of caffeine's physiological effects, which include CNS stimulation (increased alertness and insomnia), increases in heart and respiratory rates, and its diuretic effects. Caffeine is also a powerful constrictor of cerebral

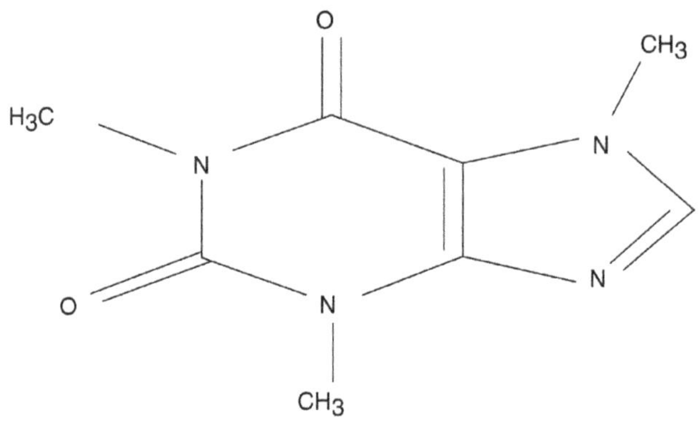

Figure 10.19 Molecular structure of caffeine.

blood vessels, making it a useful remedy for the treatment of some types of headaches, including migraines. For this reason it is added to several over-the-counter analgesics (Table 10.4). Caffeine and its active metabolite **theobromine** are also effective antiasthmatics because they relax bronchial muscles, allowing for greater airflow into the lungs. Caffeine and theobromine are mild ergogenic aids, since they increase cardiac contractility and output, and they dilate coronary arteries, allowing for greater levels of oxygen to the heart. Caffeine was listed as a banned substance by many sport organizations, including the Olympics, until 2004, when it was finally removed from the list of banned substances. It is still banned by the National Collegiate Athletic Association (NCAA), however. Whether caffeine increases athletic performance remains debatable, but numerous studies using a variety of testing protocols have found significant improvement in endurance sports (e.g., Cox et al., 2002). In addition to caffeine's effects on cardiac functioning, caffeine may also increase carbohydrate metabolism and facilitate muscle glycogen replacement both during and after prolonged exercise (Pedersen et al., 2008).

People suffering from anxiety are typically sensitive to caffeine's CNS-stimulating effects and may experience heightened anxiety following its administration. Individuals with anxiety disorders are therefore advised to abstain from caffeinated products entirely. Anxiety may also be precipitated in normal individuals who consume over 500 milligrams of caffeine over a several-hour period. Caffeine overdose, referred to as **caffeinism,** causes anxiety, irritability, muscle tremors, and insomnia, which are often referred to as caffeine jitters. Extreme caffeinism may precipitate mania, disorientation, delusions, and even temporary psychosis. Caffeine overdose may also cause cardiac arrhythmia, high heart rate and blood pressure, and gastrointestinal distress. The lethal dose of caffeine is considered to be approximately 150–200 milligrams per kilogram of body weight. This would be approximately 10,000 milligrams of caffeine, or about 100 cups of coffee. Because of the large amount of caffeinated beverage that would need to be consumed for a lethal overdose, as you must expect this would be extremely rare. However, caffeine overdose can occur with abusers of caffeine tablets. Death by caffeine overdose typically follows ventricular fibrillation.

Mechanisms of Caffeine Action: Pharmacodynamics

Caffeine exerts its effects by several mechanisms, including its effects on receptors as well as its effects within cells on cAMP metabolic pathways. Caffeine's principal mechanism of action, however, is antagonism of the neuromodulator **adenosine**. Perhaps because of the structural similarity of caffeine and the **purine** component (circled in Figure 10.20) of the adenosine compound, caffeine easily binds to adenosine receptors and inhibits adenosine effects. Adenosine is a product of normal cellular activity. It is formed during the breakdown and synthesis of adenosine monophosphate (AMP), which is a nucleotide found in all forms of ribonucleic acid (RNA) and deoxyribonucleic acid (DNA). Adenosine monophosphate is therefore a byproduct of cellular activity. As cells become more active, as a result of stimulation, adenosine is produced and released by the activated cell, and it acts upon the presynaptic cell to inhibit neurotransmitter release. Because of its backwards-acting effect, adenosine is referred to as a **retrograde neuromodulator**. Adenosine acts on presynaptic cells and inhibits their release of neurotransmitter, thereby turning down the adenosine-releasing cell's activity (see Figure 10.21). Readers who

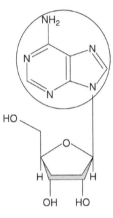

Figure 10.20 Molecular structure of adenosine. The circled purine segment resembles the structure of caffeine.

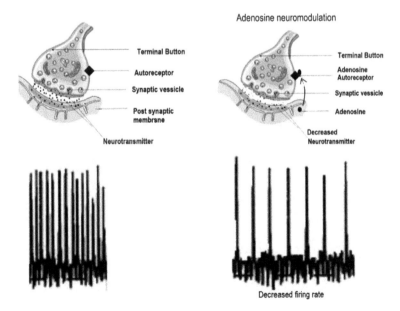

Figure 10.21 Adenosine acts as a retrograde neuromodulator inhibiting the release of neurotransmitter from presynaptic neurons, which in turn decreases the firing rate of the adenosine-releasing neuron.

see the similarities here with auto- and heteroreceptor modulation are correct. The difference here is not in the inhibitory effect, but in the origin of the inhibiting modulator. In the case of retrograde neuromodulation, the modulation of transmitter release comes from the neuron that was activated initially. High rates of cell activity increase the rate of adenosine accumulation, resulting in a decrease in its firing rate.

Adenosine receptors are present in almost all brain areas, with highest concentrations in the hippocampus, cerebral cortex, cerebellum, and the thalamus. Adenosine receptors are also found on dopaminergic cells within the striatum. Four distinct G-protein coupled adenosine receptor subtypes have been described: A_1, A_{2A}, A_{2B}, and A_3, but the A_1 and A_{2A} subtypes are considered to be the most important for understanding caffeine action. The A_{2B} and A_3 receptors appear to regulate internal metabolic pathways. The A_1 and A_{2A} subtypes modulate neurotransmitter release. Specifically, adenosine on these receptors acts to inhibit the release of the neurotransmitters dopamine, serotonin, norepinephrine, and glutamate. Caffeine appears to increase the release of these neurotransmitters by competitively blocking adenosine receptors and by reversing adenosine inhibition of intracellular cAMP-phosphodiesterase activity (Daly et al., 1998). cAMP-phosphodisterase is an essential enzyme for the cAMP second messenger pathway. Caffeine is also known to block intracellular Ca^{++} activity and to block $GABA_A$ receptors at even higher doses (see Figure 10.22). It is the increase in neural activity

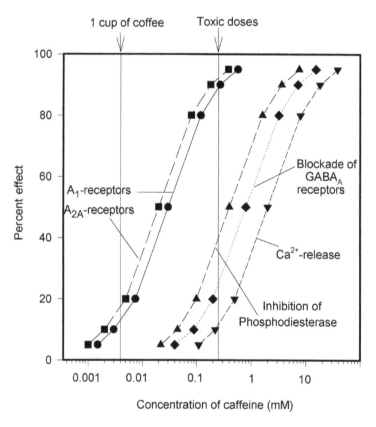

Figure 10.22 Effects of caffeine on adenosine and $GABA_A$ receptors and on intracellular messenger systems depends on concentration. At low doses, equivalent to one or two cups of coffee, caffeine primarily blocks adenosine A_1 and A_{2A} receptors. At higher, toxic doses caffeine blocks $GABA_A$ receptors, inhibits intracellular Ca^{++} release, and disrupts cAMP-phosphodiesterase activity.

Source: Daly and Fredholm (1998).

resulting from these effects that is believed to underlie caffeine's effects on arousal, cognitive performance, and motor activity as well as its effects on peripheral systems.

Caffeine Tolerance and Dependence

Tolerance to caffeine's sleep-disruptive, cardiovascular, respiratory, and motor-stimulating effects occurs quickly and can be observed after one to two weeks of moderate (400 mg/day) caffeine consumption. Other caffeine effects, including its effects on cognitive performance and mood, show little evidence of tolerance. The degree of tolerance to caffeine, therefore, depends on which caffeine effect is being investigated. Tolerance to caffeine is believed to be mediated by the upregulation of adenosine receptors, which corresponds well with the development of tolerance. All CNS and peripheral adenosine receptors do not undergo upregulation at the same rate, so tolerance across different caffeine effects is quite variable when it does occur.

Consumers of caffeinated beverages are well aware of the consequences of skipping their daily measure of caffeine. Abstinence in regular caffeine users often leads to mild-to-moderate withdrawal symptoms, which include headache, irritability, depression, drowsiness, and fatigue. These effects can begin within a few hours of abstinence but typically peak in severity between 24 and 48 hours. Withdrawal symptoms usually disappear within three to five days, corresponding to the time course of downregulation of adenosine receptors. The symptoms of withdrawal are caused in part by vasodilatation and an increase in blood flow. An increase in cerebral blood flow can cause severe headaches and is the reason why caffeine is added to several common headache remedies. A decrease in norepinephrine, dopamine, and serotonin release following the upregulation of adenosine receptors may contribute to irritability, depression, lack of motivation, and fatigue. As most of us know well, the annoying symptoms of caffeine withdrawal are quickly relieved by caffeine consumption.

The health hazards, if any, of regular caffeine consumption are negligible, even though caffeine is considered to be a dependence-producing substance. The widespread and extensive use of caffeinated beverages, therefore, does not appear to be a significant threat to the consumer or to society. Unlike the other substances covered in this chapter, caffeine is not addictive.

Glossary

Acute nicotine tolerance the first stage of nicotine tolerance resulting from rapid internalization of nACh receptors.

Adenosine an inhibitory neuromodulator and a product of normal cellular activity. Formed during the breakdown and synthesis of adenosine monophosphate (AMP).

Addiction a debilitating form of dependence resulting from exposure to drugs that rapidly increase dopamine activity and induce synaptic adaptations in the mesolimbic system.

Alcohol dehydrogenase the principal metabolite of alcohol.

Aldehyde dehydrogenase the principal enzyme involved in alcohol metabolism. See also **Nicotinamide adenine dinucleotide**.

Associative tolerance a form of Pavlovian conditioning where drug onset cues elicit cellular adaptations contributing to drug tolerance.

Behavioral sensitization an increase in motor behavior following chronic exposure to certain stimulant drugs.

Behavioral tolerance a form of operant conditioning or behavioral adaptation where training under the influence of a drug enhances performance later when under the influence of the same drug. See **State dependent learning**.

Blood alcohol concentration (BAC) the amount of alcohol in blood. Expressed as either grams per milliliter of blood or as a percent weight. The legal limit for intoxication in most states is 0.08 percent. BAC can be estimated by a breathalyzer, which measures the amount of alcohol excreted in breath.

Botox an acetylcholine antagonist derived from botulism toxin used in dermatology to decrease facial wrinkles.

Caffeine an alkaloid found in a variety of plants, including coffee shrubs, tea plants, and cocoa plants.

Caffeinism a consequence of caffeine overdose, which causes anxiety, irritability, muscle tremors, and insomnia. Extreme caffeinism may precipitate mania, disorientation, delusions, and even temporary psychosis. Caffeine overdose may also cause cardiac arrhythmia, high heart rate and blood pressure, and gastrointestinal distress.

Cellular tolerance develops as a result of cellular adaptations that decrease or downregulate cell activity.

Cotinine primary metabolite of nicotine.

Cross tolerance tolerance to a drug can occur as a consequence of tolerance being developed to a similarly acting drug. Benzodiazepine tolerance can contribute to alcohol tolerance without prior alcohol exposure.

CYP2A6 P450 liver enzyme that metabolizes nicotine into cotinine.

Delirium tremens a state characterized by confusion, agitation, fever, tachycardia, and hypertension that occurs during abstinence from chronic alcohol abuse.

Dependence a physiological state resulting from long-term exposure to certain drugs. Symptoms of dependence can include nausea, vomiting, delirium tremens, headache, sweating, nervousness, and agitation. See also **Addiction**.

Dilsufiram (Antabuse) a drug that inhibits the aldehyde dehydrogenase metabolism of acetaldehyde. Causes illness and can discourage drinking.

Ethyl alcohol (ethanol) alcohol produced during fermentation of sugars in fruits or grains.

Fetal alcohol syndrome (FAS) serious developmental disorder caused by alcohol exposure during prenatal development.

First-pass metabolism drugs that are ingested are partially metabolized by stomach and liver enzymes before the remaining unmetabolized drug enters the bloodstream.

Fluidization an increase in the fluids (alcohol) within cell membranes. Fluidization disrupts membrane processes and the ability of ions to pass through them.

Ligand-gated receptor a receptor where ion flow only occurs when the receptor is activated by a neurotransmitter or pure agonist.

Metabolic tolerance develops as a result of increased rates of drug metabolism.

Nicotinamide adenine dinucleotide a rate-limiting coenzyme involved in alcohol metabolism. See also **Alcohol dehydrogenase**.

Nicotine replacement therapy (NRP) a form of treatment for nicotine dependence where controlled doses of nicotine are administered through gums, lozenges, or transdermal patches.

Nicotinic acetylcholine receptor a subtype of the acetylcholine receptor constructed from a number of subunits referred to as alpha 2 through 10 and beta 2 through 4. The nicotinic receptor controls channels for either Na^+, K^+, or Ca^{++}.

N-methyl-D-aspartate (NMDA) a subtype of the glutamate receptor. Believed to be involved in long-term potentiation.

P450 (cytochrome P450) the liver enzyme that is essential in oxidative metabolic reactions. Many drugs are metabolized by P450.

Proof a measure of the amount of alcohol in a beverage or spirit. Proof alcohol is exactly twice the percent alcohol. Thus, 50 percent alcohol is 100 proof.

Purine a structural component of the adenosine molecule that resembles the form of caffeine.

Retrograde neuromodulator a neuromodulator that is produced and released by an activated neuron that acts backwards to inhibit the activity of the activating neuron. Adenosine is a retrograde neuromodulator.

Rimonabant (SR141716) a cannabinoid CB1 receptor antagonist. May be useful in treating substance abuse.

Ro15–4513 competitive antagonist of alcohol at GABA delta receptors.

State dependent learning a form of operant conditioning or behavioral adaptation where animals tend to perform better when tested under the same physiological or drug state as they were in during training. See **Behavioral tolerance**.

Theobromine an active metabolite of caffeine. May be used to treat asthma.

Bibliography

Abercrombie, E., Keefe, K., DiFrischia, D., & Zigmond, M. (1989). Differential effect of stress on in vitro dopamine release in striatum, nucleus accumbens, and medial frontal cortex. *Journal of Neurochemistry, 52*(5), 1655–1658.

Abi-Dargham, A., & Moore, H. (2003). Prefrontal DA transmission at D1 receptors and the pathology of schizophrenia. *The Neuroscientist, 9*(5), 404–416.

Abi-Dargham, A., Rodenhiser, J., Printz, D., Zea-Ponce, Y., Gil, R., Kegeles, L. S., Weiss, R., Cooper, T. B., Mann, J. J., Van Heertum, R. L., Gorman, J. M., & Laruelle, M. (2000). Increased baseline occupancy of D2 receptors by dopamine in schizophrenia. *Proceedings of the National Academy of Sciences of the United States of America, 97*(14), 8104–8109.

Adolphs, R., Tranel, D., Damasio, H., & Damasio, A. (1995). Fear and the human amygdala. *The Journal of Neuroscience, 15*(9), 5879–5891.

Aghajanian, G. K., & Marek, G. J. (1999). Serotonin and hallucinogens. *Neuropsychopharmacology, 21*(2), 16–23.

Agrawal, A., & Lynskey, M. T. (2008). Are there genetic influences on addiction: Evidence from family, adoption and twin studies. *Addiction, 103*(7), 1069–1081.

Alamo, C., Lopez-Munoz, F., & Garcia-Garcia, P. (2014). The effectiveness of lurasidone as an adjunct to lithium or divalproex in the treatment of bipolar disorder. *Expert Review of Neurotherapeutics, 14*(6), 593–605.

Albert, P., Vahid-Ansari, F., & Luckhart, C. (2014). Serotonin-prefrontal cortical circuitry in anxiety and depression phenotypes: pivotal role of pre- and post-synaptic 5-HT1A receptor expression. *Frontiers in Behavioral Neuroscience, 8*, 199.

Allis, D. C., Caparros, M., Jenuwein, T., & Reinberg, D. (2015). Epigenetics (2nd ed.). Cold Springs Harbor Press.

Alnefeesi, Y., Chen-Li, D., Krane, E., Jawad, M. Y., Rodrigues, N. B., & Rosenblat, J. D. (2022). Real-world effectiveness of ketamine in treatment-resistant depression: A systematic review & meta-analysis. *Journal of Psychiatric Research, 151*, 693–709.

Altar, C. A. (1999). Neurotrophins and depression. *Trends in Pharmacological Sciences, 20*(2), 59–61.

Amato, J. L., Bankson, M. G., & Yamamoto, B. K. (2007). Prior exposure to chronic stress and MDMA potentiates mesoaccumbens dopamine release mediated by the 5-HT(1B) receptor. *Neuropsychopharmacology, 32*(4), 946–954.

Amiri, S., Mohammadi, M. R., Mohammadi, M., Nouroozinejad, G. H., Kahbazi, M., & Akhondzadeh, S. (2008). Modafinil as a treatment for attention-deficit/hyperactivity disorder in children and adolescents: A double blind, randomized clinical trial. *Progress in Neuro-psychopharmacology and Biological Psychiatry, 32*(1), 145–149.

Andreatini, R., Sartori, V. A., Seabra, M. L., & Leite, J. R. (2002). Effect of valepotriates (valerian extract) in generalized anxiety disorder: A randomized placebo-controlled pilot study. *Phytotherapy Research, 16*(7), 650–654.

Antrop, I., Roeyers, H., Van Oost, P., & Buysse, A. (2000). Stimulation seeking and hyperactivity in children with ADHD. *The Journal of Child Psychology and Psychiatry and Allied Disciplines, 41*, 225–231.

APA. (2013). Diagnostic and statistical manual of mental disorders 5. American Psychiatric Association.

Appel, J. B., West, W. B., & Buggy, J. (2004). LSD, 5-HT (serotonin), and the evolution of a behavioral assay. *Neuroscience and Biobehavioral Reviews, 27*(8), 693–701.

Atmaca, M., Yildirim, H., Ozdemir, H., Tezcan, E., & Poyraz, A. K. (2007). Volumetric MRI study of key brain regions implicated in obsessive-compulsive disorder. *Progress in Neuro-Psychopharmacology and Biological Psychiatry*, *31*(1), 46–52.

Baggio, S., Mussulini, B., Losch de Oliveira, D., Cagliari, K., Emerson, Z., da Silva, S., & Pacheco Rico, E. (2017). Embryonic alcohol exposure promotes long-term effects on cerebral glutamate transport of adult zebrafish. *Neuroscience Letters*, *636*, 265–269.

Baggio, S., Zenki, K., Martins, S. A., Dos Santos, T. G., Rech, G., Lazzarotto, G., Dias, R. D., Mussulini, B. H., Rico, E. P., & de Oliveira, D. L. (2020). Fetal alcohol spectrum disorders model alters the functionality of glutamatergic neurotransmission in adult zebrafish. *Neurotoxicology*, *78*, 152–160. https://doi.org/10.1016/j.neuro.2020.03.003

Baj, G., D'Alessandro, V., Musazzi, L., Mallei, A., Satori, C., Sciancalepore, M., Tardito, D., Langone, F., Popoli, M., & Tongiorgi, E. (2012). Physical exercise and antidepressants enhance BDNF targeting in hippocampal CA3 dendrites: Further evidence of a spatial code for BDNF splice variants. *Neuropsychopharmacology*, *37*(7), 1600–1611.

Ball, K., & Slane, M. (2014). Tolerance to the locomotor-activating effects of 3, 4-methylenedioxymethamphetamine (MDMA) predicts escalation of mdma self-administration and cue-induced reinstatement of MDMA seeking rats. *Behavioural Brain Research*, *274*, 143–148.

Banaszkiewicz, M., Tarwacka, P., Krzywonos-Zawadzka, A., Olejnik, A., Laprairie, P., Noszczyk-Nowak, A., Sawicki, G., & Bil-Lula, I. (2022). Δ9-Tetrahydrocannabinol (Δ9-THC) improves ischemia/reperfusion heart dysfunction and might serve as a cardioprotective agent in the future treatment. *Frontiers in Biosciences (Landmark Ed)*, *27*(4), 114.

Barnea-Goraly, N., Kwon, H., Menon, V., Eliez, S., Lotspeich, L., & Reiss, A. L. (2004). White matter structure in autism: Preliminary evidence from diffusion tensor imaging. *Biological Psychiatry*, *55*(3), 323–326.

Basavarajappa, B. S. (2007). The endocannabinoid signaling system: A potential target for the next-generation therapeutics for alcoholism. *Mini Reviews in Medicinal Chemistry*, 7(8), 769–779.

Battista, N., Fezza, F., Finazzi-Agro, A., & Maccarrone, M. (2006). The endocannabinoid system in neurodegeneration. *The Italian Journal of Biochemistry*, *55*(3–4), 283–289.

Bechara, A., & Damasio, H. (2002). Decision-making and addiction (part 1): Impaired activation of somatic states in substance dependent individuals when pondering decisions with negative consequences. *Neuropsychologia*, *40*(10), 1675–1689.

Bechara, A., Damasio, H., & Damasio, A. (2003). Role of the amygdala in decision-making. *Annals of the New York Academy of Sciences*, *985*, 356–369.

Belin, D., & Everitt, B. J. (2008). Cocaine seeking habits depend upon dopamine-dependent serial connectivity linking the ventral with the dorsal striatum. *Neuron*, *57*(3), 432–441.

Benedetti, F., Mayberg, H. S., Wager, T. D., Stohler, C. S., & Zubieta, J. K. (2005). Neurobiological mechanisms of the placebo effect. *Journal of Neuroscience*, *25*(45), 10390–10402.

Benjamin, J., Levine, J., Fux, M., Aviv, A., Levy, D., & Belmaker, R. H. (1995). Double-blind, placebo-controlled, crossover trial of inositol treatment for panic disorder. *American Journal of Psychiatry*, *152*, 1084–1086.

Bergh, C., Eklund, T., Sodersten, P., & Nordin, C. (1997). Altered dopamine function in pathological gambling. *Psychological Medicine*, *27*(2), 473–475.

Berk, M., Hallam, K., Lucas, N., Hasty, M., McNeil, C., Conus, P., Kader, L., & McGorry, P. (2007). Early intervention in bipolar disorders: Opportunities and pitfalls. *The Medical Journal of Australia*, *187*(7), S11–14.

Beveridge, T., Smith, H., Nader, M., & Porrino, L. (2009). Abstinence from chronic cocaine self-administration alter striatal dopamine systems in rhesus monkeys. *Neuropsychopharmacology*, *34*(5). https://doi.org/10.1038/npp.2008.135

Biederman, J. (2005). Mixed amphetamine salts extended release for the treatment of ADHD. *CNS Spectrums*, *10*(12), 5.

Biederman, J., Quinn, D., Weiss, M., Markabi, S., Weidenman, M., Edson, K., Karlsson, G., Pohlmann, H., & Wigal, S. (2003). Efficacy and safety of Ritalin, a new, once daily, extended-release dosage form of methylphenidate, in children with attention deficit hyperactivity disorder. *Pediatric Drugs*, *5*(12), 833–841.

Bilge, S., & Ekici, B. (2021). CBD-enriched cannabis for autism spectrum disorder: An experience of a single center in Turkey and reviews of the literature. *Journal of Cannabis Research, 3*(1), 53. https://doi.org/10.1186/s42238-021-00108-7

Bionomics. (2007, May 29). Bionomics validates drug candidate for anxiety. *Bionomics.*

Blom, J. M., Tascedda, F., Carra, S., Ferraguti, C., Barden, N., & Brunello, N. (2002). Altered regulation of CREB by chronic antidepressant administration in the brain of transgenic mice with impaired glucocorticoid receptor function. *Neuropsychopharmacology, 26*(5), 605–614.

Bloomfield, M. A., Ashok, A. H., Volkow, N. D., & Howes, O. D. (2016). The effects of Δ^9-tetrahydrocannabinol on the dopamine system. *Nature, 539*(7629), 369–377. https://doi.org/10.1038/nature20153

Bonese, K. F., Wainer, B. H., Fitch, E. W., Rothberg, R. M., & Schuster, C. R. (1974). Changes in heroin self-administration by a rhesus monkey after morphine immunisation. *Nature, 252*(5485), 708–710.

Booij, L., Soucy, J., Young, S., Regoli, M., Gravel, P., Diksic, M., Leyton, M., Pihl, R. O., & Bebkelfat, C. (2014). Brain serotonin synthesis in MDMA (ecstasy) polydrug users: An alpha [(11)C]methyl-l-tryptophan study. *Journal of Neurochemistry, 131*(5), 634–644.

Borghese, C., Hicks, J., Lapid, D., Trudell, J., & Harris, R. (2014). GABA(A) receptor transmembrane amino acids are critical for alcohol action: Disulfide cross-linking and alkyl methanethiosulfonate labeling relative location binding sites. *Journal of Neurochemistry, 128*(3), 363–375.

Borroto, E., Romero-Fernandez, W., Narvaez, M., Oflijan, J., Agnati, L., & Fuxe, K. (2014). Hallucinogenic 5-HT2AR agonists LSD and DOI enhance dopamine D2R promoter recognition and signaling of D2-HT2A heteroreceptor complexes. *Biochemical and Biophysical Research Communications, 433*(1), 278–284.

Bortoluzzi, A., Blaya, C., Salum, G., Cappi, C., Leistner-Segal, S., & Manfro, G. (2014). Anxiety disorders and anxiety-related traits and serotonin transporter gene-linked polymorphic region (5-HTTLRP) in adolescents: case-control and trio studies. *Psychiatric Genetics, 24*(4), 176–180.

Bossert, J. M., Poles, G. C., Wihbey, K. A., Koya, E., & Shaham, Y. (2007). Differential effects of blockade of dopamine D1-family receptors in nucleus accumbens core or shell on reinstatement of heroin seeking induced by contextual and discrete cues. *The Journal of Neuroscience, 27*(46), 12655–12663.

Boyer, E., & Shannon, M. (2005). The serotonin syndrome. *The New England Journal of Medicine, 352,* 1112–1120.

Bradberry, C. W. (2000). Acute and chronic dopamine dynamics in a nonhuman primate model of recreational cocaine use. *The Journal of Neuroscience, 20*(18), 7109–7115.

Braga, R. J., & Petrides, G. (2005). The combined use of electroconvulsive therapy and antipsychotics in patients with schizophrenia. *The Journal of ECT, 21*(2), 75–83.

Brederlau, A., Correia, A., Anisimov, S., Elmi, M., Paul, G., Roybon, L., Morizane, A., Berquist, F., Riebe, I., Nannmark, U., Carta, M., Hanse, E., Takahashi, J., Sasai, Y., Funa, K., Brundin, P., Eriksson, P., & Li, J. (2006). Transplantation of human embryonic stem cell-derived cells to a rat model of Parkinson's disease: Effect of in vitro differentiation on graft survival and testoma formation. *Stem Cells, 24*(6), 1433–1440.

Bremner, J. D. (1999). Does stress damage the brain? *Biological Psychiatry, 45*(7), 797–805.

Bridge, J. A., Iyengar, S., Salary, C. B., Barbe, R. P., Birmaher, B., Pincus, H. A., Ren, L., & Brent, D. A. (2007). Clinical response and risk for reported suicidal ideation and suicide attempts in pediatric antidepressant treatment: A meta-analysis of randomized controlled trials. *Journal of American Medical Association, 297*(15), 1683–1696.

Broderick, P. A. (1992). Cocaine's colocalized effects on synaptic serotonin and dopamine in ventral tegmentum in a reinforcement paradigm. *Pharmacology, Biochemistry, and Behavior, 42*(4), 889–898.

Brunello, N. (2004). Mood stabilizers: Protecting the mood . . . protecting the brain. *The Journal of Affective Disorders, 79*(1), S15–20.

Brunello, N., & Tascedda, F. (2003). Cellular mechanisms and second messengers: Relevance to the psychopharmacology of bipolar disorders. *The International Journal of Neuropsychopharmacology, 6*(2), 181–189.

Buchanan, R. W., Javitt, D. C., Marder, S. R., Schooler, N. R., Gold, J. M., McMahon, R. P., Heresco-Levy, U., & Carpenter, W. T. (2007). The cognitive and negative symptoms in schizophrenia trial (CONSIST): The efficacy of glutamatergic agents for negative symptoms and cognitive impairments. *The American Journal of Psychiatry, 164*(10), 1593–1602.

Buchsbaum, M., & Hazlett, E. (1998). Positron emission tomography studies of abnormal glucose metabolism in schizophrenia. *Schizophrenia Bulletin, 24*(3), 343–364.

Bueno, C. H., Zangrossi, H. Jr., & Viana Mde, B. (2007). GABA/benzodiazepine receptors in the ventrome-dial hypothalamic nucleus regulate both anxiety and panic-related defensive responses in the elevated T-maze. *Brain Research Bulletin, 74*(1–3), 134–141.

Buisson, B., & Bertrand, D. (2001). Chronic exposure to nicotine upregulates the human alpha 4beta 2 nicotinic acetylcholine receptor function. *The Journal of Neuroscience, 21*(6), 1819–1829.

Burns, E. K., & Levinson, A. H. (2008). Discontinuation of nicotine replacement therapy among smoking-cessation attempters. *American Journal of Preventive Medicine, 34*(3), 212–215.

Burns, H., Van Laere, K., Sanabria, S., Hamill, T., Bormans, G., Eng, W., Gibson, R., Ryan, C., Connolly, B., Patel, S., Krause, S., Vanko, A., Van Hecken, A., Dupont, P., De Lepeleire, I., Rothenberg, P., Stoch, S. A., Cote, J., Hagmann, W. K., . . . Hargreaves, R. (2007). [18F]MK-9407, a positron emission tomography (PET) tracer for in vivo human PET brain imaging of the cannabinoid-1 receptor. *Proceeding of the Nation Academy of Sciences, 104*(23), 9800–9805.

Butterweck, V. (2003). Mechanism of action of St John's wort in depression: What is known? *CNS Drugs, 17*(8), 539–562.

Byrnes-Blake, K. A., Carroll, F. I., Abraham, P., & Owens, S. M. (2001). Generation of anti-(+)methamphetamine antibodies is not impeded by (+)methamphetamine administration during active immunization of rats. *International Immunopharmacology, 1*(2), 329–338.

Cade, J. (1949). Lithium salts in the treatment of psychotic excitement. *Medical Journal of Australia, 36*, 349.

Calabrese, J., Durgam, S., Satlin, A., Vanover, K., Davis, R., & Sachs, G. (2021). Efficacy and safety of lumateperone for major depressive episodes associated with bipolar I or bipolar II disorder: A phase 3 randomized placebo-controlled trial. *The American Journal of Psychiatry, 178*(12), 1098–1106. https://doi.org/10.1176/appi.ajp.2021.20091339.

Canli, T., Qiu, M., Omura, K., Congdon, E., Haas, B. W., Amin, Z., Hermann, M. J., Constable, R. T., & Lesch, K. P. (2006). Neural correlates of epigenesis. *Proceedings of the National Academy of Sciences of the United States of America, 103*(43), 16033–16038.

Carhart-Harris, R. L., Bolstridge, M., Day, C., Rucker, J., Watts, R., & Curran, H. V. (2018). Psicilocybin with psychological support for treatment resistant depression: Six-month follow up. *Psychopharmacology, 235*(2), 399–408.

Carlson, N. R. (2007). Physiology of behavior (9th ed.). Allyn and Bacon.

Carlson, N. R. (2010). *Physiology of behavior* (10th ed.). Pearson.

Carlsson, A., & Lindqvist, M. (1963). Effect of chlorpromazine or haloperidol on formation of 3methoxytyramine and normetanephrine in mouse brain. *Acta Pharmacologica et Toxicologica, 20*, 140–144.

Carter, L. P., Koek, W., & France, C. P. (2009). Behavioral analysis of GBH: Receptor mechanisms. *Pharmacological Therapy, 121*(1), 100–114.

Casarotto, P., Girych, M., Fred, S., Kovaleva, V., Saama, M., Vattulainen, I., & Castren, E. (2021). Antidepressant drugs act by directly binding to TRKB neurotrophin receptors. *Cell, 184*(5), 1299–1313.

Caspi, A., Sugden, K., Moffitt, T. E., Taylor, A., Craig, I. W., Harrington, H., McClay, J., Mill, J., Martin, J., Braithwaite, A., & Poulton, R. (2003). Influence of life stress on depression: Moderation by a polymorphism in the 5-HTT gene. *Science, 301*(5631), 386–389.

Cassidy, F., Zhao, C., Badger, J., Claffey, E., Dobrin, S., Roche, S., & McKeon, P. (2007). Genome-wide scan of bipolar disorder and investigation of population stratification effects on linkage: Support for susceptibility loci at 4q21, 7q36, 9p21, 12q24, 14q24, and 16p13. *American Journal of Medical Genetics. Part B, Neuropsychiatric Genetics, 144*(6), 791–801.

Castren, E., & Monteggia, L. M. (2021). Brain-derived neurotropic factor signaling in depression and anti-depressant action. *Biological Psychiatry, 90*(2), 128–136.

Castren, E., Voikar, V., & Rantamaki, T. (2007). Role of neurotrophic factors in depression. *Current Opinion in Pharmacology, 7*(1), 18–21.

CDC. (2005). Mental health in the United States: Prevalence of diagnosis and medication treatment for attention-deficit/hyperactivity disorder—United States. *Morbidity and Mortality Monthly Report, 54*(34), 842–847.

CDC. (2022). *Underlying cause of deaths occurring through 2020.* https://wonder.cdc.gov/controller/saved/D76/D266F033

Celada, P., Bortolozzi, A., & Artigas, F. (2013). Serotonin 5-HT1A receptors as targets for agents to treat psychiatric disorders: Rationale and current status of research. *CNS Drugs, 27*(9), 703–716.

Chen, B., Linke, A., Olson, L., Kohli, J., Kinnear, M., & Fishman, I. (2022). Cortical myelination in toddlers and preschoolers with autism spectrum disorder. *Developmental Neurobiology, 82*(3), 261–274.

Chen, C. Y., O'Brian, M. S., & Anthony, J. C. (2005). Who becomes cannabis dependent soon after onset of use? Epidemiological evidence from the United States: 2000–2001. *Drug and Alcohol Dependence, 79*, 11–22.

Chen, F., Ke, J., Qi, R., Xu, O., Zhong, Y., Liu, T., & Lu, G. (2018). Increased inhibition of the amygdala by the mPFC may reflect a resilience factor in post-traumatic stress disorder: A resting-state fMRI granger causality analysis. *Frontiers in Neuroscience, 9*, 516. https://doi.org/10.3389/fpsyt.2018.00516

Chen, J., Tian, C., Zhang, O., Xiang, H., Wang, R., Hu, X., & Zeng, X. (2022). Changes in volume of subregions within basal ganglia in obsessice-compulsive disorder: A study with atlas-based and VBM methods. *Frontiers in Neuroscience, 16*, 890616. https://doi.org/10.3389/fnins.2022.890616.

Chen, P. S., Peng, G. S., Yang, S., Wu, X., Wang, C. C., Wilson, B., Lu, R. B., Gean, P. W., Chuang, D. M., & Hong, J. S. (2006). Valproate protects dopaminergic neurons in midbrain neuron/glia cultures by stimulating the release of neurotrophic factors from astrocytes. *Molecular Psychiatry, 11*(12), 1116–1125.

Chen, Y., Song, R., Yang, R., Wu, N., & Li, J. (2014). A novel D3 receptor antagonist YQA14 inhibits methamphetamine self-administration and relapse to drug-seeking behavior in rats. *European Journal of Pharmacology, 743*, 126–132.

Cheng, J. K., & Chiou, L. C. (2006). Mechanisms of the antinociceptive action of gabapentin. *Journal of Pharmacological Sciences, 100*(5), 471–486.

Cheng, J. Y., Chen, R. Y., Ko, J. S., & Ng, E. M. (2007). Efficacy and safety of atomoxetine for attention-deficit/hyperactivity disorder in children and adolescents-meta-analysis and meta-regression analysis. *Psychopharmacology, 194*(2), 197–209.

Cheng, V. Y., Bonin, R. P., Chiu, M. W., Newell, J. G., MacDonald, J. F., & Orser, B. A. (2006). Gabapentin increases a tonic inhibitory conductance in hippocampal pyramidal neurons. *Anesthesiology, 105*(2), 325–333.

Chenu, F., & Bourin, M. (2006). Potentiation of antidepressant-like activity with lithium: Mechanism involved. *Current Drug Targets, 7*(2), 159–163.

Chessick, C. A., Allen, M. H., Thase, M., Batista Miralha da Cunha, A. B., Kapczinski, F. F., de Lima, M. S., & dos Santos Souza, J. J. (2006). Azapirones for generalized anxiety disorder. *Cochran Database of Systematic Reviews* (Online), *3*, CD006115.

Choi, S. (2003). Nefazodone (Serzone) withdrawn because of hepatotoxicity. *Canadian Medical Association Journal, 169*(11), 1187.

Chuang, D. M. (2005). The antiapoptotic actions of mood stabilizers: Molecular mechanisms and therapeutic potentials. *Annals of the New York Academy of Sciences, 1053*, 195–204.

Chun, Y., Chi, M., Chu, C., Chiu, N., Yao, W., Chen, P., & Yang, Y. (2019). Availability of striatal dopamine transporter in healthy individuals with and without a family history of ADHD. *Journal of Attention Disorders, 23*(7), 665–670. https://doi.org/10.1177/1087054716654570

Citrome, L., Ketter, T., Cucchiaro, J., & Loebel, A. (2014). Clinical assessment of lurasidone benefit and risk in the treatment of bipolar I depression using number needed to treat, number needed to harm, and likelihood to be helped or harmed. *Journal of Affective Disorders, 155*, 20–27.

Clayton, A. H., Croft, H., & Handiwala, L. (2014). Antidepressants and sexual dysfunction: Mechanisms and clinical implications. *Postgraduate Medicine, 126*(2), 91–99.

Clayton, A. H., & Montejo, A. L. (2006). Major depressive disorder, antidepressants, and sexual dysfunction. *The Journal of Clinical Psychiatry, 67*(Suppl 6), 33–37.

Clayton, A. H., Warnock, J. K., Kornstein, S. G., Pinkerton, R., Sheldon-Keller, A., & McGarvey, E. L. (2004). A placebo-controlled trial of bupropion SR as an antidote for selective serotonin reuptake inhibitor-induced sexual dysfunction. *Journal of Clinical Psychiatry, 65*(1), 62–67.

Colizzi, M., McGuire, P., Pertwee, R. G., & Bhattacharyya, S. (2016). Effect of cannabis on glutamate signalling in the brain: A systematic review of human and animal evidence. *Neuroscience and Biobehavioral Reviews, 64*, 359–381. https://doi.org/10.1016/j.neubiorev.2016.03.010

Collins, A. C., Romm, E., & Wehner, J. M. (1990). Dissociation of the apparent relationship between nicotine tolerance and up-regulation of nicotinic receptors. *Brain Research Bulletin, 25*, 373–379.

Comer, S. D., Collins, E. D., MacArthur, R. B., & Fischman, M. W. (1999). Comparison of intravenous and intranasal heroin self-administration by morphine-maintained humans. *Psychopharmacology, 143*, 327–338.

Comings, D. E., Rosenthal, R. J., Lesieur, H. R., Rugle, L. J., Muhleman, D., Chiu, C., Dietz, G., & Gade, R. (1996). A study of the dopamine D2 receptor gene in pathological gambling. *Pharmacogenetics, 6*(3), 223–234.

Compton, W. M., Han, B., Jones, C. M., & Blanco, C. (2019). Cannabis use disorders among adults in the United States during a time of increasing use of cannabis. *Drug Alcohol Dependence.* https://doi.org/10.1016/j.drugalcdep.2019.05.008

Connolly, C. G., Foxe, J. J., Nierenberg, J., Shpaner, M., & Garavan, H. (2012). The neurobiology of cognitive control in successful cocaine abstinence. *Drug Alcohol Dependence, 121*(1–2), 45–53.

Cooper, J. B., Jane, J. A., Alves, W., & Cooper, E. (1999). Right median nerve electrical stimulation to hasten awakening from coma. *Brain Injury, 13*(4), 261–267.

Cooper, J. C., & Knutson, B. (2008). Valence and salience contribute to nucleus accumbens activation. *NeuroImage, 39*(1), 538–547.

Cornelius, J. F., Clark, D. B., Bukstein, O. G., Birmaher, B., Salloum, I. M., & Brown, S. A. (2005). Acute phase and five-year follow-up study of fluoxetine in adolescents with major depression and a comorbid substance use disorder: A review. *Addictive Behaviors, 30*(9), 1824–1833.

Cornelius, J. R., Chung, T., Martin, C., Wood, D., & Clark, D. (2008). Cannabis withdrawal is common among treatment-seeking adolescents with cannabis dependence and major depression, and is associated with rapid relapse dependence. *Addictive Behaviors, 33*(11), 1500–1505.

Cottler, L. B. (2007). Drug use disorders in the National Comorbidity Survey: Have we come a long way? *Archives of General Psychiatry, 64*(3), 1–2.

Cowen, M. S., Adams, C., Kraehenbuehl, T., Vengeliene, V., & Lawrence, A. J. (2005). The acute anti-craving effect of acamprosate in alcohol-preferring rats is associated with modulation of the mesolimbic dopamine system. *Addiction Biology, 10*(3), 233–242.

Cox, G. R., Desbrow, B., Montgomery, P. G., Anderson, M. E., Bruce, C. R., Macrides, T. A., Martin, D. T., Moquin, A., Roberts, A., Hawley, J. A., & Burke, L. M. (2002). Effect of different protocols of caffeine intake on metabolism and endurance performance. *Journal of Applied Physiology, 93*, 990–999.

Coyle, J. T. (2006). Glutamate and schizophrenia: Beyond the dopamine hypothesis. *Cellular and Molecular Neurobiology, 26*(4–6), 365–384.

Cromberg, H., Badiani, A., Chan, J., Dell'Orco, J., Dineen, P., & Robinson, T. (2001). The ability of environmental context to facilitate psychomotor sensitization to amphetamine can be dissociated from its effect on acute drug responsiveness and on conditioned responding. *Neuropsychopharmacology, 24*, 680–690.

Cruz, F. C., Javier, R. F., Hope, B. T. (2014, November 11). Using c-Fos to study neural ensembles in corticostriatal circuitry of addiction. *Brain Research, 1628*, 157–173.

Cunningham, M. O., Woodhall, G. L., Thompson, S. E., Cooley, D. J., & Jones, R. S. (2004). Dual effects of gabapentin and pregabalin on glutamate release at rat entorhinal synapses in vitro. *The European Journal of the Neuroscience, 20*(6), 1566–1576.

Cuzon, V. C., Yeh, P. W., Yanagawa, Y., Obata, K., & Yeh, H. H. (2008). Ethanol consumption during early pregnancy alters the disposition of tangentially migrating GABAergic interneurons in the fetal cortex. *The Journal of Neuroscience, 28*(8), 1854–1864.

Czapinski, P., Blaszczyk, B., & Czuczwar, S. J. (2005). Mechanisms of action of antiepileptic drugs. *Current Topics in Medicinal Chemistry, 5*(1), 3–14.

Daghistani, N., & Rey, J. (2016). The first four times a year, long-acting injectable antipsychotic agent. *Pharmacy and Therapeutics, 41*(4), 222–227.

Daly, J. W., & Fredholm, B. B. (1998). Caffeine–an atypical drug of dependence. *Drug and Alcohol Dependence, 51*, 199–206.

Damasio, A. (1995). On some functions of the human prefrontal cortex. *Annals of the New York Academy of Sciences, 769*, 241–251.

Damasio, A., Grabowski, A., Damasio, H., Ponto, L., Parvizi, D., & Hichwa, R. (2000). Subcortical and cortical brain activity during the feeling of self-generated emotions. *Nature Neuroscience, 3*(10), 1049–1056.

Daniela, E., Gittings, D., & Schenk, S. (2006). Conditioning following repeated exposures to MDMA in rats: Role in the maintenance of MDMA self-administration. *Behavioral neuroscience, 120*(5), 1144–1150.

Dannlowski, U., Stuhmann, A., Beutelmann, V., Zwanzger, P., Lenzen, T., Grotegerd, D., Domschke, K., Hohoff, C., Ohrmann, P., Bauer, J., Lindner, C., Postert, C., Konrad, C., Arolt, V., Heindel, W., Suslow, T., & Kugel, H. (2012). Limbic scars: Long-term consequences of childhood maltreatment revealed by functional and structural magnetic resonance imaging. *Biological Psychiatry, 71*(4), 286–293.

Dariš, B., Verboten, M., Knez, Ž., & Ferk, P. (2019). Cannabinoids in cancer treatment: Therapeutic potential and legislation. *Bosnian Journal of Basic Medical Sciences, 19*(1), 14–23. https://doi.org/10.17305/bjbms.2018.3532

da Silva Lobo, D. S., Vallada, H. P., Knight, J., Martins, S. S., Tavares, H., Gentil, V., & Kennedy, J. L. (2007). Dopamine genes and pathological gambling in discordant sib-pairs. *Journal of Gambling Studies, 23*(4), 421–433.

Davidson, J. (2002). St. John's wort and depression—Reply. *Journal of the American Medical Association, 288*(4), 446–449.

Davidson, J. R. (2002). Hypericum trial study group: Effect of hypericum performatum (St. John's wort) in major depressive disorder. *Journal of the American Medical Association, 287*(14), 1807–1814.

De Gregorio, D., Posa, L., Ochoa-Sanchez, R., McLaughlin, R., Maione, S., Comai, S., & Gobbi, G. (2016). The hallucinogen d-lysergic diethylamide (LSD) decreases dopamine firing activity through 5-HT$_{1A}$, D$_2$ and TAAR$_1$ receptors. *Pharmacological Research, 133*, 81–91. https://doi.org/10.1016/j.phrs.2016.08.022

de la Mora, M., Gallegos-Cari, A., Arzmendi-Garcia, Y., Marcellino, D., & Fuex, K. (2010). Role of dopamine receptor mechanisms in the amygdaloid modulation of fear and anxiety: Structural and functional analysis. *Progress in Neurobiology, 90*(2), 198–216.

DeSanty, K. P., & Dar, M. S. (2001). Cannabinoid-induced motor incoordination through the cerebellar CB(1) receptor in mice. *Pharmacology Biochemistry and Behavior, 69*(1–2), 251–259.

De Ternay, J., Naassila, M., Nourredine, M., Louvet, A., Bailly, F., Sescousse, G., Maurage. P., Cottencin, O., Carrieri, P. M., & Rolland, B. (2019). Therapeutic prospects of cannabidiol for alcohol use disorder and alcohol-related damages on the liver and the brain. *Frontiers in Pharmacology, 10*, 627. https://doi.org/10.3389/fphar.2019.00627

Devama, S., & Duman, R. (2019). Neurotrophic mechanisms underlying rapid and sustained antidepressant actions of ketamine. *Pharmacology Biochemistry and Behavior, 188*, 172837. https://doi.org/10.1016/j.pbb.2019.172837

Devane, W. A., Dysarz, F. A., Johnson, M. R., Melvin, L. S., & Howlett, A. C. (1988). Determination and characterization of a cannabinoid receptor in rat brain. *Molecular Pharmacology, 34*(5), 605–613.

Devane, W. A., Hanus, L., Breuer, A., Pertwee, R. G., Stevenson, L. A., Griffin, G., Gibson, D., Mandelbaum, A., Etinger, A., & Mechoulam, R. (1992). Isolation and structure of a brain constituent that binds to the cannabinoid receptor. *Science, 258*(5090), 1946–1949.

de Villiers, S. H., Lindblom, N., Kalayanov, G., Gordon, S., Malmerfelt, A., Johansson, A. M., & Svensson, T. H. (2002). Active immunization against nicotine suppresses nicotine-induced dopamine release in the rat nucleus accumbens shell. *Respiration: International Review of Thoracic Diseases, 698*(3), 247–253.

Dickstein, S. G., Bannon, K., Castellanos, F. X., & Milham, M. P. (2006). The neural correlates of attention deficit hyperactivity disorder: An ALE meta-analysis. *Journal of Child Psychology and Psychiatry, and Allied Disciplines, 47*(10), 1051–1062.

DiFranza, J. R. (2008). Hooked from the first cigarette. *Scientific American, 298*(5), 82–87.

DiMarzo, V. (2008). BB(1) receptor antagonism: Biological basis for metabolic effects. *Drug Discovery Today, 13*(23), 1026–1041.

Doggrell, S. A. (2005). Fluoxetine–do the benefits outweigh the risks in adolescent major depression? *Expert Opinion on Pharmacotherapy, 6*(1), 147–150.

Doyon, W. M., Ramachandra, V., Samson, H. H., Czachowski, C. L., & Gonzales, R. A. (2004). Accumbal dopamine concentration during operant self-administration of a sucrose or a novel sucrose with ethanol solution. *Alcohol, 34*(2–3), 261–271.

D'Sa, C., & Duman, R. S. (2002). Antidepressants and neuroplasticity. *Bipolar Disorders, 4*(3), 183–194.

Dudley, M., Goldney, R., & Hadzi-Pavlovic, D. (2010). Are adolescents dying by suicide taking SSRI antidepressants? A review of observational studies. *Database of Abstracts of Reviews of Effects, 18*(3), 242–245. www.ncbi.nlm.nih.gov/books/NBK80415/

Duman, R. S., & Monteggia, L. M. (2006). A neurotrophic model for stress-related mood disorders. *Biological Psychiatry, 59*(12), 1116–1127.

Eagle, D., Noschang, C., Noble, C., Day, J., Dongelmans, M., d'Angelo, L.-S. C., Theobald, D. E., Mar, A. C., Urcelay, G. P., Morein-Zamir, S., & Robins, T. (2014). The dopamine D2/D3 receptor agonist quinpirole increases checking-like behavior in operant observing response task with uncertain reinforcement: A novel; possible model of OCD. *Behavioural Brain Research, 264*, 207–229.

Eckstein-Ludwig, U., Fei, J., & Schwarz, W. (1999). Inhibition of uptake, steady-state currents, and transient charge movements generated by the neuronal GABA transporter by various anticonvulsant drugs. *British Journal of Pharmacology, 128*(1), 92–102.

Einat, H., Yuan, P., Gould, T. D., Li, J., Du, J., Zhang, L., Manji, H. K., & Chen, G. (2003). The role of the extracellular signal-regulated kinase signaling pathway in mood modulation. *The Journal of Neuroscience, 23*(19), 7311–7316.

Eisenberg, M. J., Filion, K. B., Yavin, D., Belisle, P., Mottillo, S., Joseph, L., Gervais, A., O'Loughlin, J., Paradis, G., Rinfret, S., & Pilote, L. (2008). Pharmacotherapies for smoking cessation: A meta-analysis of randomized controlled trials. *Canadian Medical Association Journal, 179*(2), 135–144.

Elflein, J. (2022). *Adolescent drug use in the US: Statistics and facts.* www.statista.com/topics/3907/adolescent-drug-use-in-the-us/#dossierKeyfigures

El-Zein, R., Abdel-Rahman, S., Hay, M., Lopez, M., Bondy, M., Morris, D., & Legator, M. (2005). Cytogenetic effects in children treated with methylphenidate. *Cancer Letters, 230*(2), 284–291.

Engblom, D., Bilbao, A., Sanchis-Segura, C., Dahan, L., Perreau-Lenz, S., Balland, B., Parkitna, J. R., Lujan, R., Halbout, B., Mameli, M., Parlato, R., Sprengel, R., Luscher, C., Schutz, G., & Spanagel, R. (2008). Glutamate receptors on dopamine neurons control the persistence of cocaine seeking. *Neuron, 59*(3), 497–508.

Ettinger, R. H., Ettinger, W. F., & Harless, W. E. (1997). Active immunization with cocaine-protein conjugate attenuates cocaine effects. *Pharmacology, Biochemistry, and Behavior, 58*(1), 215–220.

Fadda, P., Scherma, M., Spano, M. S., Salis, P., Melis, V., Fattore, L., & Fratta, W. (2006). Cannabinoid self-administration increases dopamine release in the nucleus accumbens. *Neuroreport, 17*(15), 1629–1632.

Fagioli, A., Comandini, A., Dell'Osso, M., & Kasper, S. (2012). Rediscovering trazadone for the treatment of major depressive disorder. *CNS Drugs, 26*(12), 1033–1049.

Faraone, S. V., & Upadhyaya, H. P. (2007). The effect of stimulant treatment for ADHD on later substance abuse and the potential for medication misuse, abuse, and diversion. *The Journal of Clinical Psychiatry, 68*(11), e28.

Farsalinos, K. E., Spyrou, A., Tsimopoulou, K., Stefopoulos, C., Romanga, G., & Voudris, V. (2014). Nicotine absorption from electronic cigarette use: Comparison between first and new-generation devices. *Nature, 4*, 4133. https://doi.org/10.1038/srep04133.

Fava, M., Alpert, J., Nierenberg, A. A., Mischoulon, D., Otto, M. W., Zajecka, J., Murck, H., & Rosenbaum, J. F. (2005). A double-blind, randomized trial of St. John's wort, fluoxetine, and placebo in major depressive disorder. *Journal of Clinical Psychopharmacology, 24*(5), 441–447.

FDA. (2007). FDA proposes new warnings about suicidal thinking, behavior in young adults who take antidepressant medications. *FDA News* (PO7–77).

Fears, S., Kremeyer, B., Araya, C., Bejarano, J., Service, S. K., Araya, X., Ramirez, M., Castrillón, G., Gomez-Franco, J., Lopez, M. C., Montoya, G., Montoya, P., Aldana, I., Teshiba, T. M., Abaryan, Z., Al-Sharif, N. B., Ericson, M., Jalbrzikowski, M., Luykx, J. J., . . . Abaryan, Z. (2014). Multisystem component phenotypes of bipolar disorder for genetic investigations of extended pedigrees. *JAMA, 71*(4), 375–387.

Federici, M., Sebastianelli, L., Natoli, S., Bernardi, G., & Mercuri, N. B. (2007). Electrophysiologic changes in ventral midbrain dopaminergic neurons resulting from $(+/-)$-3,4-methylenedioxymethamphetamine (MDMA-"Ecstasy"). *Biological Psychiatry, 62*(6), 680–686.

Fehr, C., Yakushev, I., Hohmann, N., Buchholz, H. G., Landvogt, C., Deckers, H., Eberhardt, A., Klager, M., Smolka, M. N., Scheurich, A., Dielentheis, T., Schmidt, L. G., Rosch, F., Bartenstein, P., Grunder, G., & Schreckenberger, M. (2008). Association of low striatal dopamine d2 receptor availability with nicotine dependence similar to that seen with other drugs of abuse. *The American Journal of Psychiatry, 165*(4), 507–514.

Fehsel, K., Loeffler, S., Krieger, K., Henning, U., Agelink, M., Kolb-Bachofen, V., & Klimke, A. (2005). Clozapine induces oxidative stress and proapoptotic gene expression in neutrophils of schizophrenic patients. *Journal of Clinical Psychopharmacology, 25*(5), 419–426.

Fernandez-Guasti, A., Ulloa, R. E., & Nicolini, H. (2003). Age differences in the sensitivity to clomipramine in an animal model of obsessive-compulsive disorder. *Psychopharmacology, 166*(3), 195–201.

Ferrario, C. R., Shou, M., Samaha, A. N., Watson, C. J., Kennedy, R. T., & Robinson, T. E. (2008). The rate of intravenous cocaine administration alters c-fos mRNA expression and the temporal dynamics of dopamine, but not glutamate, overflow in the striatum. *Brain Research, 1209*, 151–156.

Fleisher, C., & McGough, J. (2014). Sofinicline: A novel nicotinic acetylcholine receptor agonist in the treatment of attention-deficit/hyperactivity disorder. *Expert Opinion on Investigational Drugs*, *23*(8), 1157–1163. https://doi.org/10.1517/13543784.2014.934806

Fleury-Teixeira, P., Caixeta, F. V., Ramires da Silva, L. C., Brasil-Neto, J. P., & Malcher-Lopes, R. (2019). Effects of CBD-enriched *cannabis sativa* extract on autism spectrum disorder symptoms: An observational study of 18 participants undergoing compassionate use. *Frontiers in Neurology*, *10*, 1145. https://doi.org/10.3389/fneur.2019.01145

Foley, K. F., DeSanty, K. P., & Kast, R. E. (2006). Bupropion: Pharmacology and therapeutic applications. *Expert Review of Neurotherapeutics*, *6*(9), 1249–1265.

Ford, C. P., Mark, G. P., & Williams, J. T. (2006). Properties and opioid inhibition of mesolimbic dopamine neurons vary according to target location. *The Journal of Neuroscience*, *26*(10), 2788–2797.

Fox, B. S. (1997). Development of a therapeutic vaccine for the treatment of cocaine addiction. *Drug and Alcohol Dependence*, *48*(3), 153–158.

Fredholm, B. B., Bättig, K., Holmén, J., Nehlig, A., & Zvartau, E. E. (1999). Molecular and cellular action of caffeine in the brain with special reference to factors that contribute to its widespread use. *Pharmacological Reviews*, *51*(1), 83–133.

Frey, B. N., Andreazza, A. C., Cereser, K. M., Martins, M. R., Valvassori, S. S., Reus, G. Z., Quevedo, J., & Kapczinski, F. (2006). Effects of mood stabilizers on hippocampus BCNF levels in an animal model of mania. *Life Sciences*, *79*(3), 281–286.

Fu, D., Wu, D. D., Guo, H. L., Hu, Y. H., Xia, Y., Ji, X., & Liu, Q. Q. (2022). The mechanism, clinical efficacy, safety, and dosage regimen of atomoxetine for ADHD therapy in children: A narrative review. *Frontiers in Psychiatry*, *12*, 780921. https://doi.org/10.3389/fpsyt.2021.780921

Fusar-Poli, L., Cavone, V., Tinacci, S., Concas, I., Petralia, A., Signorelli, M. S., Díaz-Caneja, C. M., & Aguglia, E. (2020). Cannabinoids for people with ASD: A systematic review of published and ongoing studies. *Brain Science*, *10*(9), 572. https://doi.org/10.3390/brainsci10090572

Gaoni, Y. E., & Mechoulam, R. (1964). Isolation, structure and partial synthesis of an active constituent of hashish. *Journal of American Chemical Society*, *86*(8), 1646–1647.

Gaudiano, B. A., & Herbert, J. D. (2003). Antidepressant-placebo debate in the media: Balanced coverage or placebo hype? *Commission for Scientific Medicine and Mental Health*, *2*(1).

Gelenberg, A. J., Shelton, R. C., Crits-Christoph, P., Keller, M. B., Dunner, D. L., Hirschfeld, R. M., Thase, M. E., Russell, J. M., Lydiard, R. B., Gallop, R. J., Todd, L., Hellerstein, D. J., Goodnick, P. J., Keitner, G. I., Stahl, S. M., Halbreich, U., & Hopkins, H. S. (2004). The effectiveness of St. John's wort in major depressive disorder: A naturalistic phase 2 follow-up in which nonresponders were provided alternate medication. *Journal of Clinical Psychiatry*, *65*(8), 1114–1119.

Gerdeman, G., & Lovinger, D. M. (2001). CB1 cannabinoid receptor inhibits synaptic release of glutamate in rat dorsolateral striatum. *Journal of Neurophysiology*, *85*(1), 468–471.

Geuze, E., vanBerckel, B., Lammertsma, A., Boellaard, R., de Kloet, C., Vermetten, E., & Westenberg, H. (2008). Reduced GABAa benzodiazepine receptor binding in veterans with post-traumatic stress disorder. *Molecular Psychiatry*, *13*, 74–83.

Gibbons, R. D., Brown, C. H., Hur, K., Marcus, S. M., Bhaumik, D. K., Erkens, J. A., Herings, R. M., & Mann, J. J. (2007). Early evidence on the effects of regulators' suicidality warnings on SSRI prescriptions and suicide in children and adolescents. *The American Journal of Psychiatry*, *164*(9), 1356–1363.

Ginovart, N., Tournier, B., Moulin-Sallanon, M., Steimer, T., Ibanez, V., & Millet, P. (2012). Chronic delta 9 tetrahydrocannabinol exposure induces a sensitization of dopamine D2/3 receptors in the mesolimbic and nigrostriatal systems. *Neuropsychopharmacology*, *37*(11), 2355–2367.

Gobbi, G., & Janiri, L. (2006). Sodium- and magnesium-valproate in vivo modulate glutamatergic and GABAergic synapses in the medial prefrontal cortex. *Psychopharmacology*, *185*(2), 255–262.

Goldberg, S. B., Pace, B. T., Nicholas, C. R., Raison, C. L., & Hutson, P. R. (2020). The experimental effects pf psilocybin on symptoms of anxiety and depression: A meta-analysis. *Psychiatry Research*, *284*, 112749. https://doi.org/10.1016/j.psychres.2020.112749

Goldstein, A. L., & Betz, G. W. (1986). The blood-brain barrier. *Cold Spring Harb Perspect Biology*, *255*(3), 74–83.

Gonzales, R. A., Job, M. O., & Doyon, W. M. (2004). The role mesolimbic dopamine in the development and maintenance of ethanol reinforcement. *Pharmacology and Therapeutics*, *103*(2), 121–146.

Gonzalez-Castro, T., Nicolini, H., Lanzagorta, N., Lopez-Narvaez, L., Genis, A., Pool Garcia, S., & Tovilla-Zarate, C. (2014). The role of brain-derived neurotropic factor (BDNF) val66met genetics polymorphism in bipolar disorder: A case-controlled study, comorbidities, and meta-analysis of 16,786 subjects. *Bipolar Disorders, 17*(1), 27–38. ISSN: 1399–5618.

González-Maeso, J., Weisstaub, N. V., Zhou, M., Chan, P., Ivic, L., Ang, R., Lira, A., Bradley-Moore, M., Ge, Y., Zhou, Q., & Sealfon, S. C. (2007). Hallucinogens recruit specific cortical 5-ht2a receptor-mediated signaling pathways to affect behavior. *Neuron, 53*, 439–452.

Goodman, A. (2008). Neurobiology of addicton. An integrative review. *Biochemical Pharmacology, 75*(1), 266–322.

Goodman, W. K., Price, L. H., Rasmussen, S. A., Mazure, C., Delgado, P., Heninger, G. R., & Charney, D. S. (1989). The Yale-Brown obsessive compulsive scale. *Archives of General Psychiatry, 48*(10), 1012–1018.

Gottschalk, M., & Domschke, K. (2017). Genetics of generalized anxiety disorder and related traits. *Dialogs in Clinical Neuroscience, 19*(2), 159–168.

Graeff, N. G., Netto, C. F., & Zangrossi, H. Jr. (1998). The elevated T-maze as an experimental model of anxiety. *Neuroscience and Biobehavioral Reviews, 23*(2), 237–246.

Gresch, P. J., Strickland, L. V., & Sanders-Bush, E. (2002). Lysergic acid diethylamide-induced Fos expression in rat brain: Role of serotonin-2A receptors. *Neuroscience, 114*(3), 707–713.

Griffiths, R. R., Johnson, M. W., Carducci, M. A., Umbricht, A., Richards, W. A., & Klinedinst, M. A. (2016). Psilocybin produces substantial and sustained decreases in depression and anxiety in patients with life-threatening cancer: A randomized double-blind trial. *Journal of Psychopharmacology, 30*(1), 1181–1197.

Griffiths, R. R., Lamb, R. J., Sannerud, C. A., Ator, N. A., & Brady, J. V. (1991). Self-injection of barbiturates, benzodiazepines and other sedative-anxiolytics in baboons. *Psychopharmacology, 103*(2), 154–161.

Griggs, E. A., & Ward, M. (1977, April). LSD toxicity: A suspected cause of death. *Journal of the Kentucky Medical Association, 75*(4), 172–173.

Grønli, J., Bramham, C., Murison, R., Kanhema, T., Fiske, E., Bjorvatn, B., Ursin, R., & Portas, C. M. (2006). Chronic mild stress inhibits BDNF protein expression and CREB activation in the dentate gyrus but not in the hippocampus proper. *Pharmacology Biochemistry and Behavior, 85*(4), 842–849.

Grover, S., Sahoo, S., Rabha, A., & Koirala, R. (2019). ECT in schizophrenia: A review of the evidence. *Acta Neuropsychiatry, 31*(3), 115–127.

Guerrero-Bautista, R., Franco-García, A., Hidalgo, J. M., Fernández-Gómez, F., Milanés, M. V., & Núñez, C. (2020). Blockade of D3 receptor prevents changes in DAT and D3R expression in the mesolimbic dopaminergic circuit produced by social stress- and cocaine prime-induced reinstatement of cocaine-CPP induced by drug priming and social stress. *International Journal of Molecular Sciences, 22*(6). https://doi.org/10.3390/ijms22063100.

Gunkelman, J. (2014). Medication prediction with electroencephalography phenotypes and biomarkers. *Biofeedback, 42*(2), 68–73.

Guzzetta, F., Tondo, L., Centorrino, F., & Baldessarini, R. J. (2007). Lithium treatment reduces suicide risk in recurrent major depressive disorder. *The Journal of Clinical Psychiatry, 68*(3), 380–383.

Hachimine, P., Seepersad, N., Ananthan, S., & Ranaldi, R. (2014). The novel dopamine D3 receptor antagonist, SR 21502, reduces cocaine conditioned place preference in rats. *Neuroscience Letters, 569*, 137–141.

Halpern, J. H., & Pope, H. G., Jr. (2002). Hallucinogen persisting perception disorder: What do we know after 50 years? *Drug and Alcohol Dependence, 69*(2003), 109–119.

Hamet, P., & Tremblay, J. (2005). Genetics and genomics of depression. *Metabolism: Clinical and Experimental/, 54*(5, Suppl. 1), 10–15.

Hamilton, M. C. (1959). The assessment of anxiety states by rating. *British Journal of Medical Psychology, 32*, 50–55.

Hanlon, C. A., Beveridge, T. J., & Porrino, L. J. (2013). Recovering from cocaine: Insights from clinical and preclinical investigations. *Neuroscience and Biobehavioral Review, 37*(9), 2037–2046.

Hardan, A. Y., Minshew, N. J., & Keshavan, M. S. (2000). Corpus callosum size in autism. *Neurology, 55*, 1033–1036.

Harlan, R. E., & Garcia, M. M. (1998). Drugs of abuse and immediate-early genes in the forebrain. *Molecular Neurobiology, 16*(3), 221–267.

Hartmann-Boyce, J., Chepkin, S. C., Ye, W., Bullen, C., & Lancaster, T. (2018). Nicotine replacement therapy versus control for smoking cessation. *Cochrane Database Systematic Reviews, 5*(5), CD000146. https://doi.org/10.1002/14651858.CD000146.pub5

Hashimoto, K., Shimizu, E., & Iyo, M. (2004). Critical role of brain-derived neurotrophic factor in mood disorders. *Brain Research. Brain Research Reviews, 45*(2), 104–114.

Hatsukami, D. K., Stead, L. F., & Gupta, P. C. (2008). Nicotine addiction: prevalence and treatment. *Lancet, 371*, 2027–2038.

Hatzidimitriou, G., McCann, U. D., & Ricaurte, G. A. (1999). Altered serotonin innervation patterns in the forebrain of monkeys treated with (+/−)3,4-methylenedioxymethamphetamine seven years previously: Factors influencing abnormal recovery. *The Journal of Neuroscience, 19*(12), 5096–5107.

Haynes, L. E., Barber, D., & Mitchell, I. J. (2004). Chronic antidepressant medication attenuates dexamethasone-induced neuronal death and sublethal neuronal damage in the hippocampus and striatum. *Brain Research, 1026*(2), 157–167.

Hazlett, E. A., Romero, M. J., Haznedar, M. M., New, A. S., Goldstein, K. E., Newmark, R. E., Siever, L. J., & Buchsbaum, M. S. (2007). Deficient attentional modulation of startle eyeblink is associated with symptom severity in the schizophrenia spectrum. *Schizophrenia Research, 93*(1–3), 288–295.

Henshaw, F. R., Dewsbury, L. S., Lim, C. K., & Steiner, G. Z. (2021). The effects of cannabinoids on pro- and anti-inflammatory cytokines: A systematic review of *In Vivo* studies. *Cannabis and Cannabinoid Research, 6*(3), 177–195. https://doi.org/10.1089/can.2020.0105

Hensler, J. G. (2003). Regulation of 5-HT1A receptor function in brain following agonist or antidepressant administration. *Life Sciences, 72*(15), 1665–1682.

Hernandez, C. M., & Terry, A. (2005). Repeated nicotine exposure in rats: Effects on memory function, cholinergic markers and nerve growth factor. *Neuroscience, 130*(4), 997–1012.

Hnasko, T. S., Sotak, B. N., & Palmiter, R. D. (2007). Cocaine-conditioned place preference by dopamine-deficient mice is mediated by serotonin. *The Journal of Neuroscience, 27*(46), 12484–12488.

Hoffman, A. F., Oz, M., Yang, R., Lichtman, A. H., & Lupica, C. R. (2007). Opposing actions of chronic Delta9-tetrahydrocannabinol and cannabinoid antagonists on hippocampal long-term potentiation. *Learning and Memory, 14*(1–2), 63–74.

Ho Pian, K. L., van Megan, H. J., Ramsey, N. F., Mandi, R., can Rijk, P. P., Wynne, H. J., & Westenberg, H. G. (2005). Decreased thalamic blood flow in obsessive-compulsive disorder patients responding to fluvoxamine. *Psychiatry Research, 138*(2), 89–97.

Hosang, G., Shiles, C., Tansey, K., McGuffin, P., & Uher, R. (2014). Interaction between stress and the BDNF Val66Met polymorphism in depression: A systematic review and meta-analysis. *BMC Medicine, 12*, 7. https://doi.org/10.1186/1741-7015-12-7

Hughes, J. R. (2007). Autism: The first firm finding = underconnectivity? *Epilepsy & Behavior, 11*(1), 20–24.

Hurley, M. J., & Jenner, P. (2006). What has been learnt from study of dopamine receptors in Parkinson's disease? *Pharmacology & Therapeutics, 111*(3), 715–728.

Hyman, S. E., Malenka, R. C., & Nestler, E. J. (2006). Neural mechanisms of addiction: The role of reward-related learning and memory. *Annual Review of Neuroscience, 29*, 565–598.

Ichikawa, J., Chung, Y. C., Dai, J., & Meltzer, H. Y. (2005b). Valproic acid potentiates both typical and atypical antipsychotic-induced prefrontal cortical dopamine release. *Brain Research, 1052*(1), 56–62.

Iqbal, U., Dringenberg, H. C., Brien, J. F., & Reynolds, J. N. (2004). Chronic prenatal ethanol exposure alters hippocampal GABA(A) receptors and impairs spatial learning in the guinea pig. *Behavioral Brain Research, 150*(1–2), 117–125.

Ivanov, A., & Aston-Jones, G. (2001). Local opiate withdrawal in locus coeruleus neurons in vitro. *The Journal of Neurophysiology, 85*, 2388–2397.

Iversen, L. L. (2000). The science of marijuana. Oxford University Press.

Izzo, A. A. (2004). Drug interactions with St. John's wort (Hypericum perforatum): A review of the clinical evidence. *International Journal of Clinical Pharmacology and Therapeutics, 42*(3), 139–148.

Javitt, D. C. (2007). Glutamate and schizophrenia: Phencyclidine, N-methyl-d-aspartate receptors, and dopamine-glutamate interactions. *International Review of Neurobiology, 78*, 69–108.

Javitt, D. C., & Coyle, J. T. (2004). Decoding schizophrenia. *Scientific American, January*, 1–4.

Jie, F., Yin, G., Yang, W., Yang, M., Gao, S., Lv, J., & Li, B. (2018). Stress in regulation of GABA amygdala system and relevance to neuropsychiatric diseases. *Frontiers in Neuroscience, 12*, 562. https://doi.org/10.3389/fnins.2018.00562

Job, M. O., Tang, A., Hall, F. S., Sora, I., Uhl, G. R., Gergeson, S. E., & Gonzales, R. A. (2007). Mu (mu) opioid receptor regulation of ethanol-induced dopamine response in the ventral striatum: Evidence of genotype specific sexual dimorphic epistasis. *Biological Psychiatry*, *62*(6), 627–634.

Joel, D. (2006). The signal attenuation rat model of obsessive-compulsive disorder: A review. *Psychopharmacology*, *186*(4), 487–503.

Johnson, M. W., & Ettinger, R. H. (2000). Active immunization attenuates cocaine's discriminative properties. *Experimental and Clinical Psychopharmacology*, *8*, 163–167.

Joyce, J. N. (1993). The dopamine hypothesis of schizophrenia: Limbic interactions with serotonin and norepinephrine. *Psychopharmacology*, *112*(1, Suppl), S16–S34.

Just, M., Cherkassky, V., Buchweitz, A., Keller, T., & Mitchell, T. (2014). Identifying autism from neural representations of social interactions: Neurocognitive markers of autism. *Plos One*. https://doi.org/10.1371/journal.pone.0113879

Just, M. A., Cherkassky, V. L., Keller, T. A., Kana, R. K., & Minshew, N. J. (2007). Functional and anatomical cortical underconnectivity in autism: Evidence from an fMRI study of an executive function task and corpus callosum morphometry. *Cerebral Cortex*, *17*(4), 951–961.

Just, M. A., Cherkassky, V. L., Keller, T. A., & Minshew, N. J. (2004). Cortical activation and synchronization during sentence comprehension in high-functioning autism: Evidence of underconnectivity. *Brain*, *127*, 1811–1821.

Just, M. A., Keller, T., Malave, V., Kana, R., & Varma, S. (2012). Autism as a neural systems disorder: A theory of frontal-posterior underconnectivity. *Neuroscience and Biobehavioral Reviews*, *36*(4), 1292–1313.

Justinova, Z., Tanda, G., Redhi, G. H., & Goldberg, S. R. (2003). Self-admininstration of Delta9-tetrahydrocannabinol (THC) by drug naive squirrel monkeys. *Psychopharmacology*, *169*, 135–140.

Kalechstein, A. D., De La Garza, R., Mahoney, J. J., Fantegrossi, W. E., & Newton, T. F. (2007). MDMA use and neurocognition: A meta-analytic review. *Psychopharmacology*, *189*(4), 531–537.

Kalivas, P. W., McFarland, K., Bowers, S., Szumlinski, K., Xi, Z. X., & Baker, D. (2003). Glutamate transmission and addiction to cocaine. *Annals of the New York Academy of Sciences*, *1003*, 169–175.

Kalivas, P. W., & Volkow, N. D. (2005). The neural basis of addiction: A pathology of motivation and choice. *The American Journal of Psychiatry*, *162*(8), 1403–1413.

Kang-Park, M. H., Kieffer, B. L., Roberts, A. J., Siggins, G. R., & Moore, S. D. (2007b). Presynaptic delta opioid receptors regulate ethanol actions in central amygdala. *The Journal of Pharmacology and Experimental Therapeutics*, *320*(2), 917–925.

Kang-Park, M. H., Wilson, W. A., Kuhn, C. M., Moore, S. D., & Swartzwelder, H. S. (2007a). Differential sensitivity of GABA A receptor-mediated IPSCs to cannabinoids in hippocampal slices from adolescent and adult rats. *Journal of Neurophysiology*, *98*(3), 1223–1230.

Kapur, S., Zipursky, R., Jones, C., Remington, G., & Houle, S. (2000). Relationship between dopamine D(2) occupancy, clinical response, and side effects: A double-blind PET study of first-episode schizophrenia. *The American Journal of Psychiatry*, *157*(4), 514–520.

Karl, A., Schaefer, M., Malta, L. S., Dorfel, D., Rohleder, N., & Werner, A. (2006). A meta-analysis of structural brain abnormalities in PTSD. *Neuroscience and Biobehavioral Reviews*, *30*(7), 1004–1031.

Kasper, S., Anghelescu, I. G., Szegedi, A., Dienel, A., & Kieser, M. (2006). Superior efficacy of St. John's wort extract WS5570 compared to placebo in patients with major depression: A randomized, double-blind, placebo-controlled, multi-center trial (ISRCTN77277298). *BMC Medicine*, *4*, 14.

Kato, T. (2007). Molecular genetics of bipolar disorder and depression. *Psychiatry and Clinical Neurosciences*, *61*(1), 3–19.

Kawahara, Y., Ohnishi, Y. N., Ohnishi, Y. H., Kawahara, H., & Nishi, A. (2021). Distinct role of dopamine in the PFC and NAc during exposure to cocaine-associated cues. *The International Journal of Neuropsychopharmacology*, *24*(12), 988–1001.

Kehoe, W. A., Jr. (2008). Substance abuse: New numbers are a cause for action. *The Annals of Pharmacotherapy*, *42*(2), 270–272.

Kendler, K. S. (1996). Major depression and generalised anxiety disorder. Same genes, (partly) different environments–revisited. *The British Journal of Psychiatry*, *30*(Suppl), 68–75.

Kendler, K. S., Gardner, C. O., Gatz, M., & Pedersen, N. L. (2007). The sources of co-morbidity between major depression and generalized anxiety disorder in a Swedish national twin sample. *Psychological Medicine*, *37*(3), 453–462.

Kessler, R. C., Berglund, P., Demler, O., Jin, R., Merikangas, K. R., & Walters, E. E. (2005). Lifetime preva-lence and age-of-onset distributions of DSM-IV disorders in the National Comorbidity Survey Replica-tion. *Archives of General Psychiatry, 62*(6), 1–11.

Khom, S., Baburin, I., Timin, E., Hohaus, A., Trauner, G., Kopp, B., & Hering, S. (2007). Valerenic acid potenti-ates and inhibits GABAa receptors: Molecular mechanism and subunit specificity. *Neuropharmacology, 20*, 1–10.

Khundakar, A. A., & Zetterstom, T. S. (2006). Biphasic change in BDNF gene expression following antide-pressant drug treatment explained by differential transcript regulation. *Brain Research, 1106*(1), 12–20.

Kim, S. W., Shin, I. S., Kim, J. M., Lee, S. H., Lee, J. H., Yoon, B. H., Yang, S. J., Hwang, M. Y., & Yoon, J. S. (2007). Amisulpride versus risperidone in the treatment of depression in patients with schizophrenia: A random-ized, open-label, controlled trial. *Progress in Neuro-Psychopharmacology and Biological Psychiatry, 31*(7), 1504–1509.

Kim, Y.-K., Lee, H.-P., Won, S.-D., Park, E.-Y., Lee, H.-Y., Lee, B.-H., Lee, S.-W., Yoon, D., Han, C., Kim, D.-J., & Choi, S.-H. (2007a). Low plasma BDNF is associated with suicidal behavior in major depression. *Progress in Neuro-Psychopharmacology and Biological Psychiatry, 31*(1), 78–85.

Kim, Y.-K., Yoon, I. Y., Shin, Y. K., Cho, S. S., & Kim, S. E. (2007b). Modafinil-induced hippocampal activation in narcolepsy. *Neuroscience Letters, 422*(2), 91–96.

Kinsey, B. M., Jackson, D. C., & Orson, F. M. (2009). Anti-drug vaccines to treat substance abuse. *Immunology and Cell Biology, 87*(4), 309–314.

Kirsch, I., & Sapirstein, G. (1998). Listening to Prozac but hearing placebo: A meta-analysis of antidepressant medication. *Prevention and Treatment, 1*(2).

Knutson, B., Adams, C. M., Fong, G. W., & Hommer, D. (2001). Anticipation of increasing monetary reward selectively recruits nucleus accumbens. *The Journal of Neuroscience, 21*(16), RC159.

Koehler, J., Feneberg, W., Meier, M., & Pollmann, W. (2014). Clinical experience with THC: CBD oromu-cosal spray in patients with multiple sclerosis-related spasticity. *The International Journal of Neuroscience, 124*(9), 652–656.

Koepp, M. J., Gunn, R. N., Lawrence, A. D., Cunningham, V. J., Dagher, A., Jones, T., Brooks, D. J., Bench, C. J., & Grasby, P. M. (1998). Evidence for striatal dopamine release during a video game. *Nature, 393*(6682), 266–268.

Kogan, M., Blumberg, S. J., Schieve, L. A., Boyle, C. A., & Perrin, J. M. (2009). Prevalence of parent-reported diagnosis of autism spectrum disorder among children in the U.U., 2007. *Pediatrics, 124*(4), 1–8.

Kogan, N. M. (2005). Cannabinoids and cancer. *Mini Reviews in Medicinal Chemistry, 5*(10), 941–952.

Kolb, B., Gorny, G., Limebeer, C., & Parker, L. (2006). Chronic treatment with Delta-9-tetrahydrocannab-inol alters the structure of neurons in the nucleus accumbens shell and medial prefrontal cortex of rats. *Synapse, 60*(6), 429–436.

Kollins, S., Schoenfelder, E., English, J., Holdaway, A., VanVoorhees, E., O'Brien, B. R., Dew, R., & Chris-man, A. (2015). An exploratory study of the combined effects of orally administered methylphenidate and delta-9-tetrahydrocannabinol (THC) on cardiovascular function, subjective effects, and performance in healthy adults. *Journal of Substance Abuse Treatment, 48*(1), 96–103.

Koponen, E., Rantamaki, T., Voikar, V., Saarelainen, T., MacDonald, E., & Castren, E. (2005). Enhanced BDNF signaling is associated with an antidepressant-like behavioral response and changes in brain mono-amines. *Cellular and Molecular Neurobiology, 25*(6), 973–980.

Kozisek, M. E., Middlemas, D., & Bylund, D. B. (2008). Brain-derived neurotrophic factor and its receptor tropomyosin-related kinase B in the mechanism of action of antidepressant therapies. *Pharmacology & Thera-peutics, 117*(1), 30–51.

Krall, C. M., Richards, J. B., Rabin, R. A., & Winter, J. C. (2008). Marked decrease of LSD-induced stimulus control in serotonin transporter knockout mice. *Pharmacology, Biochemistry, and Behavior, 88*(3), 349–357.

Kropotov, J. D., Grin-Yatsenko, V. A., Ponomarev, V. A., Chutko, L. S., Yakovenko, E. A., & Nikishena, I. S. (2005). ERPs correlates of EEG relative beta training in ADHD children. *International Journal of Psycho-physiology, 55*(1), 23–34.

Kryst, J., Kawalec, P., Mitoraj, A. M., Pilc, A., Lasoń, W., & Brzostek, T. (2020). Efficacy of single and repeated administration of ketamine in unipolar and bipolar depression: A meta-analysis of randomized clinical trials. *Pharmacological Reports, 72*(3), 543–562.

Kuan, L., Guibao, Z., Yan, X., Jiayu, G., Qiuling, C., Shouxia, X., & Junyan, W. (2022). Risk of suicidal behaviors and antidepressant exposure among children and adolescents: A meta-analysis of observational studies. *Psychiatry, 13*, 880496. https://doi.org/10.3389/fpsyt.2022.880496

Kufahl, P., Zavala, A., Akanksha, S., Singh, A., Thiel, K., Dicky, E., & Joyce, J. (2009). c-Fos expression associated with reinstatement of cocaine-seeking behavior by response-contingent conditioned cues. *Synapse*, *63*(10), 823–835. https://doi.org/10.1002/syn.20666

Kumar, S., Fleming, R. L., & Morrow, A. L. (2004). Ethanol regulation of gamma-aminobutyric acid A receptors: Genomic and nongenomic mechanisms. *Pharmacology & Therapeutics*, *101*(3), 211–226.

Kumar, S., Kralic, J. E., O'Buckley, T. K., Grobin, A. C., & Morrow, A. L. (2003). Chronic ethanol consumption enhances internalization of alpha1 subunit-containing GABAA receptors in cerebral cortex. *Journal of Neurochemistry*, *86*(8), 700–708.

Kumari, V., Antonova, E., Geyer, M. A., Ffytche, D., Williams, S. C., & Sharma, T. (2007). A fMRI investigation of startle gating deficits in schizophrenia patients treated with typical or atypical antipsychotics. *The International Journal of Neuropsychopharmacology*, *10*(4), 463–477.

Kumari, V., Soni, W., & Sharma, T. (2002). Prepulse inhibition of the startle response in risperidone-treated patients: comparison with typical antipsychotics. *Schizophrenia Research*, *44*(1–2), 139–146.

Laeng, P., Pitts, R. L., Lemire, A. L., Drabik, C. E., Weiner, A., Tang, H., Thyagarajan, R., Mallon, B. S., & Altar, C. A. (2004). The mood stabilizer valproic acid stimulates GABA neurogenesis from rat forebrain stem cells. *Journal of Neurochemistry*, *91*(1), 238–251.

LaLumiere, R. T., & Kalivas, P. W. (2008). Glutamate release in the nucleus accumbens core is necessary for heroin seeking. *The Journal of Neuroscience*, *23*(12), 3170–3177.

Landry, D. W., & Yang, G. (1997). Anti-cocaine catalytic antibodies–a novel approach to the problem of addiction. *Journal of Addictive Diseases*, *16*(3), 1–17.

Landry, D. W., Zhao, K., Yang, G., Glickman, M., & Georgiadis, T. (1993). Antibody-catalyzed degradation of cocaine. *Science*, *259*(5103), 1899–1901.

Lapidus, K., Kopell, B., Ben-Haim, S., Rezai, A., & Goodman, W. (2013). History of psychosurgery: A psychiatrist's perspective. *World Neurosurgery*, *80*, S27.e1–S27.e16.

Laruelle, M. (1998). Imaging dopamine transmission in schizophrenia. A review and meta-analysis. *The Quarterly Journal of Nuclear Medicine*, *42*(3), 211–221.

Latalova, K., Kamaradova, D., & Prasko, J. (2014). Suicide in bipolar disorder: A review. *Psychiatria Danubina*, *26*(2), 108–114.

Lecca, D., Cacciapaglia, F., Valentini, V., & Di Chiara, G. (2006). Monitoring extracellular dopamine in the rat nucleus accumbens shell and core during acquisition and maintenance of intravenous WIN 55,212-2 self-administration. *Psychopharmacology*, *188*(1), 63–74.

Lee, B.-H., Kim, H., Park, S.-H., & Kim, Y. K. (2006). Decreased plasma BDNF level in depressive patients. *Journal of Affective Disorders*, *101*(1–3), 239–244.

Lee, B.-H., & Kim, Y. K. (2010). The roles of BDNF in the pathophysiology of major depression and in antidepressant treatment. *Psychiatry Investigations*, *7*(4), 231–235.

Le Foll, B., Collo, G., Rabiner, E. A., Boileau, I., Merlo, P., & Sokoloff, P. (2014). Dopamine D3 receptor ligands for drug addiction treatment: Update on recent findings. *Progress in Brain Research*, *211*, 255–275.

Le Foll, B., & Goldberg, S. R. (2005). Cannabinoid CB1 receptor antagonists as promising new medications for drug dependence. *The Journal of Pharmacology and Experimental Therapeutics*, *312*(3), 875–883.

Lejoyeux, M., Solomon, J., & Ades, J. (1998). Benzodiazepine treatment for alcohol-dependent patients. *Alcohol and Alcoholism*, *33*(6), 563–575.

Lépicier, P., Bibeau-Poirier, A., Lagneux, C., Servant, M. J., & Lamontagne, D. (2006). Signaling pathways involved in the cardioprotective effects of cannabinoids. *Journal of Pharmacological Sciences*, *102*(2), 155–166.

Lépicier, P., Lagneux, C., Sirois, M. G., & Lamontagne, D. (2007). Endothelial CB1-receptors limit infarct size through NO formation in rat isolated hearts. *Life Sciences*, *81*(17–18), 1373–1380.

LeSage, M. G., Keyler, D. E., Hieda, Y., Collins, G., Burroughs, D., Le, C., & Pentel, P. R. (2006). Effects of a nicotine conjugate vaccine on the acquisition and maintenance of nicotine self-administration in rats. *Psychopharmacology*, *184*(3–4), 409–416.

Levin, E. D., Conners, C., Silva, D., Ninton, S., Meck, W., March, J., & Rose, J. (1998). Transdermal nicotine effects on attention. *Psychopharmacology*, *140*(2), 135–141.

Levin, G. M., Bowles, T. M., Ehret, M. J., Langaee, T., Tan, J. Y., Johnson, J. A., & Millard, W. J. (2007). Assessment of human serotonin 1A receptor polymorphisms and SSRI responsiveness. *Molecular Diagnosis & Therapy*, *11*(3), 155–160.

Levine, J. D., Gordon, N. C., & Fields, H. L. (1978). The mechanism of placebo analgesia. *Lancet, 2*(8091), 654–657.

Li, N. X., Hu, Y. R., Chen, W. N., & Zhang, B. (2022). Dose effect pf psilocybin on primary and secondary depression: A preliminary systematic review and meta-analysis. *Journal of Affective Disorders, 296*, 26–34.

Li, Z., DiFranza, J. R., Wellman, R. J., Kulkarni, P., & King, J. A. (2008). Imaging brain activation in nicotine-sensitized rats. *Brain Research, 1199*, 91–99.

Liang, J., Suryanarayanan, A., Abriam, A., Snyder, B., Olsen, R. W., & Spigelman, I. (2007). Mechanisms of reversible GABAA receptor plasticity after ethanol intoxication. *The Journal of Neuroscience, 27*(45), 12367–12377.

Licinio, J., & Wong, M. (2002). Brain-derived neurotropic factor (BDNF) in stress and affective disorders. *Molecular Psychiatry, 7*(6), 519.

Lin, P. Y. (2007). Meta-analysis of the association of serotonin transporter gene polymorphism with obsessive-compulsive disorder. *Progress in Neuro-Psychopharmacology and Biological Psychiatry, 31*(3), 683–689.

Lin, P. Y., Zack Ma, Z., Mahgoub, M., Kavalali, E., & Monteggia, L. (2021). A synaptic locus for TrkB signaling underlying ketamine rapid antidepressant action. *Cell Reports, 36*(7). https://doi.org/10.1016/j.celrep.2021.109513

Linde, K., Mulrow, C. D., Berner, M., & Egger, M. (2005). St. John's wort for depression. *Cochran Database of Systematic Reviews*, CD000448 (Online).

Line, S., Barkus, C., Coyle, C., Jennings, K., Deacon, R., Lesch, K. P., Sharp, T., & Bannerman, D. (2011). Opposing alteration in anxiety and species-typical behaviours in serotonin transporter overexpressor and knockout mice. *European Neuropsychopharmacology, 21*(1), 108–116.

Ling, S., Ceban, F., Lui, L., Lee, Y., Teopiz, K. M., Rodrigues, N. B., Lipsitz, O., Gill, H., & McIntyre, R. S. (2022). Molecular mechanisms of psilocybin and implications for the treatment of depression. *CNS Drugs, 36*(1), 17–30.

Liu, D., Tang, Q. Q., & Wang, D. (2020). Mesocortical BDNF signaling mediates antidepressive-like effects of lithium. *Neuropharmacology, 45*, 1557–1566.

Loebel, A., Cucchiaro, J., Silva, R., Kroger, H., Sarma, K., Xu, J., & Calabrese, J. (2014). Lurasidone as adjunctive therapy with lithium or valproate for the treatment of bipolar I depression: A randomized, double-blind, placebo-controlled study. *The American Journal of Psychiatry, 171*(2), 169–177.

Lohoff, F. W., Sander, T., Ferraro, T. N., Dahl, J. P., Gallinat, J., & Berrettini, W. H. (2005). Confirmation of association between the Val66Met polymorphism in the brain-derived neurotrophic factor (BDNF) gene and bipolar 1 disorder. *American Journal of Medical Genetics, Part B, Neuropsychiatric Genetics, 139*(1), 51–53.

Lombard, C., Nagarkatti, M., & Nagarkatti, P. (2007). CB2 cannabinoid receptor agonist, JWH-015, triggers apoptosis in immune cells: potential role for CB2-selective ligands as immunosuppressive agents. *Clinical Immunology, 122*(3), 259–270.

Loo, S. K., Hopfer, C., Teale, P. D., & Reite, M. L. (2004). EEG correlates of methylphenidate response in ADHD: Association with cognitive and behavioral measures. *Journal of Clinical Neurophysiology, 21*(6), 457–464.

López-Giménez, J. F., & González-Maeso, J. (2018). Hallucinogens and serotonin 5-HT$_{2A}$ receptor-mediated signaling pathways. *Current Topics in Behavioral Neuroscience, 36*, 45–73.

Ly, C., Greb, A., Cameron, L., Wong, J., Barragan, E., & Olson, D. (2018). Psychedelics promote structural and functional neural plasticity. *Cell Reports, 23*(11), 3170–3182. https://doi.org/10.1016/j.celrep.2018.05.022

Machado-Vieira, R., Dietrich, M. O., Leke, R., Cereser, V. H., Zanatto, V., Kapczinski, F., Souza, D. O., Portela, L. V., & Gentil, V. (2007). Decreased plasma brain derived neurotrophic factor levels in unmedicated bipolar patients during manic episode. *Biological Psychiatry, 61*(2), 142–144.

Mack, A. (2003). Examination of the evidence for off-label use of gabapentin. *Journal of Managed Care Pharmacy, 9*(6), 559–568.

Madras, B. K., Xie, Z., Lin, Z., Jassen, A., Panas, H., Lynch, L., Johnson, R., Livni, E., Spencer, T. J., Bonab, A. A., Miller, G. M., & Fischman, A. J. (2006). Modafinil occupies dopamine and norepinephrine transporters in vivo and modulates the transporters and trace amine activity in vitro. *The Journal of Pharmacology and Experimental Therapeutics, 319*(2), 561–569.

Maggos, C., Tsukada, H., Kakiuchi, T., Nishiyama, S., & Kreek, M. (1998). Sustained withdrawal allows normalization of in vivo [11C]N-Methylspiperone dopamine D2 receptor binding after chronic binge cocaine: A positron emission tomography study in rats. *Europsychopharmacology, 19*, 146–153.

Mai, L., Jope, R. S., & Li, X. (2002). The BDNF-mediated signal transduction is modulated by GSK3beta and mood stabilizing agents. *Journal of Neurochemistry, 82*(1), 75–83.

Marek, G. J., Martin-Ruiz, R., Abo, A., & Artigas, F. (2005). The selective 5-HT2A receptor antagonist M100907 enhances antidepressant-like behavioral effects of the SSRI fluoxetine. *Neuropsychopharmacology, 30*(12), 2205–2215.

Marona-Lewicka, D., Thisted, R., & Nichols, D. (2005). Distinct temporal phases in the behavioral pharmacology of LSD: Dopamine D2 receptor-mediated effects in the rat and implications for psychosis. *Psychopharmacology, 180*(3), 427–435.

Martell, B. A., Mitchell, E., Poling, J., Gonsai, K., & Kosten, T. R. (2005). Vaccine pharmacotherapy for the treatment of cocaine dependence. *Biological Psychiatry, 58*(2), 158–164.

Martella, D., Aldunate, N., Fuentes, L., & Sanchez-Perez, N. (2020). Arousal and executive alterations in attention deficit hyperactivity disorder (ADHD). *Frontiers in Psychology, 12*(11), 1991.

Marucci, G., Buccioni, M., Dal Ben, D., Lambertucci, C., Volpini, R., & Amenta, F. (2021). Efficacy of acetylcholinesterase inhibitors in Alzheimer's disease. *Neuropharmacology, 190*. https://doi.org/10.1016/j.neuropharm.2020.108352

Mateo, Y., Budygin, E. A., John, C. E., & Jones, S. R. (2004). Role of serotonin in cocaine effects in mice with reduced dopamine transporter function. *Proceedings of the National Academy of Sciences of the United States of America, 101*(1), 372–377.

McAlonan, G. M., Cheung, V., Cheung, C., Suckling, J., Lam, G. Y., Tai, K. S., Yip, L., Murphy, D. G. M., & Chua, S. E. (2004). Mapping the brain in autism. A voxel-based MRI study of volumetric differences and intercorrelations in autism. *Brain, 128*(2), 268–276.

McClung, C. A., & Nestler, E. J. (2003). Regulation of gene expression and cocaine reward by CREB and DeltaFosB. *Nature Neuroscience, 6*(11), Online.

McGranahan, T. M., Patzlaff, N. E., Grady, S. R., Heinemann, S. F., & Booker, T. K. (2011). α4β2 nicotinic acetylcholine receptors on dopaminergic neurons mediate nicotine reward and anxiety relief. *Journal of Neuroscience, 31*(30), 10891–11902. https://doi.org/10.1523/JNEUROSCI.0937-11.2011

McInnes, L. A., Qian, J. J., Gargeya, R. S., DeBattista, C., & Heifets, B.D, (2022). A retrospective analysis of ketamine intravenous therapy for depression in real-world care settings. *Journal of Affective Disorders, 301*, 486–495.

McKallip, R. J., Lombard, C., Martin, B. R., Nagarkatti, M., & Nagarkatti, P. S. (2002). Delta 9-tetrahydrocannabinol-induced apoptosis in the thymus and spleen as a mechanism of immunosuppression in vitro and in vivo. *Pharmacology & Experimental Therapeutics, 302*(2), 451–465.

McKinney, D. L., Cassidy, M. P., Collier, L. M., Martin, B. R., Wiley, J. L., Selley, D. E., & Sim-Selley, L. J. (2008). Dose-related differences in the regional pattern of cannabinoid receptor adaptation and in vivo tolerance development to delta9-tetrahydrocannabinol. *The Journal of Pharmacology and Experimental Therapeutics, 324*(2), 664–673.

Mechan, A., Yuan, J., Hatzidimitriou, G., Irvine, R. J., McCann, U. P., & Ricaurte, G. A. (2006). Pharmacokinetic profile of single and repeated oral doses of MDMA in squirrel monkeys: Relationship to lasting effects on brain serotonin neurons. *Neuropsychopharmacology, 31*(2), 339–350.

Mechoulam, R., & Gaoni, Y. (1965). A total synthesis of dl-delta1-tetrahydrocannabinol, the active constituent of hashish. *Journal of the American Chemical Society, 87*(14), 3273–3275.

Meier, S., Strohmaier, J., Breuer, R., Mattheisen, M., Degenhardt, F., Mühleisen, T. W., Schulze, T. G., Nöthen, M. M., Cichon, S., Rietschel, M., & Wust, S. (2013). Neuregulin 3 is associated with attention deficits in schizophrenia and bipolar disorder. *The International Journal of Neuropsychopharmacology, 16*(3), 549–556.

Mena, A., Ruiz-Salas, J., Puentes, A., Dorado, I., Ruiz-Veguilla, M., & De la Casa, L. (2016). Reduced prepulse inhibition as a biomarker of schizophrenia. *Frontiers in Behavioral Neuroscience, 10*, 202. https://doi.org/10.3389/fnbeh.2016.00202

Merikangas, K. R., Akiskal, H., Angst, J., Greenberg, P., Hirschfield, R., Petukhova, M., & Kessler, R. C. (2007). Lifetime and 12 month prevalence of bipolar spectrum disorder in the National Comorbidity Survey replication. *Archives of General Psychiatry, 64*(5), 543–552.

Michailov, G. V., Sereda, M., Brinkmann, B., Fischer, T. M., & Haug, B. (2004). Axonal neuregulin-1 regulates myelin sheath thickness. *Science, 304*, 700–703.

Miller, M. M., & McEwen, B. S. (2006). Establishing an agenda for transitional research on PTSD. *Annals of the New York Academy of Sciences, 1071*, 294–312.

Mirza, N. R., & Nielsen, E. O. (2006). Do subtype-selective gamma-aminobutyric acid A receptor modulators have a reduced propensity to induce physical dependence in mice? *The Journal of Pharmacology and Experimental Therapeutics, 316*(3), 1378–1385.

Miyasaka, L. S., Atallah, A. N., & Soares, B. G. O. (2007). Valerian for anxiety disorders. *Cochrane Database of Systematic Reviews, 2007*(4).

Moffitt, T. E., & Melchior, M. (2007). Why does the worldwide prevalence of childhood attention deficit hyperactivity disorder matter? *American Journal of Psychiatry, 164*, 856–858.

Moncrieff, J. (2003). A comparison of antidepressant trials using active and inert placebos. *International Journal of Methods in Psychiatric Research, 12*(3), 117–127.

Monteggia, L. M., Luikart, B., Barrot, M., Theobold, D., Malkovska, I., Nef, S., Parada, L. F., & Nestler, E. J. (2007). Brain-derived neurotrophic factor conditional knockouts show gender differences in depression-related behaviors. *Biological Psychiatry, 61*(2), 187–197.

Moresco, R. M., Pietra, L., Henin, M., Panzacchi, A., Locatelli, M., Bonaldi, L., Carpinelli, A., Gobbo, C., Bellodi, L., Perani, D., & Fazio, F. (2007). Fluvoxamine treatment and D2 receptors: A pet study on OCD drug-naive patients. *Neuropsychopharmacology, 32*(1), 197–205.

Mukai, T., Kishi, T., Matsuda, Y., & Iwata, N. (2014). A meta-analysis of inositol for depression and anxiety disorders. *Human Psychopharmacology, 29*(1), 55–63.

Müller, D. J., de Luca, V., Sicard, T., King, N., Strauss, J., & Kennedy, J. L. (2006). Brain-derived neurotrophic factor (BDNF) gene and rapid-cycling bipolar disorder: Family-based association study. *The British Journal of Psychiatry, 189*, 317–323.

Müller, W. E. (2003). Current St. John's wort research from mode of action to clinical efficacy. *Pharmacological Research, 47*(2), 101–109.

Murphy, K., Kubin, Z., Shepherd, J., Ettinger, R. H. (2010). Valeriana officinalis root extracts have potent anxiolytic effects in laboratory rats. *Phytomedicine, 17*, 674–678.

Murray, K. N., & Abeles, N. (2002). Nicotine's effect on neural and cognitive functioning in an aging population. *Aging and Mental Health, 6*(2), 129–138.

Musazzi, L., Cattaneo, A., Tardito, D., Barbon, A., Gennarelli, M., Barlati, S., Racagni, G., & Popoli, M. (2009). Early rise of BDNF in hippocampus suggests induction of posttranscriptional mechanisms by antidepressants. *BMC Neuroscience, 10*, 48.

Mustafa, N. S., Bakar, N. H. A., Mohamad, N., Adnan, L. H. M., Fauzi, N., Thoarlim, A., Omar, S., Hamzah, M. S., Yusoff, Z., Jufri, M., & Ahmad, R. (2020). MDMA and the brain: A short review on the role of neurotransmitters in neurotoxicity. *Basic Clinical Neuroscience, 11*(4), 381–388. https://doi.org/10.32598/bcn.9.10.485

Nair, A., Vadodaria, K. C., Banerjee, S. B., Benekareddy, M., Dias, B. G., Duman, R. S., & Vaidya, V. A. (2007). Stressor-specific regulation of distinct brain-derived neurotrophic factor transcripts and cyclic AMP response element-binding protein expression in the postnatal and adult rat hippocampus. *Neuropsychopharmacology, 32*(7), 1504–1519.

Nakata, K., Ujike, H., Sakai, A., Uchida, N., Nomura, A., Imamura, T., Katsu, T., Tanaka, Y., Hamamura, T., & Kuroda, S. (2003). Association study of the brain-derived neurotrophic factor (BDNF) gene with bipolar disorder. *Neuroscience Letters, 337*(1), 17–20.

Nasir, M., Trujillo, D., Levine, J., & Dwyer, J. (2020). Glutamate systems in DSM-5 anxiety disorders: Their role and a review of glutamate and GABA psychopharmacology. *Frontiers in Psychiatry, 11*, 548505. https://doi.org/10.3389/fpsyt.2020.548505

National Institute on Alcohol Abuse and Alcoholism. (2022). *Alcohol use in the United States.* www.niaaa.nih.gov/publications/brochures-and-fact-sheets/alcohol-facts-and-statistics

National Institute on Drug Abuse. (2020a). *High school and youth trends: Monitoring the future 2019 survey results.* https://nida.nih.gov/research-topics/trends-statistics/infographics/monitoring-future-2019-survey-results-overall-findings

National Institute on Drug Abuse. (2020b). *National survey of drug use and health.* NIH.

National Institute on Drug Abuse. (2021). https://nida.nih.gov/

Nelson, M., Saykin, A., Flashman, L., & Riordan, H. (1998). Hippocampal volume reduction in schizophrenia as assessed by magnetic resonance imaging: A meta-analytic study. *Archives of General Psychiatry, 55*(5), 433–440.

Nestler, E., & Aghajanian, G. (1997). Molecular and cellular basis of addiction. *Science, 278*, 58–63.

Niaura, R., Hays, J. T., Jorenby, D. E., Leone, F. T., Pappas, J. E., Reeves, K. R., Williams, K. E., & Billing, C. B. Jr. (2008). The efficacy and safety of varenicline for smoking cessation using a flexible dosing strategy in adult smokers: A randomized controlled trial. *Current Medical Research and Opinion, 24*(7), 1931–1941.

Nibuya, M., Nestler, E. J., & Duman, R. S. (1996). Chronic antidepressant administration increases the expression of cAMP response element binding protein (CREB) in rat hippocampus. *Journal of Neuroscience, 16*(7), 2365–2372.

Nilsson, M., Joliat, M. J., Miner, C. M., Brown, E. B., & Heiligenstein, J. H. (2004). Safety of subchronic treatment with fluoxetine for major depressive disorder in children and adolescents. *Journal of Child and Adolescent Psychopharmacology, 41*(3), 412–417.

NIMH. (2021a). Autism spectrum disorders (pervasive developmental disorders). *National Institute of Mental Health.* https://www.nimh.nih.gov/health/topics/autism-spectrum-disorders-asd

NIMH. (2021b). Mood disorders. *National Institute of Mental Health Statistics.* www.nimh.nih.gov/health/statistics/prevalence

Nyberg, S., Eriksson, B., Oxenstierna, G., Halldin, C., & Farde, L. (1999). Suggested minimal effective dose of risperidone based on PET-measured D2 and 5-HT2A receptor occupancy in schizophrenic patients. *The American Journal of Psychiatry, 156*(6), 869–875.

Olds, J., & Milner, P. (1954). Positive reinforcement produced by electrical stimulation of septal area and other regions of rat brain. *Journal of Comparative Physiological Psychology, 47*(6), 419–427.

Olié, J. P., Spina, E., Murray, S., & Yang, R. (2006). Ziprasidone and amisulpride effectively treat negative symptoms of schizophrenia: Results of a 12-week, double-blind study. *International Clinical Psychopharmacology, 21*(3), 143–151.

Olney, J. W., Newcomer, J. W., & Farber, N. B. (1999). NMDA receptor hypofunction model of schizophrenia. *Journal of Psychiatric Research, 33*(6), 523–533.

Olney, J. W., Wozniak, D. F., Jevtovic-Todorovic, V., & Ikonomidou, C. (2001). Glutamate signaling and the fetal alcohol syndrome. *Mental Retardation and Developmental Disabilities Research Reviews, 7*(4), 267–275. https://doi.org/10.1002/mrdd.1037

Olsen, R. W., Hanchar, H. J., Meera, P., & Wallner, M. (2007). GABAA receptor subtypes: The "one glass of wine" receptors. *Alcohol, 41*(3), 201–209.

Olsen, R. W., & Liang, J. (2017). Role of $GABA_A$ receptors in alcohol use disorders suggested by chronic intermittent ethanol (CIE) rodent model. *Molecular Brain, 10*(1), 45. https://doi.org/10.1186/s13041-017-0325-8

Osaka, T., & Matsumura, H. (1994). Noradrenergic inputs to sleep-related neurons in the preoptic area of the locus coeruleus and the ventromedial medulla in the rat. *Neuroscience Research, 19*(1), 39–50.

Overstreet, D. H., Commissaris, R., De La Garza, R., File, S., Knapp, D., & Seiden, L. (2003). Involvement of 5-HT1A receptors in animal tests of anxiety and depression: Evidence from genetic models. *Stress, 6*(2), 101–110.

Palatnik, A., Frolov, K., Fux, M., & Benjamin, J. (2001). Double-blind, controlled, crossover trial of inositol versus fluvoxamine for the treatment of panic disorder. *Journal of Clinical Psychopharmacology, 21*(3), 335–339.

Papakostas, G., Perlis, R., Scalia, M., Petersen, T., & Fava, M. (2006). A meta-analysis of early sustained response rates between antidepressants and placebo for the treatment of major depressive disorder. *Journal of Clinical Psychopharmacology, 26*(1), 56–60.

Park, Y., Lee, B., & Kim, S. (2014). Serum BDNF levels in relation to illness severity, suicide attempts, and central serotonin activity in patients with major depressive disorder: A pilot study. *PLoS ONE, 9*(3), e91061. https://doi.org/10.1371/journal.pone.0091061

Parsey, R. V., Oquendo, M. A., Ogden, R. T., Olvet, D. M., Simpson, N., Huang, Y. Y., Van Heertum, R. L., Arango, V., & Mann, J. J. (2006). Altered serotonin 1A binding in major depression: A{carbonyl-C-11} WAY100635 positron emission tomography study. *Biological Psychiatry, 59*(2), 106–113.

Passie, T., Seifert, J., Schneider, U., & Emrich, H. (2002). The pharmacology of psilocybin. *Addiction Biology, 7*, 357–364.

Patel, S., & Hillard, C. J. (2001). Cannabinoid CB(1) receptor agonists produce cerebellar dysfunction in mice. *The Journal of Pharmacology and Experimental Therapeutics, 297*(2), 629–637.

Patel, S., Kamil, S., Shah, M. R., Bhimanadham, N., & Imran, S. (2019). Pros and cons of marijuana in treatment of parkinson's disease. *Cureus, 11*(6). https://doi.org/10.7759/cureus.4813

Pattij, T., Groenink, L., Hijzen, T. H., Oosting, R. S., Maes, R. A. A., van der Gugten, J., & Olivier, B. (2002). Autonomic changes associated with enhanced anxiety in 5-HT1A receptor knockout mice. *Neuropsychopharmacology*, *27*, 380–390.

Payer, D., Behzadi, A., Kish, S., Houle, S., Wilson, A., & Boileau, I. (2014). Heightened D3 dopamine receptor levels in cocaine dependence and contributions to the addiction behavioral phenotype: A positron emission tomography study. *Neuropsychopharmacology*, *39*(2), 311–318.

Pedersen, D. J., Lessard, S. J., Coffey, V. G., Churchley, E. G., Wootton, A. M., Ng, T., Watt, M. J., & Hawley, J. A. (2008). High rates of muscle glycogen resynthesis after exhaustive exercise when carbohydrate is coingested with caffeine. *Journal of Applied Physiology*, *105*, 7–13.

Pentel, P. R., & LeSage, M. G. (2014). New directions in nicotine vaccine design and use. *Advances in Pharmacology*, *69*, 553–580.

Pentel, P. R., Malin, D. H., Ennifar, S., Hieda, Y., Keyler, D. E., Lake, J. R., Milstein, J. R., Basham, L. E., Coy, R. T., Moon, J. W., Naso, R., & Fattom, A. (2000). A nicotine conjugate vaccine reduces nicotine distribution to brain and attenuates its behavioral and cardiovascular effects in rats. *Pharmacology, Biochemistry, and Behavior*, *65*(1), 191–198.

Phend, C. (2007, May 8). Bipolar disorder prevalence hidden by diagnostic thresholds. *Medpage Today*.

Philip, N. S., Carpenter, L. L., Tyrka, A. R., & Price, L. H. (2008). Augmentation of antidepressants with atypical antipsychotics: A review of the current literature. *Journal of Psychiatric Practice*, *14*(1), 34–44.

Pianezza, M. L., Sellers, E., & Tyndale, R. (1998). Nicotine metabolism defect reduces smoking. *Nature*, *393*(6687), 750.

Ping, A., Xi, J., Prasad, B. M., Wang, M. H., & Kruzich, P. J. (2008). Contributions of nucleus accumbens core and shell GluR1 containing AMPA receptors in AMPA- and cocaine-primed reinstatement of cocaine-seeking behavior. *Brain Research*, *1215*, 173–182.

Pinna, G., Agis-Balboa, R. C., Zhubi, A., Matsumoto, K., Grayson, D. R., Costa, E., & Guidotti, A. (2006). Imidazenil and diazepam increase locomotor activity in mice exposed to protracted social isolation. *Proceedings of the National Academy of Sciences of the United States of America*, *103*(11), 4275–4280.

Plaze, M., Bartres-Faz, D., Martinot, J. L., Januel, D., Bellivier, F., De Beaurepaire, R., Chanraud, S., Andoh, J., Lefaucheur, J. P., Artiges, E., Pallier, C., & Paillere-Martinot, M. L. (2006). Left superior temporal gyrus activation during sentence perception negatively correlates with auditory hallucination severity in schizophrenia patients. *Schizophrenia Research*, *87*(1–3), 109–115.

Pliszka, S. R. (2007). Pharmacologic treatment of attention-deficit/hyperactivity disorder: Efficacy, safety and mechanisms of action. *Neuropsychology Review*, *17*(1), 61–72.

Pobbe, R. L., & Zangrossi, H., Jr. (2005). 5-HT(1A) and 5-HT(2A) receptors in the rat dorsal periaqueductal gray mediate the antipanic-like effect induced by the stimulation of serotonergic neurons in the dorsal raphe nucleus. *Psychopharmacology*, *183*(3), 314–321.

Porrino, L. J. (1993). Functional consequences of acute cocaine treatment depend on route of administration. *Psychopharmacology*, *112*(2–3), 343–351.

Porsolt, R. D., Bertin, A., & Jalfre, M. (1977). Behavioural despair in mice: A primary screening test for antidepressants. *Archives of International Pharmacodynamics and Therapeutics*, *229*, 327–336.

Post, R. M. (2007). Role of BDNF in bipolar and unipolar disorder: Clinical and theoretical implications. *Journal of Psychiatric Research*, *41*(12), 979–990.

Posternak, M. A., & Zimmerman, M. (2007). Therapeutic effect of follow-up assessments on antidepressant and placebo response rates in antidepressant efficacy trials. *The British Journal of Psychiatry*, *190*, 287–292.

Potkin, S., Saha, A., Kujawa, M., Carson, W., Ali, M., Stock, E., Stringfellow, J., Ingenito, G., & Marder, S. (2003). Aripiprazole, an antipsychotic with a novel mechanism of action, and risperidone vs placebo and schizoaffective disorder. *Archives of General Psychiatry*, *60*, 681–690.

Potter, A. S., & Newhouse, P. (2008). Acute nicotine improves cognitive deficits in young adults with attention-deficit/hyperactivity disorder. *Pharmacological Biochemical Behavior*, *88*(4), 407–417.

Preet, A., Ganju, R. K., & Groopman, J. E. (2008). Delta9-Tetrahydrocannabinol inhibits epithelial growth factor-induced lung cancer cell migration in vitro as well as its growth and metastasis in vivo. *Oncogene*, *27*(3), 339–346.

Preller, K., Razi, A., Zeidman, P., Stampfi, P., Friston, K., & Vollenweider, F. (2019). Effective connectivity changes in LSD-induced altered states of consciousness in humans. *PNAS*, *116*(7), 2743–2748. https://doi.org/10.1073/pnas.1815129116

Punch, L. J., Self, D. W., Nestler, E. J., & Taylor, J. R. (1997). Opposite modulation of opiate withdrawal behaviors on microinfusion of a protein kinase a inhibitor versus activator into the locus coeruleus or periaqueductal gray. *The Journal of Neuroscience, 17*(21), 8520–8527.

Randrup, A., & Munkvad, I. (1965). Special antagonism of amphetamine-induced abnormal behavior. Inhibition of stereotyped activity with increase of some normal activities. *Psychopharmacologia, 7*, 416–422.

Ranganathan, M., & D'Souza, D. C. (2006). The acute effects of cannabinoids on memory in humans: A review. *Psychopharmacology, 188*(4), 425–444.

Rao, Y., Liu, Z. W., Borok, E., Rabenstein, R. L., Shanabrough, M., Lu, M., Picciotto, M. R., Harvath, T. L., & Gao, X. B. (2007). Prolonged wakefulness induces experience-dependent synaptic plasticity in mouse hypocretin/orexin neurons. *The Journal of Clinical Investigation, 117*(2), 4022–4033.

Rasmussen, K., Beitner-Johnson, D. B., Krystal, J. H., Aghajanian, G. K., & Nestler, E. J. (1990). Opiate withdrawal and the rat locus coeruleus: Behavioral, electrophysiological, and biochemical correlates. *The Journal of Neuroscience, 10*, 2308–2317.

Reif, A., Richter, J., Straube, B., Hofler, M., Lueken, U., Gloster, A. T., Weber, H., Domschke, K., Fehm, L., Ströhle, A., Jansen, A., Gerlach, A., Pyka, M., Reinhardt, I., Konrad, C., Wittmann, A., Pfleiderer, B., Alpers, G. W., Pauli, P., . . . Deckert, J. (2014). MAOA and mechanisms of panic disorder revisited: from bench to molecular psychotherapy. *Molecular Psychiatry, 19*(1), 122–128.

Reite, M., Reite, E., Collins, D., Rojas, D., & Sandburg, E. (2010). Brain size and brain/intracranial volume ratio in major depression. *BMC Psychiatry, 10*, 79.

Rekand, T. (2014). THC: CBD spray and MS plasticity symptoms: Data from latest studies. *European Neurology, 71*(1), 4–9.

Resnick, R. B., Kestenbaum, R. S., & Schwartz, L. K. (1977). Acute systemic effects of cocaine in man: A controlled study by intranasal and intravenous route. *Science, 195*(4279), 695–698.

Rial, D., Lemos, C., Pinheiro, H., Duarte, J., & Cunha, R. (2016). Depression as a glial-based synaptic dysfunction. *Frontiers in Cell Neuroscience, 9*, 521. https://doi.org/10.3389/fncel.2015.00521

Richardson, K., Baillie, A., Reid, S., Morley, K., Teesson, M., Sannibale, C., Weltman, M., & Haber, P. (2008). Do acamprosate or naltrexone have an effect on daily drinking by reducing craving for alcohol? *Addiction, 103*(6), 953–959.

Robbins, T. W., & Murphy, E. R. (2006). Behavioral pharmacology: 40 years of progress, with a focus on glutamate receptors and cognition. *Trends in Pharmacological Sciences, 27*(3), 141–148.

Rocca, P., Beoni, A. M., Eva, C., Ferrero, P., Zanalda, E., & Ravizza, L. (1998). Peripheral benzodiazepine receptor messenger RNA is decreased in lymphocytes of generalized anxiety disorder patients. *Biological Psychiatry, 43*(10), 767–773.

Rodd, Z. A., Melendez, R. I., Bell, R. L., Kuc, K. A., Zhang, Y., Murphy, J. M., & McBride, W. J. (2004). Intracranial self-administration of ethanol within the ventral tegmental area of male Wistar rats: Evidence for involvement of dopamine neurons. *The Journal of Neuroscience, 24*(5), 1050–1057.

Rogawski, M. A., & Loscher, W. (2004). The neurobiology of antiepileptic drugs for the treatment of non-epileptic conditions. *Nature Medicine, 10*(7), 685–692.

Rogóz, Z., Skuza, G., & Legutko, B. (2005). Repeated treatment with mirtazepine induces brain-derived neurotrophic factor gene expression in rats. *Journal of Physiology and Pharmacology, 56*(4), 661–671.

Rojas, D. C., Peterson, E., Winterrowd, E., Reite, M. L., Rogers, S. J., & Tregellas, J. R. (2006). Regional gray matter volumetric changes in autism associated with social and repetitive behavior symptoms. *BMC Psychiatry, 6*, 56.

Rosack, J. (2002). Switching drug classes benefits treatment-resistant patients. *Psychiatric News, 37*(9), 31.

Rose, J. E., Behm, F. M., Westman, E. C., & Johnson, M. (2000). Dissociating nicotine and nonnicotine components of cigarette smoking. *Pharmacology, Biochemistry, and Behavior, 67*, 71–81.

Rowe, D. L., Robinson, P. A., Lazzaro, I. L., Powles, R. C., Gordon, E., & Williams, L. M. (2005). Biophysical modeling of tonic cortical electrical activity in attention deficit hyperactivity disorder. *The International Journal of Neuroscience, 115*(9), 1273–1305.

Roz, N., Mazur, Y., Hirshfeld, A., & Rehavi, M. (2002). Inhibition of vesicular uptake of monoamines by hyperforin. *Life Sciences, 71*(19), 2227–2237.

Roz, N., & Rehavi, M. (2004). Hyperforin depletes synaptic vesicles content and induces compartmental redistribution of nerve ending monoamines. *Life Sciences, 75*(23), 2841–2850.

Ruelaz, A. R. (2006). Treatment-resistant depression: Strategies for management. *Psychiatric Times, 23*(11).

Russo-Neustadt, A., Beard, R. C., & Cotman, C. W. (1999). Exercise, antidepressant medications, and enhanced brain derived neurotrophic factor expression. *Nueropsychopharmacology*, *21*, 679–682.

Rybakowski, J. K., Suwalska, A., Skibinska, M., Dmitrzak-Weglarz, M., Leszczynska-Rodziewicz, A., & Hauser, J. (2007). Response to lithium prophylaxis: Interaction between serotonin transporter and BDNF genes. *American Journal of Medical Genetics. Part B, Neuropsychiatric Genetics*, *144*(6), 820–823.

Sagredo, O., Garcia-Arencibia, M., de Lago, E., Finetti, S., Decio, A., & Fernandez-Ruiz, J. (2007). Cannabinoids and neuroprotection in basal ganglia disorders. *Molecular Neurobiology*, *36*(1), 82–91.

Sahay, A., & Hen, R. (2007). Adult hippocampal neurogenesis in depression. *Nature Neuroscience*, *10*(9), 1110–1115.

Sakae, D. Y., Marti, F., Lecca, S., Vorspan, F., Martín-García, E., Morel, L. J., Henrion, A., Gutiérrez-Cuesta, J., Besnard, A., Heck, N., Herzog, E., Bolte, S., Prado, V. F., Prado, M. A. M., Bellivier, F., Eap, C. B., Crettol, S., Vanhoutte, P., Caboche, J., . . . El Mestikawy, S. (2015). The absence of VGLUT3 predisposes to cocaine abuse by increasing dopamine and glutamate signaling in the nucleus accumbens. *Molecular Psychiatry*, *20*(11), 1448–1459.

Sallette, J., Bohler, S., Benoit, P., Soudant, M., Pons, S., Le Novere, N., Changeux, J. P., & Corringer, P. J. (2004). An extracellular protein microdomain controls up-regulation of neuronal nicotinic acetylcholine receptors by nicotine. *Journal of Biological Chemistry*, *279*(18), 18767–18775.

Samaha, A.-N., Mallet, N., Ferguson, S. M., Gonon, F., & Robinson, T. E. (2004). The rate of cocaine administration alters gene regulation and behavioral plasticity: Implications for addiction. *The Journal of Neuroscience*, *24*(28), 6362–6370.

Samaha, A.-N., & Robinson, T. E. (2005). Why does the rapid delivery of drugs to the brain promote addiction? *Trends in Pharmacological Sciences*, *26*(2), 82–87.

Samat, A., Tomlinson, B., Taheri, S., & Thomas, G. N. (2008). Rimonabant for the treatment of obesity. *Recent Patents on cardiovascular Drug Discovery*, *3*(3), 187–193.

SAMHSA (Substance Abuse and Mental Health Services Administration). (2021). *Substance abuse disorders*. www.samhsa.gov/disorders/substance-use

SAMHSA (Substance Abuse and Mental Health Services Administration). (2022). *National survey on drug use and health*. www.samhsa.gov/data/data-we-collect/nsduh-national-survey-drug-use-and-health

Sanchez-Mateo, C., Bonkanka, C., & Rabanal, R. (2007). Antidepressant activity of some hypercium reflexum l: Fil extracts in the forced swimming task in mice. *Journal of Ethnopharmacology*, *112*(1), 115–121.

Sanna, E., Busonero, F., Talani, G., Mostallino, M. C., Mura, M. L., Pisu, M. G., Maciocco, E., Serra, M., & Biggio, G. (2005). Low tolerance and dependence liabilities of etizolam: Molecular, functional, and pharmacological correlates. *European Journal of Pharmacology*, *519*(1–2), 31–42.

Santhakumar, V., Wallner, M., & Otis, T. S. (2007). Ethanol acts directly on extrasynaptic subtypes of GABAA receptors to increase tonic inhibition. *Alcohol*, *41*(3), 211–221.

Sarai, S. K., Mekala, H. M., & Lippmann, S. (2018). Lithium suicide prevention: A brief review and reminder. *Innovation in Clinical Neuroscience*, *15*(11–12), 30–32.

Sato, K. (2020). Why is prepulse inhibition disrupted in schizophrenia? *Med Hypotheses*, *143*, 109901. https://doi.org/10.1016/j.mehy.2020.109901

Saxena, S., Brody, A. L., Schwartz, J. M., & Baxter, L. R. (1998). Neuroimaging and frontal-subcortical circuitry in obsessive-compulsive disorder. *The British Journal of Psychiatry, Supplement*, *1998*(35), 26–37.

Saxena, S., Brody, A. O., Ho, M. L., Zohrabi, N., Maidment, K. M., & Baxter, L. R. Jr. (2003). Differential brain metabolic predictors of response to paroxetine in obsessive-compulsive disorder versus major depression. *The American Journal of Psychiatry*, *160*(3), 522–532.

Schotanus, S. M., & Chergui, K. (2008). Dopamine D1 receptors and group l metabotropic glutamate receptors contribute to the induction of long-term potentiation in the nucleus accumbens. *Neuropharmacology*, *54*(5), 837–844.

Schule, C., Zill, P., Baghai, T. C., Eser, D., Zwanzger, P., Wenig, N., Rupprecht, R., & Bondy, B. (2006). Brain-derived neurotrophic factor Val66Met polymorphism and dexamethasone/CRH test results in depressed patients. *Psychoneuroendocrinology*, *31*(8), 1019–1025.

Sciascia, J., Mendoza, J., & Chaudhri, N. (2014). Blocking dopamine d1-like receptors attenuates context-induced renewal of pavlovian-conditioned alcohol-seeking in rats. *Alcoholism, Clinical and Experimental Research*, *38*(2), 418–427.

Sciotto, M. J. (2007). Evaluating the evidence for and against the overdiagnosis of ADHD. *Journal of Attention Disorders, 11*(2), 106–113.

Scotton, E., Antqueviezc, B., Vasconcelos, M. F., Dalpiaz, G., Paul Géa, L., Ferraz Goularte, J., Colombo, R., & Ribeiro Rosa, A. (2022). Is ®-ketamine a potential therapeutic agent for treatment-resistant depression with less detrimental side effects? A review of molecular mechanisms underlying ketamine and its enantiomers. *Biochemical Pharmacology, 198*. https://doi.org/10.1016/j.bcp.2022.114963

Scragg, R., Wellman, R. J., Laugesen, M., & DiFranza, J. R. (2008). Diminshed autonomy over tobacco can appear with the first cigarettes. *Addictive Behaviors, 33*(5), 389–398.

Seeman, P. (2002). Atypical antipsychotics: mechanism of action. *Canadian Journal of Psychiatry, 47*(1), 27–38.

Seeman, P., Schwarz, J., Chen, J. F., Szechtman, H., Perreault, M., McKnight, G. S., Roder, J. C., Quirion, R., Boksa, P., Srivastava, L. K., Yanai, K., Weinshenker, D., & Sumiyoshi, T. (2006). Psychosis pathways converge via D2high dopamine receptors. *Synapse, 60*(4), 319–346.

Seeman, P., & Tallerico, T. (1998). Antipsychotic drugs which elicit little or no parkinsonism bind more loosely than dopamine to brain D2 receptors, yet occupy high levels of these receptors. *Molecular Psychiatry, 3*(2), 123–134.

Sena, L. M., Bueno, C., Pobbe, R. L., Andrade, T. G., Zangrossi, H. Jr., & Viana, M. B. (2003). The dorsal raphe nucleus exerts opposed control on generalized anxiety and panic-related defensive responses in rats. *Behavioral Brain Research, 142*(1–2), 125–133.

Shafer, R. A., & Levant, B. (1998). The D3 dopamine receptor in cellular and organismal function. *Psychopharmacology, 135*(1), 1–16.

Sharkey, K. A., Cristino, L., Oland, L. D., Van Sickle, M. D., Starowicz, K., Pittman, Q. J., Guglielmotti, V., Davison, J. S., & Di Marzo, V. (2007). Arvanil, anandamide and N-arachidonoyl-dopamine (NADA) inhibit emesis through cannabinoid CB1 and vanilloid TRPV1 receptors in the ferret. *The European Journal of the Neuroscience, 25*(9), 2773–2782.

Shaw, P., Eckstrand, K., Sharp, W., Blumenthal, J., Lerch, J. P., Greenstein, D., Clasen, L., Evans, A., Giedd, J., & Rapoport, J. L. (2007). Attention-deficit/hyperactivity disorder is characterized by a delay in cortical maturation. Proceedings of the National Academy of Sciences of the United States of America, *104*(49), 19649–19654.

Shelton, R. C. (2007). The molecular neurobiology of depression. *The Psychiatric Clinics of North America, 30*(1), 1–11.

Shelton, R. C., Keller, M. B., Gelenberg, A., Dunner, D., Hirschfield, R., Thase, M., Russell, J., Lydiard, R., Crits, P., Gallop, R., Todd, L., Hellerstein, D., Goodnick, P., Keitner, G., Stahl, S., & Halbreich, U. (2001). Effectiveness of St. John's wort in major depression: A randomized controlled trial. *Journal of the American Medical Association, 285*(15), 1978–1986.

Sheth, S., Neal, J., Tangherlini, F., Mian, M., Gentil, A., Cosgrove, G. R., Eskandar, E. N., & Dougherty, D. (2013). Limbic system surgery for treatment-refractory obsessive-compulsive disorder: A prospective long-term follow-up of 64 patients. *Journal of Neurosurgery, 118*(3), 491–497.

Shin, L. M., Rauch, S. L., & Pitman, R. K. (2006). Amygdala, medial prefrontal cortex, and hippocampal function in PTSD. *Annals of the New York Academy of Sciences, 1071*, 67–79.

Shiroma, P., Thuras, P., Wels, J., Albott, C., Erbes, C., Tye, S., & Lim, K. (2020). A randomized, double-blind, active placebo-controlled study of efficacy, safety, and durability of repeated vs single subanesthetic ketamine for treatment-resistant depression. *Translational Psychiatry, 10*, 206. https://doi.org/10.1038/s41398-020-00897-0

Siegel, S. (1975). Evidence from rats that morphine tolerance is a learned response. *Journal of Comparative and Physiological Psychology, 89*, 498–506.

Siegel, S. (1987). Pavlovian conditioning of ethanol tolerance. *Alcohol and Alcoholism, 1*, 25–36.

Silk, T. J., Rinehart, N., Bradshaw, J. L., Tonge, B., Egan, G., O'Boyle, M. W., & Cunnington, R. (2006). Visuospatial processing and the function of prefrontal-parietal networks in autism spectrum disorders: A functional MRI study. *The American Journal of Psychiatry, 163*(8), 1440–1443.

Simpson, H., Foa, E., Liebowitz, M., Huppert, J., Cahill, S., Maher, M. J., McLean, C. P., Bender, J., Jr., Marcus, S. M., Williams, M. T., Weaver, J., Vermes, D., Van Meter, P. E., Rodriguez, C. I., Powers, M., Pinto, A., Imms, P., Hahn, C.-G., & Campeas, R. (2013). Cognitive-behavioral therapy vs risperidone for augmenting serotonin reuptake inhibitors in obsessive-compulsive disorder: A randomized clinical trial. *JAMA Psychiatry, 70*(11), 1190–1199.

Siu, E. C., & Tyndale, R. F. (2008). Selegiline is a mechanism-based inactivator of CYP2A6 inhibiting nicotine metabolism in humans and mice. *The Journal of Pharmacology and Experimental Therapeutics, 324*(3), 992–999.

Siu, E. C., Wildenauer, D. B., & Tyndale, R. F. (2006). Nicotine self-administration in mice is associated with rates of nicotine inactivation by CYP2A5. *Psychopharmacology, 184*(3), 401–408.

Slatkin, N. E. (2007). Cannabinoids in the treatment of chemotherapy-induced nausea and vomiting: Beyond prevention of acute emesis. *The Journal of Supportive Oncology, 5*(Suppl. 3), 1–9.

Snead, O. C. (2000). Evidence for a G protein-coupled gamma-hydroxybutyric acid receptor. *Journal of Neurochemistry, 75*(5), 1986–1996.

Snyder, J. L., & Bowers, T. G. (2008). The efficacy of acamprosate and naltrexone in the treatment of alcohol dependence: a relative benefits analysis of randomized controlled trials. *The American Journal of Drug and Alcohol Abuse, 34*(4), 449–461.

Snyder, S. M., & Hall, J. R. (2006). A meta-analysis of quantitative EEG power associated with attention-deficit hyperactivity disorder. *Journal of Clinical Neurophysiology, 23*(5), 440–455.

Solinas, M., Goldberg, S. R., & Piomelli, D. (2008). The endocannabinoid system in brain reward processes. *British Journal of Phamacology, 154*(2), 369–383.

Solís, O., García-Sanz, P., Martín, A. B., Granado, N., Sanz-Magro, A., Podlesniy, P., Trullas, R., Murer, M. G., Maldonado, R., & Moratalla, R. (2021). Behavioral sensitization and cellular responses to psychostimulants are reduced in D2R knockout mice. *Addiction Biology, 26*(1), e12840. https://doi.org/10.1111/adb.12840

Song, D. H., Shin, D. W., Jon, D. I., & Ha, E. H. (2005). Effects of methylphenidate on quantitative EEG of boys with attention-deficit hyperactivity disorder in continuous performance test. *Yonsei Medical Journal, 46*(1), 34–41.

Song, R., Zhang, H., Peng, X., Su, R., Yang, R., Li, J., Xi, Z., & Gardner, E. (2013). Dopamine D3 receptor deletion or blockade attenuates cocaine-induced conditioned place preference. *Neuropharmacology, 72,* 82–87.

Sora, I., Hall, F. S., Andrews, A. M., Itokawa, M., Li, X.-F., Wei, H.-B., Wichems, C., Lesch, K.-P., Murphy, D. L., & Uhl, G. R. (2001). Molecular mechanisms of cocaine reward: Combined dopamine and serotonin transporter knockouts eliminate cocaine place preference. *Proceedings of the National Academy of Sciences of the United States of America, 98*(9), 5300–5305.

Soyka, M., Koller, G., Schmidt, P., Lesch, O. M., Leweke, M., Fehr, C., Gann, H., & Mann, K. F. (2008). Cannabinoid receptor 1 blocker rimonabant (SR 141716) for treatment of alcohol dependence: Results from a placebo-controlled, double-blind trial. *Journal of Clinical Pyschopharmacology, 28*(3), 317–324.

Spencer, T. J., Biederman, J., Madras, B. K., Dougherty, D. D., Bonab, A. A., Livini, E., Meltzer, P. C., Martin, J., Rauch, S., & Fischman, A. J. (2007). Further evidence of dopamine transporter dysregulation in ADHD: A controlled PET imaging study using altropane. *Biological Psychiatry, 62*(9), 1059–1061.

Spencer, T. J., Heiligenstein, J. H., Biederman, J., Faries, D. E., Kratochvil, C. J., Conners, C. K., & Potter, W. Z. (2002). Results from 2 proof-of-concept, placebo-controlled studies of atomoxetine in children with attention-deficit/hyperactivity disorder. *Journal of Clinical Psychiatry, 63,* 1140–1147.

Stahl, S. M. (2009). Mechanisms of action of trazodone: a multifunctional drug. *CNS Spectrums, 14*(10), 536–546.

Stahl, S. M., Pradko, J. F., Haight, B. R., Modell, J. G., Rockett, C. B., & Learned-Coughlin, S. (2004). A review of the neuropharmacology of bupropion, a dual norepinephrine and dopamine reuptake inhibitor. *Primary Care Companion Journal of Clinical Psychiatry, 6*(4), 159–166.

Stein, M. B., Seedat, S., & Gelernter, J. (2006). Serotonin transporter gene promoter polymorphism predicts SSRI response in generalized social anxiety disorder. *Psychopharmacology, 187*(1), 68–72.

Stokes, P., Mehta, M., Curran, H., Breen, G., & Gransby, P. (2009). Can recreational doses of THC produce significant dopamine release in the human striatum? *Neuroimage, 48*(1), 186–190.

Stolerman, I. P., Fink, R., & Jarvik, M. (1973). Acute and chronic tolerance to nicotine measured by activity in rats. *Psychopharmacologia, 30*(4), 329–342.

Stone, J. M., Morrison, P. D., & Pilowsky, L. S. (2007). Glutamate and dopamine dysregulation in schizophrenia–a synthesis and selective review. *Journal of Psychopharmacology, 21*(4), 440–452.

Strakowski, S. M., DelBello, M. P., & Adler, C. M. (2005). The functional neuroanatomy of bipolar disorder: a review of neuroimaging findings. *Molecular Psychiatry, 10*(1), 105–116.

Strakowski, S. M., DelBello, M. P., Zimmerman, M. E., Getz, G. E., Mills, N. P., Ret, J., Shear, P., & Adler, C. M. (2002). Ventricular and periventricular structural volumes in first-versus multiple-episode bipolar disorder. *The American Journal of Psychiatry, 159*(11), 1841–1847.

Suh, J. J., Pettinati, H. M., Kampman, K. M., & O'Brien, C. P. (2006). The status of disulfiram: A half of a century later. *Journal of Clinical Psychopharmacology, 26*(3), 290–302.

Suzdak, P. D., Glowa, J. R., Crawley, J. N., Schwartz, R. D., Skolnick, P., & Paul, S. M. (1986). A selective imidazobenzodiazepine antagonist of ethanol in the rat. *Science, 234*(4781), 1243–1247.

Swanson, J. M., Kinsbourne, M., Nigg, J., Lanphear, B., Stefanatos, G. A., Volkow, N., Taylor, E., Casey, B. J., Castellanos, F. X., & Wadhwa, P. D. (2007). Etiologic subtypes of attention-deficit/hyperactivity disorder: brain imaging, molecular genetic and environmental factors and the dopamine hypothesis. *Neuropsychology Review, 17*(1), 39–59.

Swerdlow, N. R., Light, G. A., Cadenhead, K. S., Sprock, J., Hsieh, M. H., & Braff, D. L. (2006). Startle gating deficits in a large cohort of patients with schizophrenia: Relationship to medications, symptoms, neurocognition, and level of function. *Archives of General Psychiatry, 63*(12), 1325–1335.

Szabo, B., Siemes, S., & Wallmichrath, I. (2002). Inhibition of GABAergic neurotransmission in the ventral tegmental area by cannabinoids. *The European Journal of the Neuroscience, 15*(12), 2057–2061.

Szechtman, H., Sulis, W., & Eilam, D. (1998). Quinpirole induces compulsive checking behavior in rats: A potential animal model of obsessive-compulsive disorder (OCD). *Behavioral Neuroscience, 112*(6), 1475–1485.

Tabet, N. (2006). Acetylcholine inhibitors for Alzheimer's disease: Anti-inflamatories in acetylcholine clothing! *Age and Aging, 34*(4), 336–338.

Tadic, A., Rujescu, D., Szegedi, A., Giegling, I., Singer, P., Moller, H. J., & Dahmen, N. (2003). Association of a MAOA gene variant with generalized anxiety disorder, but not with panic disorder or major depression. *American Journal of Medical Genetics, Part B, Neuropsychiatric Genetics, 117*(1), 1–6.

Tao, X., Finkbeiner, S., Arnold, D. B., Shaywitz, A. J., & Greenberg, M. E. (1998). Ca2+ Influx regulates BDNF transcription by a CREB family transcription factor-dependent mechanism. *Neuron, 20*(4), 709–726.

Tapper, A. R., McKinney, S. L., Nashmi, R., Schwarz, J., Deshpande, P., Labarca, C., Whiteaker, P., Marks, M. J., Collins, A. C., & Lester, H. A. (2004). Nicotine Activation of a4* Receptors: Sufficient for reward, tolerance, and sensitization. *Science, 306*(5698), 1029–1032.

Taylor, J., Borckardt, J., & George, M. (2012). Endogenous opioids mediate left dorsolateral prefrontal cortex rTMS-induced analgesia. *Pain, 153*(6), 1219–1225.

Taylor, W. D., & Doraiswamy, P. M. (2003). A systematic review of antidepressant placebo-controlled trials for geriatric depression: Limitations of current data and directions for the future. *Neuropsychopharmacology, 29*, 2285–2299.

Thalemann, R., Wolfling, K., & Grusser, S. M. (2007). Specific cue reactivity on computer game-related cues in excessive gamers. *Behavioral Neuroscience, 121*(3), 614–618.

Thanos, P. K., Michaelides, M., Benvenista, H., Wang, G. J., & Volkow, N. D. (2008). The effects of cocaine on regional brain glucose metabolism is attenuated in dopamine transporter knockout mice. *Synapse, 62*(5), 319–324.

Thase, M. E., Jonas, A., Khan, A., Bowden, C. L., Wu, X., McQuade, R. D., Carson, W. H., Marcus, R. N., & Owen, R. (2008). Aripiprazole monotherapy in nonpsychotic bipolar I depression: results of 2 randomized, placebo-controlled studies. *Journal of Clinical Psychopharmacology, 28*(1), 13–20.

Theile, J. W., Morikawa, H., Gonzales, R. A., & Morrisett, R. A. (2008). Ethanol enhances GABAergic transmission onto dopamine neurons in the ventral tegmental area of the rat. *Alcoholism, Clinical and Experimental Research, 32*(6), 1040–1048.

Thomas, M. J., Kalivas, P. W., & Shaham, Y. (2008). Neuroplasticity in the mesolimbic dopamine system and cocaine addiction. *British Journal of Pharmacology, 154*(2), 327–342.

Thomas, R. M., & Peterson, D. A. (2003). A neurogenic theory of depression gains momentum. *Molecular Interventions, 3*, 441–444.

Thome, J., Sakai, N., Shin, K.-H., Steffen, C., Zhang, Y.-J., Impey, S., Storm, D., & Duman, R. S. (2000). cAMP response element-mediated gene transcription is upregulated by chronic antidepressant treatment. *Journal of Neuroscience, 20*(11), 4030–4036.

Ticku, M. K., & Mehta, A. K. (2008). Characterization and pharmacology of the GHB receptor. *Annals of the New York Academy of Science, 1139*, 374–385.

Tiihonen, J., Lonnqvist, J., Wahlbeck, K., Klaukka, T., Tanskanen, A., & Haukka, J. (2006). Antidepressants and the risk of suicide, attempted suicide, and overall mortality in a nationwide cohort. *Archives of General Psychiatry*, *63*(12), 1358–1367.

Tiraboschi, E., Tardito, D., Kasahara, J., Moraschi, S., Pruneri, P., Gennarelli, M., Racagni, G., & Popoli, M. (2004). Selective phosphorylation of nuclear CREB by fluoxetine is linked to activation of CaM kinase IV and MAP kinase cascades. *Neuropsychopharmacology*, *29*, 1831–1840.

Torrens, M., Fonseca, F., Mateu, G., & Farre, M. (2005). Efficacy of antidepressants in substance use disorders with and without comorbid depression. A systematic review and meta-analysis. *Drug and Alcohol Dependence*, *78*(1), 1–22.

Tsai. (2005). Diagnostic confusion in asperger disorder. *Paper presented at the ASC-US Annual Conference*, Orlando, FL.

Tuominen, H. J., Tiihonen, J., & Wahlbeck, K. (2006). Glutamatergic drugs for schizophrenia. *Cochrane Database of Systematic Reviews*, *2006*(2), CD003730.

Turner, T. (2007). Chlorpromazine: Unlocking psychosis. *British Medical Journal (Clinical Research Ed.)*, *334*(Suppl 1), S7.

Uhl, G., Koob, G., & Cable, J. (2019). The neurobiology of addiction, *Annals of the New York Academy of Science*, *1415*(1), 5–28.

Uno, Y., & Coyle, J. (2019). Glutamate hypothesis in schizophrenia. *Psychiatry and Clinical Neuroscience*, *73*(5), 204–215. https://doi.org/10.1111/pcn.12823

Vallance, A. K. (2006). Something out of nothing: The placebo effect. *Advances in Psychiatric Treatment*, *12*, 287–296.

Vallejo, Y. F., Buisson, B., Bertrand, D., & Green, W. N. (2005). Chronic nicotine exposure upregulates nicotinic receptors by a novel mechanism. *Journal of Neuroscience*, *25*(23), 5563–5572.

Vanelle, J. M., & Douki, S. (2006). A double-blind randomised comparative trial of amisulpride versus olanzapine for 2 months in the treatment of subjects with schizophrenia and comorbid depression. *European Psychiatry*, *21*(8), 523–530.

Vann, R. E., James, J. R., Rosecrans, J. A., & Robinson, S. E. (2006). Nicotinic receptor inactivation after acute and repeated in vivo nicotine exposures in rats. *Brain Research*, *1086*, 98–103.

van Rossum, J. M. (1966). The significance of dopamine-receptor blockade for the mechanism of action of neuroleptic drugs. *Archives Internationales de Pharmacodynamie et de Therapie*, *160*(2), 492–494.

Van Sickle, M. D., Oland, L. D., Ho, W., Hillard, C. J., Mackie, K., Davison, J. S., & Sharkey, K. A. (2001). Cannabinoids inhibit emesis through CB1 receptors in the brainstem of the ferret. *Gastroenterology*, *121*(4), 767–774.

Varvel, S. A., Martin, B. R., & Lichtman, A. H. (2007). Lack of behavioral sensitization after repeated exposure to THC in mice and comparison to methamphetamine. *Psychopharmacology*, *193*, 511–519.

Vasconcelos, M. M., Werner, J., Jr., Malheiros, A. F., Lima, D. F., Santos, I. S., & Barbosa, J. B. (2003). Attention deficit/hyperactivity disorder prevalence in an inner city elementary school. *Arq Neuropsiquiatr*, *61*(1), 67–73.

Velazquez-Sanchez, C., Ferragud, A., Ramos-Miguel, A., Garcia-Sevilla, J., & Canales, J. (2013). Substituting a long-acting dopamine uptake inhibitor for cocaine prevents relapse to cocaine seeking. *Behavioral Neuroscience*, *18*(4), 633–643.

Verly, M., Verhoeven, J., Zink, I., Mantini, D., Van Oudenhove, L., Lagae, L., Sunaert, S., & Rommel, N. (2014). Structural and functional underconnectivity as a negative predictor for language in autism. *Human Brain Mapping*, *35*(8), 3602–3615.

Villanueva, R. (2013). Neurobiology of major depressive disorder. *Neural Plasticity*, *2013*, 873278. https://doi.org/10.1155/2013/873278

Viswanathan, V., Yu, C., Sambursky, J. A., Kaur, S., & Simpkins, A. N. (2019). Acute cerebral ischemia temporally associated with marijuana use. *Cureus*, *11*(7). https://doi.org/10.7759/cureus.5239

Volkow, N. D., Chang, L., Wang, G., Fowler, J., Franceschi, D., & Logan, J. (2001). Loss of dopamine transporters in methamphetamine abusers recovers with protracted abstinence. *The Journal of Neuroscience*, *21*(23), 9414–9418.

Volkow, N. D., Fowler, J. S., Wang, G., & Goldstein, R. Z. (2002). Role of dopamine, the frontal cortex and memory circuits in drug addiction: insight from imaging studies. *Neurobiology of Learning and Memory*, *78*(3), 610–624.

Volkow, N. D., & Swanson, J. (2003). Variables that affect the clinical use and abuse of methylphenidate in the treatment of ADHD. *The American Journal of Psychiatry*, *160*(11), 1909–1918.

Volkow, N. D., Wang, G.-J., Fischman, M. W., Foltin, R. W., Fowler, J. S., Abumrad, N. N., Vitkun, S., Logan, J., Gatley, S. J., Pappas, N., Hitzemann, R., & Shea, C. E. (1997). Relationship between subjective effects of cocaine and dopamine transporter occupancy. *Nature*, *396*, 827–830.

Volkow, N. D., Wang, G. J., Fowler, J., Logan, J., Gerasimov, M., & Franceschi, D. (2001). Therapeutic doses of oral methylphenidate significantly increase extracellular dopamine in the human brain. *Neuroscience*, *21*(2), RC121. https://doi.org/10.1523/JNEUROSCI.21-02-j0001.2001

Volkow, N. D., Wang, G. J., Newcorn, J., Telang, F., Solanto, M. V., Fowler, J. S., Logan, J., Ma, Y., Schulz, K., Pradhan, K., Wong, C., & Swanson, J. M. (2007). Depressed dopamine activity in caudate and preliminary evidence of limbic involvement in adults with attention-deficit/hyperactivity disorder. *Archives of General Psychiatry*, *64*(8), 932–940.

Volkow, N. D., Wang, G. J., Telang, F., Fowler, J. S., Logan, J., Childress, A. R., Jayne, M., Ma, Y., & Wong, C. (2008). Dopamine increases in striatum do not elicit craving in cocaine abusers unless they are coupled with cocaine cues. *NeuroImage*, *39*(3), 1266–1273.

Volkow, N. D., Wang, G. J., Telang, F., Fowler, J. S., Logan, J., Childress, A. R., Jayne, M., & Wong, C. (2006). Cocaine cues and dopamine in dorsal striatum: Mechanism of craving in cocaine addiction. *The Journal of Neuroscience*, *26*(24), 6583–6588.

Vyas, A., Mitra, R., Shankaranarayana Roa, B. S., & Chattarji, S. (2002). Chronic stress induces contrasting patterns of dendritic remodeling in hippocampal and amygdaloid neurons. *The Journal of Neuroscience*, *22*(15), 6810–6818.

Walitza, S., Werner, B., Romanos, M., Warnke, A., Gerlach, M., & Stopper, H. (2007). Does methylphenidate cause a cytogenetic effect in children with attention deficit hyperactivity disorder? *Environmental Health Perspect*, *115*(6), 936–940.

Walsh, B. T., Seidman, S. N., Sysko, R., & Gould, M. (2002). Placebo response in studies of major depression. *Journal of the American Medical Association*, *287*, 1840–1847.

Walsh, H., Govind, A. P., Mastro, R., Hoda, J. C., Bertrand, D., Vallejo, Y., & Green, W. N. (2008). Up-regulation of nicotinic receptors by nicotine varies with receptor subtype. *The Journal of Biological Chemistry*, *283*(10), 6022–6032.

Walsh, S. (2007). FDA proposes new warnings about suicidal thinking, behavior in young adults who take antidepressant medications. *FDA News*.

Wang, D., Li, H., Du, X., Zhou, J., Yuan, L., & Chen, X. (2020). Circulating brain-derived neurotrophic factor, antioxidant enzymes activities, and mitochondrial DNA in bipolar disorder: An exploratory report. *Frontiers in Psychiatry*, *11*, 514658. https://doi.org/10.3389/fpsyt.2020.514658

Wang, J., Michelhaugh, S. K., & Bannon, M. (2007). Valproate robustly increases Sp transcription factor-mediated expression of the dopamine transporter gene within dopamine cells. *The European Journal of the Neuroscience*, *25*(7), 1982–1986.

Wang, M., Liu, H., & Ma, Z. (2022). Roles of the cannabinoid system in the basal ganglia in Parkinson's Disease. *Frontiers in Cell Neuroscience*, *16*, 832854. https://doi.org/10.3389/fncel.2022.832854

Wang, Z., Faith, M., Patterson, F., Tang, K., Kerrin, K., Wileyto, E. P., Detre, J. A., & Lerman, C. (2007). Neural substrates of abstinence-induced cigarette cravings in chronic smokers. *The Journal of Neuroscience*, *27*(51), 14036–14040.

Weeland, C., Kasprzak, S., de Joode, N., Abe, Y., Alonso, P., Ameis, S., & Vriend, C. (2022). The thalamus and its subnuclei—a gateway to obsessive-compulsive disorder. *Translational Psychiatry*, *12*(1), 70. https://doi.org/10.1038/s41398-022-01823-2

Weeland, C. J., Vriend, C., van der Werf, Y., Tiemeier, H., White, T., & van den Heuvel, O. (2021). Thalamic subregions and obsessive-compulsive disorder symptoms in 2500 children from the general population. *Child and Adolescent Psychiatry*, *61*(2), 321–330.

Wenger, J. R., Tiffany, T. M., Bombardier, C., Nicholis, K., & Woods, S. C. (1981). Ethanol tolerance in the rat is learned. *Science*, *213*(4507), 575–577.

Westenberg, H. G., Fineberg, N. A., & Denys, D. (2007). Neurobiology of obsessive-compulsive disorder: serotonin and beyond. *CNS Spectrums*, *12*(2, Suppl 3), 14–27.

White, J. D. (1999). Review personality, temperament and ADHD: A review of the literature. *Personality and Individual Differences*, *27*(4), 589–598.

Wikgren, J., Lavond, D. G., Ruusuvita, T., & Korhonen, T. (2006). Cooling of the cerebellar interpositus nucleus abolishes somatosensory cortical learning-related activity in eyeblink conditioned rabbits. *Behavioural Brain Research*, *170*(1), 94–98.

Wilens, T., McBurnett, K., Stein, M., Lerner, M., Spencer, T., & Wolraich, M. (2005). ADHD treatment with once-daily OROS methylphenidate: Final results from a long-term open-label study. *Journal of the American Child Adolescent Psychiatry*, *44*(10), 1015–1023.

Wilson, L. D., & French, S. (2002). Cocaethylene's effects on coronary artery blood flow and cardiac function in a canine model. *Journal of Toxicology-Clinical Toxicology*, *40*(5), 535–546.

Wisor, J. P., & Eriksson, S. (2005). Dopaminergic-adrenergic interactions in the wake promoting mechanism of modafinil. *Neuroscience*, *132*(4), 1027–1034.

Wolf, M. E., Sun, X., Mangiavacchi, S., & Chao, S. Z. (2004). Psychomotor stimulants and neuronal plasticity. *Neuropharmacology*, *47*(1), 61–79.

Wu, D. F., Yang, L. Q., Goschke, A., Stumm, R., Brandenburg, L. O., Liang, Y. J., Hollt, V., & Koch, T. (2008). Role of receptor internalization in the agonist-induced desensitization of cannabinoid type 1 receptors. *Journal of Neurochemistry*, *104*(4), 1132–1143.

Wynn, J. K., Green, M. F., Sprock, J., Light, G. A., Widmark, C., Reist, C., Erhart, S., Marder, S. R., Mintz, J., & Braff, D. L. (2007). Effects of olanzapine, risperidone and haloperidol on prepulse inhibition in schizophrenia patients: A double-blind, randomized controlled trial. *Schizophrenia Research*, *95*(1–3), 134–142.

Xi, Z., Li, X., Li, J., Peng, X., Somg, R., Gaal, J., & Gardner, E. (2013). Blockade of dopamine D3 receptors in the nucleus accumbens and central amygdala inhibits incubation of cocaine craving in rats. *Addiction Biology*, *18*(4), 665–677.

Xiao, C., Zhang, J., Krnjevic, K., & Ye, J. H. (2007). Effects of ethanol on midbrain neurons: Role of opioid receptors. *Alcoholism, Clinical and Experimental Research*, *31*(7), 1106–1113.

Xiaoshan, T., Junjie, Y., Wenqing, W., Yunong, Z., Jiaping, L., & Kui, C. (2020). Immunotherapy for treating methamphetamine, heroin and cocaine use disorders. *Drug Discovery Today*, *25*(3), 610–619. https://doi.org/10.1016/j.drudis.2019.07.009

Xing, B., Liu, P., Jiang, W., Liu, F., Zhang, H., Cao, G., Chen, T., & Dang, Y. (2013). Effects of immobilization stress on emotional behaviors in dopamine D3 receptor knockout mice. *Behavioural Brain Research*, *243*, 261–266.

Xu, A., & Kosten, T. R. (2021). Current status of immunotherapies for addiction. *Annals of the New York Academy of Sciences*, *1489*(1), 3–16.

Yang, T., Nie, Z., Shu, H., Kuang, Y., Chen, X., & Liu, H. (2020). The role of BDNF on neural plasticity in depression. *Frontiers of Cell Neuroscience*, *14*, 82. https://doi.org/10.3389/fncel.2020.00082

Yerevanian, B. I., Koek, R. J., & Mintz, J. (2007). Bipolar pharmacotherapy and suicidal behavior. Part I: Lithium, divalproex and carbamazepine. *Journal of Affective Disorders*, *103*(1–3), 5–11.

Yolkow, N. D., Wang, G. J., Newcorn, J., Telang, F., Solanto, M. V., Fowler, J. S., Logan, J., Schulz, K., Pradhan, K., Wong, C., & Swanson, J. M. (2007). Depressed dopamine activity in caudate and preliminary evidence of limbic involvement in adults with attention-deficit/hyperactivity disorder. *Archives of General Psychiatry*, *64*(8), 932–940.

Yoo, H. J., Woo, R. S., Cho, S., Kim, B., & Shin, M. (2015). Genetic association analysis of neuregulin 1 gene polymorphism with endophenotype for sociality of Korean autism spectrum disorders family. *Psychiatry Research*, *227*(2), 366–368.

Yoshida, K., Higuchi, H., Kamata, M., Takashashi, H., Inoue, K., Susuki, T., Itoh, K., & Ozaki, N. (2007). The G196A polymorphism of the brain-derived neurotrophic factor gene and the antidepressant effect of milnacipran and fluvoxamine. *Journal of Psychopharmacology*, *21*(6), 650–656.

Yoshimura, R., Mitoma, M., Sugita, A., Hori, H., Okamoto, T., Umene, W., Ueda, N., & Nakamura, J. (2007). Effects of paroxetine or milnacipran on serum brain-derived neurotrophic factor in depressed patients. *Progress in Neuro-Psychopharmacology and Biological Psychiatry*, *31*(5), 1034–1037.

Yuan, C.-S., Mehendale, S., Xiao, Y., Aung, H. H., Xie, J.-T., & Ang-Lee, M. K. (2004). The Gamma-aminobutyric acidergic effects of valerian and valerenic acid on rat brainstem neuronal activity. *Anesthesia and Analgesia*, *98*, 353–358.

Zakzanis, K. K., Campbell, Z., & Jovanovski, D. (2007). The neuropsychology of ecstasy (MDMA) use: A quantitative review. *Human Psychopharmacology*, *22*(7), 427–435.

Zang, Y. F., He, Y., Zhu, C. Z., Cao, Q. J., Sui, M. Q., Liang, M., Tian, L. X., Jiang, T. Z., & Wang, Y. F. (2007). Altered baseline brain activity in children with ADHD revealed by resting-state functional MRI. *Brain & Development, 29*(2), 83–91.

Zangrossi, H., Jr., & Graeff, F. G. (1997). Behavioral validation of the elevated T-maze, a new animal model of anxiety. *Brain Research Bulletin, 44*(1), 1–5.

Zanoli, P. (2004). Role of hyperforin in the pharmacological activities of St. John's wort. *CNS Drug Reviews, 10*(3), 203–218.

Zanoli, P., Rivasi, M., Baraldi, C., & Baraldi, M. (2002). Pharmacological activity of hyperforin acetate in rats. *Behavioral Pharmacology, 13*(8), 645–651.

Zhang, J., Zhang, L., Jiao, H., Zhang, Q., Zhang, D., Lou, D., Katz, J. L., & Xu, M. (2006). c-Fos facilitates the acquisition and extinction of cocaine-induced persistent changes. *The Journal of Neuroscience, 26*(51), 13287–13296.

Zhang, Y., Yang, H., Yang, S., Liang, W., Dai, P., & Wang, C. (2013). Antidepressdants for bipolar disorder: A meta-analysis of randomized, double-blind, controlled trials. *Neural Regulation Research, 8*(31), 2962–2974.

Zikopoulos, B., & Barbas, H. (2006). Prefrontal projections to the thalamic reticular nucleus form a unique circuit for attentional mechanisms. *The Journal of Neuroscience, 26*(28), 7348–7361.

Zimmerman, M., & Thongy, T. (2007). How often do SSRIs and other new-generation antidepressants lose their effect during continuation treatment? Evidence suggesting the rate of true tachyphylaxis during continuation treatment is low. *Journal of Clinical Psychiatry, 68*(8), 1271–1276.

Zubieta, J. K., Bueller, J. A., Jackson, L. R., Scott, D. J., Xu, Y., Koeppe, R. A., Nichols, T. E., & Stohler, C. S. (2005). Placebo effects mediated by endogenous opioid activity on mu-opioid receptors. *The Journal of Neuroscience, 24*(34), 7754–7762.

Index

Note: Page locators in **bold** indicate a table. Page locators in *italics* indicate a figure.

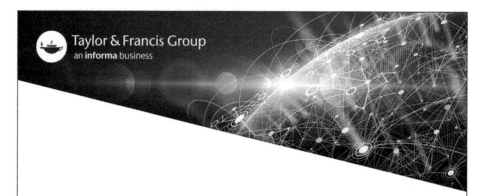

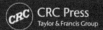

For Product Safety Concerns and Information please contact our EU
representative GPSR@taylorandfrancis.com
Taylor & Francis Verlag GmbH, Kaufingerstraße 24, 80331 München, Germany